D1020030

ETHICAL CONDUCT OF CLINICAL RESEARCH INVOLVING CHILDREN

Committee on Clinical Research Involving Children
Board on Health Sciences Policy

Marilyn J. Field and Richard E. Behrman, *Editors*

INSTITUTE OF MEDICINE
OF THE NATIONAL ACADEMIES

THE NATIONAL ACADEMIES PRESS
Washington, D.C.
www.nap.edu

THE NATIONAL ACADEMIES PRESS 500 Fifth Street, NW Washington, DC 20001

NOTICE: The project that is the subject of this report was approved by the Governing Board of the National Research Council, whose members are drawn from the councils of the National Academy of Sciences, the National Academy of Engineering, and the Institute of Medicine. The members of the committee responsible for the report were chosen for their special competences and with regard for appropriate balance.

This study was supported by Contract No. N01-OD-4-2139, TO #115 between the National Academy of Sciences and the National Institute of Child Health and Development and also the U.S. Food and Drug Administration. Any opinions, findings, conclusions, or recommendations expressed in this publication are those of the author(s) and do not necessarily reflect the view of the organizations or agencies that provided support for this project.

Library of Congress Cataloging-in-Publication Data

Ethical conduct of clinical research involving children / Marilyn J. Field and Richard E. Behrman, editors ; Committee on Clinical Research Involving Children, Board on Health Sciences Policy, Institute of Medicine of the National Academies.
   p. ; cm.
  Includes bibliographical references and index.
  ISBN 0-309-09181-0 (hardcover)
  1. Pediatrics—Research—Moral and ethical aspects. 2. Human experimentation in medicine.
  [DNLM: 1. Biomedical Research—ethics—Child. 2. Human Experimentation. 3. Research Subjects. W 20.5 E838 2004] I. Field, Marilyn J. (Marilyn Jane) II. Behrman, Richard E., 1931- III. Institute of Medicine (U.S.). Committee on Clinical Research Involving Children.
  RJ85.E85 2004
  174.2'8—dc22

                              2004008514

Additional copies of this report are available from the National Academies Press, 500 Fifth Street, NW, Lockbox 285, Washington, DC 20055; (800) 624-6242 or (202) 334-3313 (in the Washington metropolitan area); Internet, http://www.nap.edu.

For more information about the Institute of Medicine, visit the IOM home page at: **www.iom.edu.**

The serpent has been a symbol of long life, healing, and knowledge among almost all cultures and religions since the beginning of recorded history. The serpent adopted as a logotype by the Institute of Medicine is a relief carving from ancient Greece, now held by the Staatliche Museen in Berlin.

*"Knowing is not enough; we must apply.
Willing is not enough; we must do."*
—Goethe

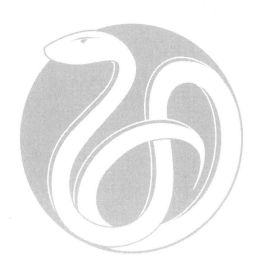

INSTITUTE OF MEDICINE
OF THE NATIONAL ACADEMIES

Adviser to the Nation to Improve Health

THE NATIONAL ACADEMIES
Advisers to the Nation on Science, Engineering, and Medicine

The **National Academy of Sciences** is a private, nonprofit, self-perpetuating society of distinguished scholars engaged in scientific and engineering research, dedicated to the furtherance of science and technology and to their use for the general welfare. Upon the authority of the charter granted to it by the Congress in 1863, the Academy has a mandate that requires it to advise the federal government on scientific and technical matters. Dr. Bruce M. Alberts is president of the National Academy of Sciences.

The **National Academy of Engineering** was established in 1964, under the charter of the National Academy of Sciences, as a parallel organization of outstanding engineers. It is autonomous in its administration and in the selection of its members, sharing with the National Academy of Sciences the responsibility for advising the federal government. The National Academy of Engineering also sponsors engineering programs aimed at meeting national needs, encourages education and research, and recognizes the superior achievements of engineers. Dr. Wm. A. Wulf is president of the National Academy of Engineering.

The **Institute of Medicine** was established in 1970 by the National Academy of Sciences to secure the services of eminent members of appropriate professions in the examination of policy matters pertaining to the health of the public. The Institute acts under the responsibility given to the National Academy of Sciences by its congressional charter to be an adviser to the federal government and, upon its own initiative, to identify issues of medical care, research, and education. Dr. Harvey V. Fineberg is president of the Institute of Medicine.

The **National Research Council** was organized by the National Academy of Sciences in 1916 to associate the broad community of science and technology with the Academy's purposes of furthering knowledge and advising the federal government. Functioning in accordance with general policies determined by the Academy, the Council has become the principal operating agency of both the National Academy of Sciences and the National Academy of Engineering in providing services to the government, the public, and the scientific and engineering communities. The Council is administered jointly by both Academies and the Institute of Medicine. Dr. Bruce M. Alberts and Dr. Wm. A. Wulf are chair and vice chair, respectively, of the National Research Council.

www.national-academies.org

Contents

Preface xiii

Acknowledgments xv

Reviewers xvii

Summary 1

1 INTRODUCTION 25
  Origins of Study and Overview of Report, 30
  Definitions: Research, Clinical Research, and Human Subjects
   or Research Participants, 31
  A Systems Perspective on Protecting Human Participants in
   Research, 35
  Ethical Principles for a System to Protect Human
   Research Participants, 39
  Historical Evolution of Policies for Protecting Human
   Participants in Research, 44

2 THE NECESSITY AND CHALLENGES OF CLINICAL
  RESEARCH INVOLVING CHILDREN 58
  Context, 59
  Definitions: Infants, Children, and Adolescents, 62

The Rationale for Pediatric Drug Research, 66
Implications for Pediatric Investigation, 72
Challenges of Designing and Conducting Pediatric Studies, 74
Data on the Extent of Children's Participation in
    Clinical Research, 87
Initiatives to Increase Involvement of Children in Research, 89
Conclusion, 92

3   REGULATORY FRAMEWORK FOR PROTECTING
    CHILD PARTICIPANTS IN RESEARCH   93
    Federal Regulations to Protect Child Participants in Research, 95
    Additional Federal Policies for Monitoring Safety of
        Participants in Clinical Research, 105
    Federal Rules for Research Conducted in Other Countries, 110
    Conclusion, 112

4   DEFINING, INTERPRETING, AND APPLYING CONCEPTS
    OF RISK AND BENEFIT IN CLINICAL RESEARCH
    INVOLVING CHILDREN   113
    Basic Concepts of Risk, Harm, and Benefit, 114
    Assessing the Level of Risk Posed by a Research Protocol, 117
    Other Issues Related to the Assessment of Risk, 136
    Conclusion, 145

5   UNDERSTANDING AND AGREEING TO CHILDREN'S
    PARTICIPATION IN CLINICAL RESEARCH   146
    Ethical Principles and Legal Requirements, 147
    Research Relevant to Parents' Comprehension of Children's
        Participation in Research, 159
    Children's and Adolescents' Comprehension of
        Research Participation, 178
    IRB and Investigator Policies and Practices, 193
    Improving Processes for Requesting Permission and Assent, 195
    Conclusion, 209

6   PAYMENTS RELATED TO CHILDREN'S
    PARTICIPATION IN CLINICAL RESEARCH   211
    Types of Payments Related to Research Participation, 212
    Ethical Principles and Regulatory Policies, 213
    Use of Payments in Research Involving Children, 217
    IRB Policies and Practices, 220
    Statements of Professional Organizations, 221

Other Concerns About Payment Related to Children's
    Research Participation, 221
Improving Practices and Policies on Payment Related to
    Children's Participation in Research, 223
Conclusion, 228

7   REGULATORY COMPLIANCE, ACCREDITATION, AND
    QUALITY IMPROVEMENT   229
    Continued Concern About Oversight of Research
        Involving Humans, 230
    Government Oversight of Regulations Protecting Child
        Participants in Research, 234
    Compliance in the Context of Voluntary Action, Quality
        Improvement, and Accreditation, 239
    Conclusion, 245

8   RESPONSIBLE RESEARCH INVOLVING CHILDREN   246
    Roles and Responsibilities, 248
    Conclusion, 275

REFERENCES   277

APPENDICES

A   STUDY ORIGINS AND ACTIVITIES   311
B   STATE REGULATION OF MEDICAL RESEARCH WITH
    CHILDREN AND ADOLESCENTS: AN OVERVIEW
    AND ANALYSIS   320
    Amy T. Campbell
C   HEALTH CARE PRIVACY AND CONFLICT-OF-INTEREST
    REGULATIONS RELEVANT TO PROTECTION OF
    HUMAN PARTICIPANTS IN RESEARCH   388
D   GLOSSARY, ACRONYMS, AND LAWS AND
    REGULATIONS   394
E   COMMITTEE BIOGRAPHICAL STATEMENTS   402

INDEX   409

BOXES, FIGURES, AND TABLES

Boxes

S.1   Summary of Categories of Research Involving Children That Are Approvable Under Subpart D of 45 CFR 46, 4

S.2   Questions Parents May Want to Ask When Considering Their Children's Participation in Clinical Research, 12

S.3   Key Responsibilities of Investigators for the Ethical Conduct of Clinical Research Involving Infants, Children, and Adolescents, 13

S.4   Key Ethical and Legal Responsibilities of IRBs and Research Institutions Involved with Clinical Research That Includes Infants, Children, and Adolescents, 14

1.1   Ethical Principles for Human Research Identified in the *Belmont Report*, 41

1.2   Summary of Discussion of Pediatric Research in the 1950s, 49

3.1   General Criteria That Research Must Meet to Be Approved Under Federal Regulations, 98

3.2   Definitions in Subpart D That Have Also Been Adopted by the FDA, 101

3.3   Research Involving Children That DHHS Is Permitted to Conduct or Support, 102

3.4   General Responsibilities of Data and Safety Monitoring Boards and Data Monitoring Committees, 109

4.1   Determinations Related to Research Risks and Potential Benefits Required by Regulation for Federally Supported, Conducted, or Regulated Research Involving Children, 118

4.2   Guidelines for Considering Risk and Risk Minimization in Research That Includes Children, 144

5.1   Selected Regulatory Provisions for Informed Consent That Also Apply Generally to Parental Permission for a Child's Participation in Research, 152

5.2   Questions Parents May Want to Ask When Considering Their Child's Participation in Clinical Research, 178

5.3   Questions and Information for Investigators Seeking Waiver of Parental Permission for Adolescent's Participation in Research, 202

7.1   Potential Data for a Federal Database on the System for Protecting Adult and Child Participants in Research, 240

7.2   Examples of What Might Be Included in a Quality Assurance
       Database Related to Studies Involving Infants, Children, and
       Adolescents, 243

8.1   Key Responsibilities of Investigators for the Ethical
       Conduct of Clinical Research Involving Infants, Children, and
       Adolescents, 249
8.2   Key Ethical and Legal Responsibilities of IRBs and Research
       Institutions Involved with Clinical Research That Includes
       Infants, Children, and Adolescents, 252
8.3   Suggested Elements of IRB and Research Institution
       Guidance on Clinical Research Involving Infants, Children,
       and Adolescents, 256
8.4   Example of Protocol Checklist for Investigators That
       Highlights Requirements for IRB Approval of Research
       Involving Children, 259
8.5   Key Responsibilities of Federal Agencies for the Ethical
       Conduct of Clinical Research Involving Infants, Children, and
       Adolescents, 268
8.6   Examples of Protocols Referred for Review by the Secretary
       of DHHS Under 45 CFR 46.407, by Year of Referral and
       Institution, 271

Figures

1.1   Simplified representation of a system for protecting human
       research participants (2002, 2003), 38

4.1   Algorithm for making assessments of research protocols
       as required by 45 CFR 46.404-407 and 21 CFR 50.51-54
       (2003), 119

Tables

4.1   Common Research Procedures by Category of Risk (2002), 135

5.1   Developmental Differences Influencing a Child's Participation in
       Research (1999), 180

8.1   Example 1—Variability in IRB Approval of a Multicenter Research
       Protocol That Includes Children, 263
8.2   Example 2—Variability in IRB Approval of a Multicenter Research
       Protocol That Includes Children, 264

B.1   State Education-Related Provisions for Research with
        Children and Adolescents (in School Settings) (2003), 340
B.2   Age of Majority (2003), 342
B.3   Emancipation Conditions (2003), 344
B.4   Mature Minor Provisions (2003), 347
B.5   Minor Consent for Certain Conditions/Disorders (2003), 354
B.6   Regulation of Research with Children and Adolescents in
        State Custody: Responses from Child Welfare or Social Services
        Personnel (2003), 364

PREFACE

Those who care about and for children currently face a dilemma. We want children to benefit from the dramatic and accelerating rate of progress in medical care that is fueled by scientific research. At the same time, we do not want to place any children at risk of being harmed by participating in such research, even though their very involvement may be essential to improving the overall medical care of children. We also want to discourage research that is of minimal value. The concern is how best to balance these potentially conflicting objectives. Five important considerations should guide us as we seek to resolve our dilemma.

First, because of the inherent vulnerabilities arising from their immaturity, infants, children, and adolescents need additional protections beyond what is provided to competent adults when they participate in research. This principle underlies all others.

Second, the design of the research required to improve the health and well-being of infants, children, and adolescents must consider their physical, cognitive, emotional, and social development. Similarly, when children of any age become participants in such research, the protections provided must be appropriate to their stages of development.

Third, sharing in the advances in medical care for this vulnerable group includes a special emphasis on protecting them from harm caused by standard medical procedures and treatments based on research with adults when the benefits and risks for children of different ages have not been established through scientific research involving these populations. Except when it is not feasible or reasonable, research with animals, and adults should precede studies with children to minimize research risks.

Fourth, the system for protecting infants, children, and adolescents involved in research, while ensuring such protection, should not unreasonably impede research that may benefit them. The contribution of rules and regulations to desired outcomes as well as possible unintended negative consequences should be considered.

Finally, all of those responsible for research involving infants, children, and adolescents need to understand the special ethical issues that are relevant to the conduct of such research and the additional protection that must be provided. In certain cases, ethical standards will preclude some otherwise desirable research.

Overall, a satisfactory resolution of our dilemma can be achieved. Children involved in research can be appropriately protected as well as share fairly in the increasing benefits of biomedical science. This report suggests ways to balance sometimes conflicting objectives in ways that will contribute to children's health and well-being now and in the future.

Richard E. Behrman, M.D., J.D.
Committee Chair

Acknowledgments

The committee and staff are indebted to a number of individuals and organizations for their assistance in the development of this report. The committee learned much through workshops and public meetings it organized to obtain information and perspectives from groups and individuals knowledgeable and concerned about research involving infants, children, and adolescents. Appendix A includes the meeting agendas and participant lists and also cites the organizations that provided written statements to the committee.

Special thanks go to Carolyn Brokowski, Maureen and Joseph Lilly, Joan and Sarah Lippincott, Andrell Vaughn, and Lise Yasui, who were willing to share their experiences with the committee. Consultants Eric Kodish and Myra Bluebond-Langner provided valuable guidance in addition to their presentations to the committee. The committee also appreciates the contributions of Amy Campbell, who prepared the background paper on state policies relevant to children's participation in research. Mark Green, a Greenwall Foundation Fellow who served as a summer intern, assisted in developing the discussion of pediatric drug research.

A number of people at the Office for Human Research Protections (OHRP), the Food and Drug Administration (FDA), and the National Institute of Child Health and Human Development (NICHD) contributed to this study. Duane Alexander and Gilman Graves at NICHD, which sponsored this study, were unfailingly constructive in their support for the committee's work. Michael Carome, Leslie Ball, and Kate Gottfried at OHRP provided useful information about the office's policies, practices, and databases. David Lepay, Rosemary Roberts, and Susan Cummins at FDA helped the committee understand FDA policies on the protection of human participants in research and also relevant policies involving other aspects of the agency's mission. In addition, the committee appreciates the information and insights offered by David Wendler and Benjamin Wilfond at the Department of Clinical Bioethics of the National Institutes of Health Clinical Center.

Meetings with researchers and institutional review board members and administrators at the Children's Hospital of Philadelphia and Children's National Medical Center (arranged with much appreciated assistance from John Sever) helped provide additional perspective on the practical realities of administering federal and institutional policies to protect child participants in research. Allison Clarke-Stewart and Virginia Allhusen from the University of California, Irvine, generously shared the knowledge and insights into long-term research gained through their Study of Early Child Care and Youth Development. Among the many others who helped the committee clarify issues, find important information, or otherwise complete its work are Laura Rodriguez, Ellen Wright Clayton, Marion Broome, Scott Powers, George Retsch Bogart, Lisya VanHousen, Adam Fried, Suzanne Rivera, Steven Joffe, Rosemary Galvin, Juliette Schlucter, Jane Burns, Judith Argon, Lea Ann Hansen, James Chamberlain, Jackie Moran, and Stacey Berg.

Many within the Institute of Medicine were, as usual, helpful to the study staff. The committee would especially like to thank Jessica Aungst, Natasha Dickson, Judy Estep, Alex Ommaya, Sally Stanfield, Bronwyn Schrecker, and Jennifer Bitticks.

REVIEWERS

This report has been reviewed in draft form by individuals chosen for their diverse perspectives and technical expertise, in accordance with procedures approved by the Report Review Committee of the National Research Council (NRC). The purpose of this independent review is to provide candid and critical comments that will assist the institution in making its published reports as sound as possible and to ensure that the report meets institutional standards for objectivity, evidence, and responsiveness to the study charge. The review comments and draft manuscript remain confidential to protect the integrity of the deliberative process. The committee wishes to thank the following individuals for their review of this report:

MARION E. BROOME, University of Alabama at Birmingham
ELLEN WRIGHT CLAYTON, Vanderbilt University
RONALD E. DAHL, University of Pittsburgh Medical Center
REBECCA S. DRESSER, Washington University in St. Louis
ABIGAIL ENGLISH, Center for Adolescent Health & the Law
PAUL L. GELSINGER, Citizens for Responsible Care and Research
PAUL W. GOEBEL, Chesapeake Research Review, Inc.
DALE HAMMERSCHMIDT, University of Minnesota
GREGORY L. KEARNS, Children's Mercy Hospitals and Clinics, University of Missouri–Kansas City
MICHELE D. KIPKE, University of Southern California and Childrens Hospital Los Angeles

JEFFREY L. PLATT, Mayo Clinic
GREGORY H. REAMAN, Children's Oncology Group and
George Washington University
LISE YASUI, Children's Oncology Group and New Approaches to
Neuroblastoma Therapy Consortium

Although the reviewers listed above have provided many constructive comments and suggestions, they were not asked to endorse the conclusions or recommendations, nor did they see the final draft of the report before its release. The review of this report was overseen by **THOMAS F. BOAT,** Cincinnati Children's Hospital Medical Center and University of Cincinnati, and **BERNARD LO,** University of California, San Francisco. Appointed by the NRC Report Review Committee, these individuals were responsible for making certain that an independent examination of this report was carried out in accordance with the institutional procedures and that all review comments were carefully considered. Responsibility for the final content of this report rests entirely with the authoring committee and the institution.

ETHICAL CONDUCT
OF CLINICAL RESEARCH
INVOLVING CHILDREN

Summary

In recent decades, advances in biomedical research have, each year, helped to save or lengthen the lives of tens of thousands of children around the world, prevent or reduce illness or disability in many more, and improve the quality of life for countless others. Beyond the infants, children, and adolescents directly affected, the benefits of research extend to the families, friends, and communities who love and care for them. Since the 1950s, for example, researchers have created vaccines against polio, measles, mumps, and a number of other childhood infections that have dramatically cut deaths, disability, and discomfort from these diseases. Children and their families have also benefited from research demonstrating the harm or ineffectiveness of what were once standard therapies, for instance, high-dose oxygen for premature infants.

Despite these advances, pediatricians and others have argued that infants, children, and adolescents have not shared equally with adults in advances in biomedicine. In particular, many drugs with potential pediatric uses have not been tested in studies that include children. These drugs may

1

still be prescribed for children based on physicians' judgment about how data from studies with adults might be extrapolated to children. Because children differ physiologically from adults in myriad ways that can affect how drugs work in the body, extrapolation based on adult drug doses and children's weight or age can be dangerous and lead to underdosing, overdosing, or specific adverse effects not evident in adults.

The U.S. Congress, the Food and Drug Administration (FDA), and the National Institutes of Health (NIH) have acted in recent years to expand research involving children. Notwithstanding the expected benefits of these efforts, some caution is appropriate. Unlike most adults, children usually lack the legal right and the intellectual and emotional maturity to consent to research participation on their own behalf. Their vulnerability demands special consideration from researchers and policymakers and additional protections beyond those provided to mentally competent adult participants in research.

In the United States, research that is supported, conducted, or regulated by the U.S. Department of Health and Human Services (DHHS) is now subject to a (mostly) common set of regulations to protect adult and child participants in research. Nonetheless, deficiencies in the conduct of human research—most of which are fairly minor but some of which result in deaths or serious injuries—continue to be revealed.

Concerns about the adequacy of the system for protecting child participants in research, combined with the public commitment to expanding clinical research involving children, provided the impetus for this Institute of Medicine (IOM) report, which was requested in the Best Pharmaceuticals for Children Act of 2002 (P.L. 107-109). The legislation charged the IOM with preparing a report that reviewed federal regulations, reports, and research and that made recommendations about desirable practices in clinical research involving children. Specifically designated topics were (1) the appropriateness of the regulations for children of various ages, (2) the interpretation of regulatory criteria for approving research, (3) the processes for securing parents' and children's agreement to a child's participation in research, (4) the expectations and comprehension of children and parents about participating in research, (5) the appropriateness of payments related to the child's participation in research, (6) compliance with and enforcement of federal regulations, and (7) the unique roles and responsibilities of institutional review boards (IRBs).

The report, prepared by a 14-member committee of the Institute of Medicine, focuses primarily on clinical research involving preventive, diagnostic, treatment, or similar interventions and direct interactions with children. It stresses three broad themes:

*   Well-designed and well-executed clinical research involving children is essential to improve the health of future children—and future adults—in the United States and worldwide.* Children should not be routinely excluded from clinical studies. No subgroups of children should be either unduly burdened as research participants or unduly excluded from involvement.

*   A robust system for protecting human research participants in general is a necessary foundation for protecting child research participants in particular.* An efficiently administered, effectively performing system with adequate resources must, however, commit additional resources and attention to meet ethical and legal standards for protecting infants, children, and adolescents who participate in research.

*   Effective implementation of policies to protect child participants in research requires appropriate expertise in child health at all stages in the design, review, and conduct of such research.* This expertise includes knowledge of infant, child, and adolescent physiology and development as well as awareness of the unique scientific, psychosocial, and ethical requirements and challenges of pediatric clinical care and research.

REGULATORY CONTEXT

In 1983, DHHS published the first regulations specifically governing federally supported or conducted research involving children (Subpart D of 45 CFR 46). This was 10 years after the first general departmental regulations on protecting human participants in research were published (now Subpart A of 45 CFR 46, also called the "Common Rule"). Similar but not identical regulations for research regulated by FDA are found at 21 CFR 50 and 56. (For simplicity in making comparisons, the regulations at 45 CFR 46 are termed DHHS regulations, even though the FDA is part of DHHS.)

Subpart A of the regulations sets forth basic requirements for all covered research, including provisions that the risk to research participants be minimized, that the risks be reasonable in relation to the anticipated benefits, that the selection of research participants be equitable, and that informed consent be obtained from participants. Subpart D provides that parents must, under most circumstances, provide permission before children (usually those under age 18 as defined by state laws) can participate in research. It also provides that, when appropriate, children should affirmatively agree or assent to participate in research.

In addition, Subpart D establishes four categories under which research involving children can be approved. Omitting reference to specific requirements for parents' permission and children's assent, these categories of approvable research are summarized in Box S.1.

The committee concluded that the federal regulations providing special

---

BOX S.1
Summary of Categories of Research Involving Children That Are Approvable Under Subpart D of 45 CFR 46

Section 46.404: Research that involves no greater than minimal risk to children

Section 46.405: Research that involves greater than minimal risk but the risk is justified by the anticipated benefit to the participants and the relation of the anticipated benefit to the risk is at least as favorable as that presented by available alternative approaches.

Section 46.406: Research that involves greater than minimal risk and no prospect of direct benefit to research participants but (a) the risk represents only a minor increase over minimal risk, (b) the research involves experience reasonably commensurate with those inherent in the child's medical, dental, psychological, social, or educational situations, and (c) the research is likely to yield generalizable, vitally important knowledge about the child's disorder or condition.

Section 46.407: Research that is not otherwise approvable but that the IRB and the Secretary of DHHS determine presents an opportunity to understand, prevent, or alleviate a serious problem affecting children's health or welfare and will be conducted in accordance with sound ethical principles.

NOTE: The corresponding regulations for the FDA are found at 21 CFR 50.51 to 50.54.

---

protections for child participants are, in general, appropriate for children of different ages. They reasonably defer to state laws that define both the age at which individuals become entitled to make medical care decisions and the special circumstances under which minors may make such decisions in their own right (e.g., for care related to sexually transmitted diseases).

For the most part, the problems with the regulations relate to insufficient government guidance about their interpretation and implementation, shortfalls in data about implementation and compliance, and variability in investigator and IRB interpretations of the criteria for approving research involving children. Some of these criteria include inherently subjective elements that the committee doubts would be substantially and predictably clarified by revising the regulations. As discussed below, one change that the committee does recommend is that FDA make its policies consistent with those of DHHS that allow the waiver of parental permission for children's, especially adolescents', participation in research when permission is not a reasonable requirement to protect a child. Another recommendation is that all research that includes infants, children, and adolescents should occur under the umbrella of a formal program for the protection of human research participants (Recommendation 8.1). Because the federal government may not have the authority to require this, state governments should consider exercising their authority to regulate research in ways that are consistent with federal regulations and supportive of multistate studies. All federal agencies that support or conduct research involving children can, however, adopt the protections in Subpart D of 45 CFR 46.

INTERPRETING RESEARCH RISK AND
OTHER REGULATORY CONCEPTS

Categorizing, evaluating, and weighing the risks of proposed research are among the most challenging and subjective tasks for those charged with reviewing research that includes infants, children, and adolescents. The committee was specifically asked to consider the regulatory definition of "minimal risk" in the context of research involving children. It also examined several other closely related concepts in the regulations.

For purposes of approving human research, federal regulations define the term *minimal risk* as meaning "that the probability and magnitude of harm or discomfort anticipated in the research are not greater in and of themselves than those ordinarily encountered in daily life or during the performance of routine physical or psychological examinations or tests" (45 CFR 46.102(i); 21 CFR 50.3(k)). That this standard invites variable interpretations has long been clear, especially for studies involving multiple sites and multiple IRBs.

Consistent with the conclusions of a number of other groups, the committee rejected an interpretation of minimal risk that would allow greater research risk for children exposed to higher than average risk of harm in their personal lives (e.g., because they are ill or live in unsafe neighborhoods). This "relative" interpretation misinterprets the minimal risk standard and undercuts its moral and social purposes for pediatric studies, which are to guide judgments about when risks are low enough to safely and ethically enroll children in studies that are not designed to benefit them. The assessment of risk should be compared or indexed to the experiences of average, normal, healthy children.

Recommendation 4.1: In evaluating the potential harms or discomfort posed by a research protocol that includes children, investigators, and reviewers of research protocols should

• interpret *minimal risk* in relation to the normal experiences of average, healthy, normal children;
• focus on the equivalence of potential harms or discomfort anticipated in research with the harms or discomfort that average, healthy, normal children may encounter in their daily lives or experience in routine physical or psychological examinations or tests;

- consider the risk of harms or discomfort in relation to the ages of the children to be studied; and
- assess the duration as well as the probability and magnitude of potential harms or discomfort in determining the level of risk.

In Section 406 of 45 CFR 46, federal regulations permit research that involves a minor increase over minimal risk without the prospect of direct benefit if the research involves children with a disorder or condition, is likely to yield vital knowledge about that disorder or condition, and entails research experiences that are reasonably similar to those that such children encounter in certain other situations. Consistent with the interpretation of minimal risk, the interpretation of this level of research risk should *not* allow a higher threshold of risk for children who are exposed to more risk in other aspects of their lives (Recommendation 4.2). Also, consistent with the language of the National Commission for the Protection of Human Subjects of Biomedical and Behavioral Research, which defined this standard in 1977, the risk allowed under this category can be only *slightly* above minimal risk.

In the context of IRB determinations about whether a study can be approved under Section 406 of 45 CFR 46, the term *condition* is also ambiguous. If a characteristic of a group of children is to be designated as a condition that allows children to be exposed to a higher level of risk without a prospect of benefit, the link between the characteristic and a deficit in children's health or well-being should be supported by scientific evidence or clinical knowledge.

> Recommendation 4.3: In determining whether proposed research involving a minor increase over minimal risk and no direct benefit can be approved, the term *condition* should be interpreted as referring to a specific (or a set of specific) physical, psychological, neurodevelopmental, or social characteristic(s) that an established body of scientific evidence or clinical knowledge has shown to negatively affect children's health and well-being or to increase their risk of developing a health problem in the future.

The committee further recommends that IRBs make (and record in their minutes) explicit determinations about each of the regulatory criteria that must be met for the approval of research involving children (Recommendation 4.4). To assist investigators and IRBs, the committee recommends that the DHHS Office for Human Research Protections (OHRP) develop explicit guidance and examples for IRBs and investigators based on the findings presented in this IOM report and the work that it cites (Recommendation 4.5). In addition, the Secretary's Advisory Committee on Human Research Protection is encouraged to continue work to develop consensus assessments about the risk of common research procedures, including rationales for the categorization of procedures judged to involve either minimal risk or a minor increase over minimal risk (Recommendation 4.5).

UNDERSTANDING AND AGREEING TO CHILDREN'S PARTICIPATION IN RESEARCH

Informed consent is widely regarded as a cornerstone of ethical research. Because children (except for adolescents under certain conditions) do not have the legal capacity to provide informed consent, the concepts of parental *permission* and child *assent* have been developed as standards for ethical research involving children. (The term *parent* is used here to include guardians as well.)

Parents asked for permission for a child's participation in clinical research are often making decisions under great stress and time pressure. Some prefer to trust the physician's assessment rather than make their own, and investigators must be acutely sensitive to the influence that they wield in discussions with parents of ill or injured children. As is also the case for adults considering their own participation in research, a significant minority of parents may misunderstand the purpose of the research, especially when the research tests a therapy for a serious medical condition. Nonetheless, the goal of informed agreement by parents remains an important protection for children, both when participation in research is initially sought and throughout the course of a study.

The capacity to make voluntary, informed decisions clearly evolves from birth through adolescence and into adulthood. It also clearly varies among individuals of the same age. The committee found some disagreement and mixed evidence about the age at which children can be meaningfully involved in discussions and decisions about their research participation given various research contexts. Again, despite this uncertainty, the goal should be to involve children in discussions and decisions about research participation as appropriate given their cognitive and emotional maturity and psychological state. Involving children in discussions and decision making respects their emerging maturity, helps them prepare for participation in research, gives them an opportunity to express their concerns and objections and, possibly, allows them to influence what happens to them.

As many others have argued, informed consent—and, by extension, permission and assent—should be viewed as a process and not a form. This goal remains less a reality than an aspiration. IRBs should focus more of their attention on the adequacy of the process for securing permission and assent in proposed research protocols. Discussions with parents and, as appropriate, children should allow sufficient time for questions and, if necessary, further explanations. Such discussions should precede the presentation of a permission or assent form.

> Recommendation 5.1: To focus attention on the process of requesting parents' permission and children's assent to research participation, investigators should provide and IRBs should review protocol descriptions of
>
> • who will request permission and assent;
> • how and when permission and assent will be requested;
> • who should be contacted if parents have questions or concerns about the research; and
> • for studies that extend over considerable periods of time, when and how permission and assent may be requested again, for example, as children reach important developmental milestones.

Although the research literature is limited and not entirely consistent, it supports a gradual expansion of the involvement of children in discussions and decisions about their participation in research. For younger children, the emphasis should be on providing basic information about what will happen, responding to their questions and concerns, and—particularly when the research does not offer the prospect of direct benefit—recognizing when children do not want to participate. As children mature, they can participate more fully in discussions and decisions about their participation in research. Older adolescents may not have the legal capacity to make decisions in their own right, but research generally suggests that the substance of the assent process can be similar to the substance of the consent process for adults *if* that process is properly designed to accommodate people of various educational, social, and cultural backgrounds.

> Recommendation 5.6: In designing and reviewing procedures for seeking a child's assent to participation in research, investigators and institutional review boards should aim to create assent processes that consider and respect the child and the family as a unit as well as individually. The process for requesting assent should
>
> • be developmentally appropriate given the ages and other characteristics of the children to be approached;
> • provide opportunities for children to express and discuss their willingness or unwillingness to participate;
> • clarify for parents and children (as appropriate) the degree of control that each will have over the participation decision; and
> • when appropriate, describe to children and parents the kinds of information about the child that will or will not be shared with the parents.

One particularly sensitive issue is when adolescents should be free to consent to research participation without parental permission. Certain studies that are important to adolescent health and well-being will not be feasible without such a waiver. The research reviewed here suggests that the DHHS regulations appropriately provide for waivers, including a requirement that a suitable mechanism is provided to protect children when parental permission is waived. FDA should revise its rule on the waiver of parental permission to be consistent with DHHS rules (Recommendation 5.4).

PAYMENT RELATED TO RESEARCH PARTICIPATION

Ethical standards for participation in research require that the agreement to participate be freely given; that is, it should not be either coerced or unduly influenced by psychological, financial, or other pressure. The major concern about payments related to research participation is that they may unduly influence and distort decisions about research participation made by individuals in their own right or by parents on behalf of their child.

Survey and other information available to the committee suggested that many IRBs and research institutions do not have written policies to guide reviews of research payment practices. By developing written policies on payments to parents and children, IRBs can consider ethical issues outside of the context of an individual protocol. Such deliberation will help achieve a fairer and more consistent approach to making decisions on appropriate payments. In general, these policies should provide that payment be discussed during the process of seeking parents' permission and the child's assent to participation in research.

Recommendation 6.1: Institutional review boards, research institutions, and sponsors of research that includes children and adolescents should adopt explicit written policies on acceptable and unacceptable types and amounts of payments related to research participation. These policies should specify that investigators

- disclose the amount, the recipient, the timing, and the purpose (e.g., an expense reimbursement or a token of appreciation to a child) of any payments as part of the process of seeking parents' permission and, as appropriate, children's assent to research participation;
- avoid emphasis on payments or descriptions of payments as benefits of participating in research during the permission or assent process; and
- obtain institutional review board approval for the disclosure of information about payments in advertisements and in permission and assent forms and procedures.

Certain types of payments to parents or adolescents are usually, if not always acceptable, for example, reimbursement for reasonable expenses that are necessary for participation in research. Other payments are never appropriate, for example, paying parents for permitting their child to be exposed to a greater research risk. Compensation to parents for lost wages or time may be appropriate under carefully scrutinized circumstances. One objective of IRB and institutional policies on payments related to children's participation in research should be to encourage equal access to study participation, regardless of a family's economic status, while avoiding practices that risk exerting undue influence over the parents' and children's consideration of the child's participation in research (Recommendation 6.2). To respond to the diverse barriers to children's participation in research, nonfinancial alternatives that equalize participation opportunities should also be considered, for example, adjusting the times or places for research visits for parents who cannot take time off from work.

REGULATORY COMPLIANCE, QUALITY IMPROVEMENT, AND ACCCREDITATION

The dearth of information about human research protection programs in general and about protections for child research participants in particular makes it impossible to describe adequately the implementation and enforcement of federal regulations and, likewise, hinders evaluation and improvement efforts. As one of its recommendations for strengthening the system for protecting human participants in research, the 2003 IOM report *Responsible Research* proposed that DHHS commission studies to gather basic information about the current system as needed to identify problems and track improvements. This committee agrees.

Recommendation 7.1: To help identify what further guidance, education, or other steps may be needed to protect child participants in research, the U.S. Department of Health and Human Services—with direction from the U.S. Congress, if necessary—should develop and implement a plan for gathering and reporting data on

• research involving children, including the categorization of studies by the relevant section of federal regulations (45 CFR 46.404 to 407 and 21 CFR 50.51 to 54), and
• implementation of the regulations that govern research involving children, including data from the Office for Human Research Protections and the Food and Drug Administration on their inquiries, investigations, and sanctions related to such research.

The committee recognizes that such data collection responsibilities will require a considerable investment of resources by OHRP and, particularly, FDA, given the latter's more extensive oversight activities. Nonetheless, in calling for the present IOM study, the U.S. Congress has already recognized the concerns presented by research involving children and the regulations applicable to that research. If necessary, it should be prepared to direct and fund the collection of data on research involving children.

For most public policies, including those related to the protection of child participants in research, the path to desired results depends in large measure on the voluntary actions of private individuals and organizations. Within the arena of human research protections, voluntary quality improvement efforts should, if successful and sustained, strengthen the overall system of human research protections within which the policies for children are embedded.

Consistent with recommendations in earlier IOM reports, the committee supports the further development and systematic evaluation of accreditation for human research participant protection programs. For accrediting organizations to assess programs that encompass research involving children, these organizations themselves need expertise in child health and research involving children (Recommendation 7.2).

ROLES AND RESPONSIBILITIES IN PROTECTING CHILDREN INVOLVED IN RESEARCH

The benefits to the health of children collectively from involving more children individually in clinical research are compelling. Also compelling are the moral and legal obligations of all involved in research to specially protect children who are not able to provide informed, reasoned, and voluntary consent to their participation in research in their own right.

This report focuses on those who conduct, review, regulate, and fund research, but the central role of parents must be recognized and respected. Parents have a most intimate and profound duty and desire to protect and promote their child's safety and well-being in research, as in all realms of life. By improving the initial and continuing process for securing parental agreement to a child's participation in research, investigators, IRBs, research institutions, and others can support parents in fulfilling their responsibilities and, thereby, help them feel that they have done the right thing for their child, whatever their decisions about research participation. Box S.2 summarizes some questions that parents may want to ask about their child's participation in research.

BOX S.2
Questions Parents May Want to Ask When Considering Their Child's Participation in Clinical Research

- What is the purpose of the research? Who is paying for it?
- Where will the research be done? How long will it last?
- What kinds of procedures and/or tests will be involved? How will they differ from what will happen if my child doesn't participate?
- What are the possible short-term and long-term harms and benefits (if any) of the study? How do they compare with treatments that my child is receiving or might receive without being in the research?
- Will the research procedure(s) hurt? If so, for how long? What can be done to prevent or limit pain? Are there other side effects?
- What will I have to do? What will my child have to do?
- Will I have to pay anything if my child is part of the study? Will my child or I be paid anything for participating?
- Who do I call with questions or in an emergency? What will happen if something goes wrong?
- What will I be told during the study and after it is finished?
- How can I withdraw my child from the study? Will that affect my child's care?
- Who will know that my child is in the study? What information will they get?

Investigators

In clinical research, the investigator has the ultimate responsibility for ensuring the safety, rights, and welfare of individuals participating in research and for seeing that all members of the research team adhere to the requirements for valid, ethical research. This is the case whether the investigator has a major role in designing the research or uses a design developed by a research sponsor or others. Likewise, he or she is responsible for the safety and welfare of child participants in research, whether the study includes only children or also includes adults.

Box S.3 summarizes some of the major responsibilities of clinical investigators who conduct research that includes infants, children, or adolescents. To varying degrees, research institutions, sponsors of research, and regulators understand—or should understand—that investigators' success in fulfilling their responsibilities depends significantly on supportive administrative, financial, educational, and other systems, both local and national. The infrastructure provided by these systems should stretch from the initial education of investigators through the eventual dissemination of research findings and likewise should extend to all settings and types of practice.

BOX S.3
Key Responsibilities of Investigators for the
Ethical Conduct of Clinical Research Involving
Infants, Children, and Adolescents

• Achieve and maintain appropriate training, credentials, and skills to perform or supervise all clinical and research procedures required for a study that includes children.
• Achieve and maintain appropriate training and knowledge to meet the ethical and regulatory requirements for conducting research that includes children.
• Ensure that research protocols involving children conform to ethical and scientific standards for such research.
• Submit proposals and proposal amendments for scientific and ethical review and approval before beginning or modifying research and, as required, during the course of research.
• Conduct the study in accord with the approved protocol.
• Disclose potential conflicts of interest to appropriate parties.
• Ensure that the processes for securing parents' permission and children's assent to research participation meet ethical and regulatory standards and are effective and active through the duration of the study. Provide the rationale and propose appropriate protections consistent with federal and state laws if a waiver of parental permission is sought.
• Communicate with children participating in research in developmentally appropriate ways—and with guidance from their parents—about what will happen to them throughout the course of the research.
• Support appropriate safety monitoring and reporting of adverse events.
• Report protocol violations, errors, and problems as required to research sponsors, regulators, or IRBs.
• Disclose research results to the scientific community and the public.
• Communicate research results, as appropriate, to research participants or participant communities.

SOURCE: Adapted from IOM, *Responsible Research: A Systems Approach to Protecting Research Participants.* Washington, D.C.: The National Academies Press, 2003a.

Institutional Review Boards and Research Institutions

Much of the administrative infrastructure and activity that contribute to competent and ethical IRB and research institution performance will support equally the protection of adult and child participants in research. Beyond this foundation, research institutions that conduct studies that include children and IRBs that review such studies have further ethical and legal responsibilities that require special attention. Box S.4 summarizes these responsibilities, which begin with educating IRB members, investigators, and others about their ethical and legal obligations to protect child participants in research.

> **BOX S.4**
> **Key Ethical and Legal Responsibilities of IRBs and Research Institutions Involved with Clinical Research That Includes Infants, Children, and Adolescents**
>
> • Educate IRB members and, as needed, IRB pediatric consultants about the ethical, legal, and scientific standards for approving research involving children and their appropriate interpretation.
> • Educate investigators who conduct research that includes infants, children, or adolescents about their special ethical, legal, and scientific responsibilities.
> • Apply ethical and regulatory standards for the initial and continuing review and approval of research protocols involving children, including careful evaluation and categorization of research risks.
> • Provide for adequate expertise in child health and research in the review of protocols that include children, including assessment of whether those conducting the studies have adequate pediatric expertise.
> • Make available reference materials and resources on research involving children, including information on research ethics, as part of IRB or research administration web sites and educational programs.
> • Conduct ongoing assessments to guide improvements in IRB performance in reviewing and monitoring research involving children.
> • Develop explicit policies or guidelines on important topics for which additional guidance to IRB members or investigators is needed (see Box 8.3).

A critical obligation of IRBs is to bring appropriate expertise to the review of research involving infants, children, and adolescents. As more children participate in clinical trials and other research, the need grows for both investigator and IRB expertise in the biological, medical, behavioral, and emotional development and needs of children. The following recommendation applies to independent, central, and other IRBs as well as to those affiliated with biomedical and social science research institutions and children's hospitals:

Recommendation 8.3: Institutional review boards (IRBs) that review protocols for clinical research involving infants, children, and adolescents should have adequate expertise in child health care and research. They should have at least three individuals with such expertise present as members or alternates during meetings in which a research protocol involving children is reviewed. Among them, these individuals—who may be generalists or specialists—should have expertise in pediatric clinical care and research, the psychosocial dimensions of child and adolescent health care and research, and the ethics of research involving children. As appropriate for specific studies, IRBs should consult with other child health experts and with parents, children, adolescents, and community members who can provide relevant family or community perspectives.

Publicly accessible information about IRB procedures and guidance related to the design and review of protocols that include children is limited and highly variable, which makes it difficult to judge this dimension of IRB and institutional performance. Some publicly accessible IRB websites display little readily identifiable information or guidance for investigators or IRB members related to research that includes children. For example, some websites have protocol checklists or application forms that include no items or an incomplete list of items that highlight requirements for research involving children (and no obvious alternative document with the relevant items). Federal agencies have found deficiencies in IRB practices related to the review of research involving children, particularly in the description of the bases for IRB decisions in the meeting minutes. More complete and specific protocol checklists or application forms would help highlight the ethical and regulatory standards for approving and conducting research involving children and should improve compliance with those standards.

> **Recommendation 8.4:** For their policy manuals, websites, and other resources, institutional review boards (IRBs) and research institutions should provide easily understood and easily located information that directs investigator and IRB member attention to the ethical principles and special regulatory requirements that apply to the conduct and review of research that includes infants, children, and adolescents.

Federal Policymakers and Regulators

For approximately a half-century, federal agencies responsible for conducting and sponsoring biomedical research and for regulating medical products have—sometimes directed by Congress—played a major role in developing policies to protect human participants in research. In recent years, they have paid increasing attention to the application of those policies by investigators, IRBs, and research institutions and to the education of these parties about their responsibilities.

The guidance and other resources that OHRP and FDA have made available strongly shape if not dominate local IRB policy manuals and resource links. Although investigators and IRB members at research institutions should have good local support as recommended above, they and others—including policymakers and others interested in ethical and regulatory standards for clinical research—should also find it easy to locate guidance and information on government websites. FDA, which now has an Office of Pediatric Therapeutics within the Center for Drug Evaluation and Research, has a web page dedicated to pediatric research with links to a variety of resources, including FDA regulations and guidelines for such research. The OHRP website has limited resources relevant to research involving children and they can be difficult to locate.

Recommendation 8.6: The Office for Human Research Protections, the Food and Drug Administration, the National Institutes of Health, and other agencies with relevant responsibilities that include research involving children should each provide—in an easily identifiable document or set of linked documents—comprehensive, consistent, periodically updated guidance to investigators, institutional review boards, and others on the interpretation and application of federal regulations for the protection of child participants in research.

DHHS has moved to significantly improve the process for reviewing proposals for research involving children that IRBs have referred to the Secretary for approval under the provisions of 45 CFR 46.407. That effort, with support from the Secretary's Advisory Committee on Human Research Protections, should continue with the objective of establishing an open and publicly accessible process for reviewing referred protocols (Recommendation 8.7). DHHS should also develop guidance to help IRBs determine when it is appropriate to refer protocols for review. The referral of proposed research for "national" review should be reserved for "exceptional situations" and research of "major significance" and protocols should only be approved if they are expected to produce vitally important knowledge.

The committee encourages the continued investment by OHRP in its quality improvement initiative, with attention to the special requirements and challenges of research involving children. OHRP, FDA, and other agencies should also continue to cooperate in the development of educational programs for use by government agencies, IRBs, research institutions, pediatric academic societies, and other groups.

In addition, agencies should fund research and demonstration projects to expand the knowledge base for improving the performance of the system for protecting child participants in research. They can, for example, test strategies to improve the quality and consistency of reviews for multisite research projects and reduce unnecessary burdens and frustrations for their investigators and sponsors. Such improvements will not eliminate tensions between the goal of protecting today's children from research harms and the goal of advancing research that improves the health and well-being of tomorrow's children. They can, however, help all parties feel more confident that policymakers and IRBS are trying to identify and remove needless burdens on researchers.

The full list of committee recommendations follows.

Ethical Conduct of Clinical Research Involving Children: Complete List of Recommendations

Recommendation 4.1 In evaluating the potential harms or discomfort posed by a research protocol that includes children, investigators, and reviewers of research protocols should

- interpret *minimal risk* in relation to the normal experiences of average, healthy, normal children;
- focus on the equivalence of potential harms or discomfort anticipated in research with the harms or discomfort that average, healthy, normal children may encounter in their daily lives or experience in routine physical or psychological examinations or tests;
- consider the risk of harms or discomfort in relation to the ages of the children to be studied; and
- assess the duration as well as the probability and magnitude of potential harms or discomfort in determining the level of risk.

Recommendation 4.2 In evaluating the potential harms or discomfort posed by a research protocol that includes children who have a disorder or condition but no prospect of benefiting from participation, investigators and reviewers of research protocols should

- interpret *minor increase over minimal risk* to mean a slight increase in the potential for harms or discomfort beyond minimal risk (as defined in relation to the normal experiences of average, healthy, normal children);
- assess whether the research procedures or interventions present experiences that are commensurate with, that is, reasonably comparable to experiences already familiar to the children being studied on the basis of their past tests or treatments or their knowledge and understanding of the treatments that they might undergo in the future;
- consider risks of harms or discomfort in relation to the ages of the children to be studied; and
- assess the duration as well as the probability and magnitude of potential harms or discomfort in determining the level of risk.

Recommendation 4.3 In determining whether proposed research involving a minor increase over minimal risk and no direct benefit can be approved, the term *condition* should be interpreted as referring to a specific (or a set of specific) physical, psychological, neurodevelopmental, or social characteristic(s) that an established body of scientific evidence or clinical knowledge has shown to negatively affect children's health and well-being or to increase their risk of developing a health problem in the future.

Recommendation 4.4 For purposes of determining whether proposed research involving a minor increase over minimal risk and no direct benefit can be approved, institutional review boards should make a determination that

• the children to be included in the research have a disorder or condition;

• the research is likely to generate vital knowledge about the children's disorder or condition;

• the research procedures or interventions present experiences that are commensurate with, that is, reasonably comparable to, experiences already familiar to the children being studied on the basis of their past tests or treatments or on their knowledge and understanding of the treatments that they might undergo in the future; and

• the research does not unjustly single out or burden any group of children for increased exposure to research risk on the basis of their social circumstances.

Recommendation 4.5 The Secretary's Advisory Committee on Human Research Protections (U.S. Department of Health and Human Services) should continue the work of its predecessor committee by developing additional consensus descriptions of procedures or interventions that present minimal risk or no more than a minor increase over minimal risk. In addition, the Office for Human Research Protections and the Food and Drug Administration should cooperate to develop and disseminate guidance and examples for investigators and institutional review boards to clarify important regulatory concepts and definitions (including definitions of minimal risk, minor increase over minimal risk, condition, and prospect of direct benefit).

Recommendation 4.6 Institutional review boards should assess the potential harms and benefits of each intervention or procedure in a pediatric protocol to determine whether each conforms to the regulatory criteria for approving research involving children. When some procedures present the prospect of direct benefit and others do not, the potential benefits from one component of the research should not be held to offset or justify the risks presented by another.

Recommendation 5.1 To focus attention on the process of requesting parents' permission and children's assent to research participation, investigators should provide and IRBs should review protocol descriptions of

• who will request permission and assent;

• how and when permission and assent will be requested;

• who should be contacted if parents have questions or concerns about the research; and

• for studies that extend over considerable periods of time, when and how permission and assent may be requested again; for example, as children reach important developmental milestones.

Recommendation 5.2 When appropriate for research involving children with acute illnesses or injuries, investigators and institutional review boards should provide for ongoing processes for permission and assent that will accommodate a family's evolving understanding of the child's condition, the child's emotional state and decision-making capacity, and the child's changing medical and psychological status. These processes are not matters of signing or updating forms but, rather, of continuing communication based on appreciation of the difficult and even overwhelming circumstances in which parents may be asked to make grave decisions about their child's future.

Recommendation 5.3 Investigators—with assistance and oversight from institutional review boards, research institutions, and research sponsors—should design procedures for seeking parental permission for a child's participation in research that are sensitive to educational, cultural, and other differences among families and include provisions for
- educating—not merely presenting information to—parents about issues critical to informed decision making and, as appropriate, assessing the degree to which these critical issues are understood;
- writing consent and permission materials in the simplest language that still conveys essential information about the study; and
- providing competent, trained translators and interpreters, when needed, and otherwise assisting parents with limited English-language proficiency with making informed decisions.

Recommendation 5.4 Institutional review boards should consider granting waivers of parental permission for adolescent participation in research when
- the research is important to the health and well-being of adolescents and it cannot reasonably or practically be carried out without the waiver (consistent with 45 CFR 46.116(d) and 45 CFR 408(c)) or
- the research involves treatments that state laws permit adolescents to receive without parental permission (consistent with the definition of children at 46 CFR 402(a))
and when
- the investigator has presented evidence that the adolescents are capable of understanding the research and their rights as research participants and
- the research protocol includes appropriate safeguards to protect the interests of the adolescent consistent with the risk presented by the research.

Recommendation 5.5 The Food and Drug Administration should adopt policies consistent with federal regulations at 45 CFR 46.408(c) that allow institutional review boards with appropriate expertise to waive requirements for parental permission in research, provided that additional, appropriate safeguards are in place to protect the child's or the adolescent's welfare.

Recommendation 5.6 In designing and reviewing procedures for seeking a child's assent to participation in research, investigators and institutional review boards should aim to create assent processes that consider and respect the child and the family as a unit as well as individually. The process for requesting assent should

• be developmentally appropriate given the ages and other characteristics of the children to be approached;

• provide opportunities for children to express and discuss their willingness or unwillingness to participate;

• clarify for parents and children (as appropriate) the degree of control that each will have over the participation decision; and

• when appropriate, describe to children and parents the kinds of information about the child that will or will not be shared with the parents.

Recommendation 5.7 Guidance and education for investigators and members of institutional review boards should make clear that federal regulations allow discretion—based on children's developmental maturity—about the way in which information is presented to children and the manner in which assent is documented. Investigators and institutional review board members should apply that knowledge in determining what procedures will best serve the goals of assent for particular research protocols and populations.

Recommendation 5.8 To increase investigator competence in communicating with children and parents about research participation, educational programs for investigators and research staff who expect to do research involving children should include training and evaluation in developmentally appropriate and family-sensitive processes for seeking permission and assent.

Recommendation 5.9 Federal agencies, private foundations, and advocacy groups should encourage and support research on existing and innovative permission and assent processes and information materials to support improvements in these processes and guide the education of investigators and institutional review board members.

Recommendation 6.1 Institutional review boards, research institutions, and sponsors of research that includes children and adolescents should adopt explicit written policies on acceptable and unacceptable types and amounts of payments related to research participation. These policies should specify that investigators

- disclose the amount, the recipient, the timing, and the purpose (e.g., an expense reimbursement or a token of appreciation to a child) of any payments as part of the process of seeking parents' permission and, as appropriate, children's assent to research participation;
- avoid emphasis on payments or descriptions of payments as benefits of participating in research during the permission or assent process; and
- obtain institutional review board approval for the disclosure of information about payments in advertisements and in permission and assent forms and procedures.

Recommendation 6.2 In addition to offering small gifts or payments to parents and children as gestures of appreciation, investigators may also—if they minimize the potential for undue influence—act ethically to reduce certain barriers to research participation when they

- reimburse reasonable expenses directly related to a child's participation in research;
- provide reasonable, age-appropriate compensation for children based on the time involved in research that does not offer the prospect of direct benefit; and
- offer evening or weekend hours, on-site child care, and other reasonable accommodations for parental work and family commitments.

Recommendation 6.3 Research organizations and sponsors should pay the medical and rehabilitation costs for children injured as a direct result of research participation, without regard to fault. Consent and permission documents should disclose to parents (and adolescents, if appropriate) the child's right to compensation and the mechanisms for seeking such compensation.

Recommendation 6.4 Investigators and their staffs may appropriately be reimbursed for the costs associated with conducting research. Payments in the form of finder's fees or bonuses for enrolling a specific number of children or adolescents are unethical and should not be permitted.

Recommendation 7.1 To help identify what further guidance, education, or other steps may be needed to protect child participants in research, the U.S. Department of Health and Human Services—with direction from the

U.S. Congress, if necessary—should develop and implement a plan for gathering and reporting data on

- research involving children, including the categorization of studies by the relevant section of federal regulations (45 CFR 46.404 to 407 and 21 CFR 50.51 to 54), and
- implementation of the regulations that govern research involving children, including data from the Office for Human Research Protections and the Food and Drug Administration on their inquiries, investigations, and sanctions related to such research.

Recommendation 7.2 Organizations that accredit human research protection programs should

- provide for expertise in child health in their own activities;
- develop explicit provisions for evaluating whether institutional review boards are appropriately constituted and are prepared to review research involving children; and
- involve parents, children, and adolescents who have experience with pediatric clinical research in discussions to identify their concerns with the conduct of research.

Recommendation 8.1 Federal law should require that all clinical research involving infants, children, and adolescents be conducted under the oversight of a formal program for protecting human participants in research.

Recommendation 8.2 To strengthen the base of qualified pediatric clinical investigators, federal and state policymakers and research institutions should support

- education in the fundamentals of pediatric clinical research, including research ethics, in all educational programs for pediatric subspecialists and
- additional advanced education in pediatric clinical research, including research ethics, for those who seek careers in this field of research.

Recommendation 8.3 Institutional review boards (IRBs) that review protocols for clinical research involving infants, children, and adolescents should have adequate expertise in child health care and research. They should have at least three individuals with such expertise present as members or alternates during meetings in which a research protocol involving children is reviewed. Among them, these individuals—who may be generalists or specialists—should have expertise in pediatric clinical care and research, the psychosocial dimensions of child and adolescent health care and research, and the ethics of research involving children. As appropriate for specific studies, IRBs should consult with other child health experts and with parents, children, adolescents, and community members who can provide relevant family or community perspectives.

Recommendation 8.4 For their policy manuals, websites, and other resources, institutional review boards (IRBs) and research institutions should provide easily understood and easily located information that directs investigator and IRB member attention to the ethical principles and special regulatory requirements that apply to the conduct and review of research that includes infants, children, and adolescents.

Recommendation 8.5 The federal government, research institutions, research sponsors, and groups of institutional review boards should continue to test and evaluate means to improve the efficiency as well as the quality and consistency of reviews of multicenter studies, including those involving infants, children, and adolescents.

Recommendation 8.6 The Office for Human Research Protections, the Food and Drug Administration, the National Institutes of Health, and other agencies with relevant responsibilities that include research involving children should each provide—in an easily identifiable document or set of linked documents—comprehensive, consistent, periodically updated guidance to investigators, institutional review boards, and others on the interpretation and application of federal regulations for the protection of child participants in research.

Recommendation 8.7 The Office for Human Research Protections and the Food and Drug Administration should
- continue their activities to establish an open and publicly accessible review process for considering research protocols referred by institutional review boards for review under 45 CFR 46.407 and 21 CFR 50.54;
- create a standing panel that would meet as needed to consider such proposals; and
- provide detailed guidance on the interpretation of the federal regulations governing research involving children to reduce unnecessary referrals of protocols.

1

INTRODUCTION

> *The level of trust that has characterized science and its relationship with society has contributed to a period of unparalleled scientific productivity. But this trust will endure only if the scientific community devotes itself to exemplifying and transmitting the values associated with ethical scientific conduct.*
>
> National Academy of Sciences (NAS, 1995, p. v)

The scientific community today recognizes how crucial it is to understand and to honor ethical research conduct as well as scientific progress if it is to sustain the trust placed in it by policymakers and the public, including parents who are considering whether to enroll their child in clinical research. This report examines how this recognition has been demonstrated in the development of policies and practices to protect the safety and well-being of the children who participate today in research that advances the future prevention, diagnosis, and treatment of child health problems. It also describes continuing problems and concerns and makes recommendations for further action by policymakers and those who sponsor, conduct, review, and monitor research.

The benefits that biomedical research has brought to infants, children, and adolescents are remarkable. In recent decades, research has helped change medical care and public health practices in ways that, each year, save or lengthen the lives of tens of thousands of children around the world, prevent or reduce illness or disability in many more, and improve the quality of life for countless others. Beyond the infants, children, and adolescents directly affected, the benefits of research extend to the families, friends, and communities who love and care for them.

Since the 1950s, research has led to polio, measles, and other vaccines that have dramatically cut child deaths, disability, and discomfort from communicable diseases (CDC, 1999). Similarly, many premature babies with underdeveloped lungs who once would have died now survive with the use of mechanical ventilators and surfactants (substances that make breathing easier). Statistical analyses of clinical trial data have suggested a 30 to 40 percent absolute decrease in the number of deaths among affected infants after the adoption of surfactant therapy (Jobe, 1993). With improved therapies, the rate of mortality from acute lymphocytic leukemia (formerly called acute lymphoblastic leukemia) dropped by 65 percent between 1975 and 1999 for children under age 20 years (Ries et al., 2003).

Children and their families have also benefited from research identifying the unanticipated harms or ineffectiveness of what were once standard therapies. For example, in the 1940s and early 1950s, an epidemic of blindness occurred among premature newborns who were routinely treated with high-dose oxygen, which at that time was almost universally viewed as reducing the risk of anoxic brain injury (Silverman, 1977). Three controlled clinical trials demonstrated oxygen's toxic effects on the developing retina (James and Lanman, 1976). Another once widely used practice that long-term follow-up studies showed to be dangerous was irradiation for purported thymus enlargement in young children (see, e.g., Shore et al., 1985, 1993).

Despite many advances, pediatricians have argued that infants, young children, and adolescents have not shared equally with adults in the achievements of biomedicine (see, e.g., AAP, 1977, 1995). Most attention has focused on pharmaceutical research. Surveys of the *Physician's Desk Reference* (a comprehensive guide to pharmaceuticals that includes prescribing information) found in 1973 and again in 1991 that approximately 80 percent of the medications listed had no prescription information for children (Wilson, 1975; Gilman and Gal, 1992; both cited in AAP, 1995). These analyses did not assess which drugs were realistically candidates for use with children, but they nonetheless suggested an information gap for clinicians and families who were searching for safe and effective medications for sick children. This information gap leaves physicians with the choice of not prescribing such medications for children (and thus potentially undertreating them) or using the medications based on their or their colleagues' experience and judgment about whether and how data from studies with adults might apply to children of different ages.

In fact, children differ physiologically from adults in myriad ways that can affect how drugs work in the body. Extrapolation based on adult drug doses can be dangerous and lead to underdosing, overdosing, or specific adverse effects that do not occur in adults. Such extrapolation and unsystematic "experimentation" thus may expose children to risk while simultaneously failing to generate a trustworthy knowledge base for future care. For example, the drug cyclosporine was approved for adults in 1982 to counter immune system rejection of transplanted organs. The drug was then used in children without testing in clinical trials and without the same degree of success as achieved in adults. Eventually, researchers discovered that young children metabolize cyclosporine much more quickly than adults and thus need more frequent dosing to maintain therapeutic levels of the drug. For more recent immunosuppressive agents, the National Institutes of Health (NIH) and pharmaceutical companies have sponsored clinical trials to test the agents' action and effectiveness in children prospectively (Hoppu et al., 1991; Harmon, 2003; Schachter et al., 2004).

Another example of problems created by lack of pediatric studies is the undertreatment of children with schizophrenia because many drugs that have helped adults have not been tested in studies with children (Quintana and Keshavan, 1995; Findling et al., 2000). Additional examples of research shortfalls are cited in Chapter 2.[1]

Laboratory experiments, animal studies, and research involving adults helped lay the foundation for many of the research advances cited above, but most ultimately required studies involving children. Some advances, for example, the use of surfactants to treat hyaline membrane disease, required studies that could not be done initially with adults because only infants have the disease. Other advances (e.g., those involving chloramphenicol) required participation in research by children in several age groups to identify different developmental effects. Often, the research involved ill children, including premature babies. Sometimes, it depended on participation by healthy children, for example, in vaccine studies.

In recent years, both NIH and the Food and Drug Administration (FDA) have adopted policies to increase the amount of clinical research involving children. These policies are discussed in Chapter 2.

Notwithstanding the expected benefits of policies to increase the amount of research involving infants, children, and adolescents, some cau-

---

[1]Sometimes the concern is not the lack of pediatric studies *per se* but the choice of research sponsors not to disclose unfavorable research findings to clinicians and the public. Recent warnings by British and American regulatory agencies that a popular antidepressant might increase suicide-related behaviors among children prompted controversy following reports that several manufacturers of antidepressants had refused to publish results from a number of clinical studies involving children (Vedantam, 2004; see also, Boseley, 2003; Neergaard, 2003; FDA, 2003c). The FDA has requested that manufacturers of antidepressants approved for adults to submit additional analyses of the data from studies of the drugs with children.

tion is appropriate. Unlike most adults, children usually lack the legal right and the intellectual and emotional maturity to consent to research participation on their own behalf. Their vulnerability demands special consideration from researchers and policymakers and additional protections beyond those provided to mentally competent adult participants in research.

As discussed later in this chapter, instances of unethical research practices involving children have prompted public criticism and concern that has contributed to the development of current federal regulations to protect both child and adult participants in research. Since the 1960s, policymakers, researchers, research institutions, and research sponsors have taken a number of steps to strengthen ethical standards and policies for human research and to create formal programs, including institutional review boards (IRBs), to approve and monitor research. Clinical studies funded, conducted, or regulated by the government are now subject to a (mostly) common set of provisions for the protection of human participants in research, including special protections for children. One result is that some potentially important clinical studies that would be approved for adult participation cannot be approved for participation by children.

At the same time, the challenges in implementing human research protection policies consistently and effectively have multiplied as clinical research has increased in size, scope, and complexity. For example, multisite studies are now the norm for much research involving children, with a consequent increase in opportunities for delays and variations in protocol reviews and approvals across different sites.

Scientific advances, such as those emerging from the Human Genome Project, have created new challenges for the assessment of risk and benefit in research involving children. As new knowledge about genetic risk emerges, the psychological consequences of knowledge may become more or less serious for children and families, as may the social and economic harms that could follow a breach of confidentiality.

Despite the strengthening of human research protection policies and programs and in the face of highly complex advances in biomedical science, deficiencies in the conduct of research—some resulting in deaths or serious injuries—continue to be exposed. The 1999 death of 18-year-old Jesse Gelsinger, legally an adult, in a gene transfer trial at the University of Pennsylvania led to widely publicized investigations and discoveries of numerous deficiencies in gene transfer trials (see, e.g., Thompson, 2000a and Weiss and Nelson, 2000). These deficiencies included the substantial underreporting of serious health problems involving participants in the trials. As one recent report concluded, "the system intended to protect [Jesse Gelsinger] from unacceptable risks in research instead failed him" (IOM, 2001, p. 4).

Less dramatic examples of deficiencies in the conduct or review of research, some involving children, have also been identified. For example, the federal Office for Human Research Protections (OHRP) has cited several major research universities for deficiencies in their oversight of studies involving children. (The letters of determination for the years since 2000 can be viewed at http://ohrp.osophs.dhhs.gov/detrm_letrs/lindex.htm.)

These and other problems make clear that the design of standards, policies, and formal programs to protect research participants must be matched by consistent, effective implementation. As a consequence, recent years have seen more efforts to monitor policy implementation, to match responsibilities with adequate resources, and to hold investigators and institutions accountable for fulfilling their responsibilities. Still, concerns persist about the adequacy, interpretation, and application of standards and policies for research involving humans, including infants, children, and adolescents. Another area of concern is whether the various administrative and other burdens or costs imposed by protective regulations are, in all cases, justified by the contribution that they make to the goal of protecting children from unethical or harmful research.

These concerns, combined with the public commitment to expanding clinical research to benefit children, provided the impetus for this study. The major themes of this report are

• *Well-designed and well-executed clinical research involving children is essential to improve the health of future children—and future adults—in the United States and worldwide.* Failure to undertake such research can deny children timely access to effective new therapies and expose them to harm from therapies not specifically demonstrated to be safe and effective for children, including infants and adolescents. Children should not be routinely excluded from potentially beneficial clinical studies, and no subgroup of children should be either unduly burdened as research participants or unduly excluded from involvement.

• *A robust system for protecting human participants in research in general is a necessary foundation for protecting child research participants in particular.* An efficiently administered, effectively performing system with adequate resources must, however, commit additional resources and attention to meet ethical and legal standards for protecting infants, children, and adolescents who participate in research. All investigators conducting studies that include infants, children, and adolescents should work under the umbrella of a formal program for the protection of human research participants.

• *Effective implementation of policies to protect child participants in research requires appropriate expertise in child health at all stages in the design, review, and conduct of such research.* This expertise includes knowledge of infant, child, and adolescent physiology and development as well as awareness of the unique requirements and challenges of pediatric clinical care and research. It also includes understanding of ethical principles and regulatory requirements specific to child participants in research and appreciation of the family systems in which decisions about children's clinical care and research participation are made.

ORIGINS OF STUDY AND OVERVIEW OF REPORT

This report was provided for in the Best Pharmaceuticals for Children Act of 2002 (P.L. 107-109). The broad purpose of the legislation was to improve the safety and efficacy of drugs for children. One key provision renewed incentives for pharmaceutical manufacturers to test drugs in studies with children to establish the safe doses of medications that had been approved as safe and effective in adults. The legislation also called for a study by the Institute of Medicine (IOM) of research involving children.

The IOM, which is the health policy arm of the National Academy of Sciences, was to prepare a report that reviewed federal regulations, reports, and research and made recommendations about desirable practices in ethical research involving children. Appendix A describes the specific topics to be considered and the information strategies used in developing the report. The IOM appointed an expert committee of 14 members to prepare this report, which covers children of all ages, including infants and adolescents. In its work, the committee focused primarily on research that involved preventive, diagnostic, treatment, or similar interventions and direct interactions with children. It examined, but less intensively, research that involved only observation, questionnaires, medical records, or stored samples of blood or other biologic material. The committee also did not consider in depth other important questions, including financial and other conflicts of interest, standards for pediatric research in developing countries, priorities for pediatric research, scientific methods, scientific misconduct, and appropriate review of low-risk social science research. Past reports from the IOM and the National Research Council have examined a number of these issues as well as the topics that are the primary focus of this report.[2] As far as the

---

[2]These reports include *The Responsible Conduct of Research in the Health Sciences* (IOM, 1989); *Responsible Science, Volume 1: Ensuring the Integrity of the Research Process* (NAS, 1992); *On Being a Scientist: Responsible Conduct in Research* (NAS, 1995); *Protecting Data Privacy in Health Services Research* (IOM, 2000a); *Rational Therapeutics for Infants and Children: Workshop Summary* (IOM, 2000b); *Preserving Public Trust: Accreditation and Human Research Participant Protection Programs* (IOM, 2001); *Integrity in Scientific Research: Creating an Environment That Promotes Responsible Conduct* (IOM/NRC, 2002); *Responsible Research: A Systems Approach to Protecting Research Participants* (IOM, 2003a); and *Protecting Participants and Facilitating Social and Behavioral Sciences Research* (NRC, 2003). In addition, a study is currently under way to investigate protection of child participants in housing research.

committee could determine, this is one of very few comprehensive reports on ethical issues in research involving children since the first major report on this topic in 1977 (National Commission, 1977).

This report presents the committee's analysis and recommendations. It is written for a broad audience that may not be familiar with the technical aspects of clinical research nor the intricacies of federal regulations.

The remainder of this chapter offers arguments for a systems perspective on human research protection, summarizes core principles for ethical research involving humans, and reviews the evolution of policies based on these principles. Chapter 2 examines the necessity for clinical research involving children, the challenges in undertaking such research, and initiatives to encourage pediatric research. It also discusses how different government agencies and private groups or individuals conceptualize the periods of infancy, childhood, and adolescence. Chapter 3 reviews the regulations governing human research generally and pediatric research specifically.

In Chapter 4, the focus is on the interpretation and application of ethical principles and federal regulations relating to the assessment of risks and potential benefits in pediatric research. The chapter includes several recommendations intended to encourage greater consistency in the interpretation of the regulations. Chapter 5 turns to the question of what children and parents understand about participation in research; it makes recommendations about processes for seeking parent's permission and children's assent to research participation. Chapter 6 examines the question of paying for children's participation in research and makes recommendations for IRBs.

Chapter 7 considers compliance with the regulations governing pediatric research. The chapter also discusses accreditation and quality improvement as strategies for improving performance. The final chapter discusses the roles and responsibilities of IRBs as well as investigators, regulators, and others whose actions affect the safety and well-being of child participants in research.

Appendix B presents an in-depth review of state laws relating to children's agreement to medical care and research participation. Appendix C briefly considers other protections for research participants beyond those emphasized in the text of the report. Appendix D includes a glossary, and Appendix E contains short biographies of committee members.

DEFINITIONS: RESEARCH, CLINICAL RESEARCH, AND HUMAN SUBJECTS OR RESEARCH PARTICIPANTS

As defined in federal regulations, *research* is "a systematic investigation, including research development, testing and evaluation, designed to develop or contribute to generalizable knowledge" (45 CFR 46.102(d)).

The regulations also refer more specifically to research that either generates data through intervention or interaction with the individual or obtains identifiable private information about an individual (45 CFR 46.102(f)).

What constitutes an effort to develop generalizable knowledge is the subject of some disagreement and confusion (see, e.g., NBAC, 2001b). For example, student "research" projects involving questionnaires or observation are often intended to teach students about research design and techniques, statistical analysis, scientific methods, and, more broadly, scientific thinking. Some may qualify as research, whereas others are clearly learning exercises that hold no promise of creating generalizable knowledge.

Questions have also arisen about certain kinds of institutional projects to improve the quality of their medical care by systematically assessing the link between processes of care and health or other outcomes (see, e.g., Brett and Grodin, 1991; Casarett et al., 2000; Bellin and Dubler, 2001; and NBAC, 2001b). These quality improvement projects use systematic planning, control, assessment, and intervention methods that rely on many scientific precepts, methods, and analytic strategies that are also used in health services and other kinds of research (see, e.g., Berwick et al., 1990; Batalden et al., 1994; Nelson et al., 1998; and IOM, 2000a). Some projects are undertaken from the outset with the intent to generalize and publish findings and so qualify as research. Many other projects have only internal, institutional goals and do not constitute research. Like other routine management decisions and actions that are clearly not research, quality improvement activities may cause harm, be monitored for consequences, and even be described in trade publications. Drawing the line between research and certain health care management strategies continues to be a challenge and suggests the need for better communication between human research protection programs and institutional quality improvement activities (see, e.g., Bellin and Dubler, 2001).

Some questions also arise about the boundary between clinical research and clinical practice innovations by individual physicians. Typical examples of such innovations include a surgeon's modification of an existing surgical technique or trying different mechanical ventilation strategies for patients with respiratory distress. The general view is that radically new procedures should "be made the object of formal research at an early stage in order to determine whether they are safe and effective" (National Commission, 1978a, p. 3). The definitions of "radically new" and "early stage" are, however, controversial.

For purposes of regulatory oversight, the National Bioethics Advisory Commission (NBAC) recommended that research should be considered to involve human participants "when individuals (1) are exposed to manipulations, interventions, observations, or other types of interactions with investigators or (2) are identifiable through research using biological materials, medical and other records, or databases" (NBAC, 2001b, p. 40). Thus, research involving human biological materials, medical record data, or other information that cannot be linked to identifiable individuals is not human research in this context. NBAC also recommended that federal policy explicitly identify research activities that are not subject to federal regulations.

Clinical research is commonly viewed as research that uses human participants to test the safety or effectiveness of medical interventions (e.g., drugs or diagnostic tests) or to study the diagnosis or pathophysiology of diseases, disorders, or injuries. Synonyms include clinical study and clinical investigation. A clinical experiment is one kind of clinical research. Consistent with the FDA's statutory mandate, agency regulations on the protection of human subjects define clinical investigation as "any experiment that involves a test article [e.g., a drug or medical device] and one or more human subjects and that either is subject to requirements for prior submission to the Food and Drug Administration. . . [or] . . . the results of which are intended to be submitted later to, or held for inspection by, the Food and Drug Administration as part of an application for a research or marketing permit" (21 CFR 50.3(c)).[3] More broadly conceived, "clinical investigation . . . includes all studies intended to produce knowledge valuable to the prevention, diagnosis, prognosis, treatment, or cure of human disease" (IOM, 1994a, p. 35). Disease, in this context, can be interpreted to include disorders and injuries. This broad definition encompasses biomedical research and certain kinds of psychosocial, health services, and epidemiological studies, as well as laboratory research involving, for example, tissues, cells, and genes. As explained earlier, the emphasis in this report is on clinical research that involves direct interactions with child participants in research.

Some statements of ethical principles for research have made an implicit or explicit distinction between therapeutic and nontherapeutic research.[4] The former category of research would, for example, include the

---

[3]In other FDA regulations related specifically to drugs, clinical investigation is defined as "any experiment in which a drug is administered or dispensed to, or used involving, one or more human subjects. For the purposes of this part, an experiment is any use of a drug except for the use of a marketed drug in the course of medical practice" (21 CFR 312.3(b)).

[4]The Declaration of Helsinki has been criticized on this point, and the National Commission on the Protection of Human Subjects in Research has been commended for clearly rejecting the distinction in its 1977 and 1978 reports (see, e.g., discussion in Jonsen, 1998a, and Levine, 1999). The federal regulations on protection of human participants in research follow the National Commission's lead. FDA has, however, issued as guidance the International Conference of Harmonisation's guidelines on good clinical practice, which makes the distinction (ICH, 1996). These documents are further discussed in later sections of this report.

administration of a new combination of chemotherapeutic agents for the treatment of leukemia to test the hypothesis that the experimental agents will provide a benefit over standard therapy. In contrast, a study involving various tests intended solely to increase knowledge of the pathophysiology of a disease would be nontherapeutic, although the knowledge gained might contribute to the development of a therapy that might subsequently benefit those who had participated in the study. Federal regulations on protection of human subjects in research do not use therapeutic-nontherapeutic distinction but refer to *interventions* with the *prospect of direct benefit* or with *no prospect of direct benefit* to participants (45 CFR 46.405 and 46.406). This wording, which is also adopted in this report, puts the focus not on the research as a whole but rather on the characteristics of the specific interventions that are included in a study. Some of the interventions may have the prospect of direct benefit whereas others may not. Under federal regulations, these distinctions can affect what aspects of a research protocol are approvable by an IRB. Another problem with the characterization of studies as therapeutic or nontherapeutic is that such labeling may contribute to the common confusion between clinical care and clinical research. Chapters 4 and 5 discuss these distinctions further.

Federal regulations define a *human subject* of research as "a living individual about whom an investigator (whether professional or student) conducting research obtains (1) data through intervention or interaction with the individual, or (2) identifiable private information. Intervention includes both physical procedures by which data are gathered (for example, venipuncture) and manipulations of the subject or the subject's environment that are performed for research purposes)" (45 CFR 46.102(f)). This report generally follows the practice of recent IOM and other reports in referring to *research participants* rather than subjects (see, e.g., IOM, 2001; 2003a; and NBAC, 2001b). This usage recognizes the subjects of research as members of a research project who may, depending on their maturity and capacities, have their own special responsibilities, for example, adhering to drug, diet, exercise, or other intervention protocols. It also conveys a more respectful stance. Although the 2001 NBAC report also supported the use of the term participants, it noted that the term *subject* portrays more accurately than any other "the relationship and the unequal balance of power between the investigator and the individual in the research" (NBAC, 2001b, p. 33).

Parents sometimes participate with their children in clinical studies, for instance, when a study assesses the health knowledge, beliefs, or practices of both. Even when parents are not research participants in this direct way, they may be "surrogate" participants in certain respects; for example, when outcome measurements rely in whole or in part on parental assessments of aspects of the child's quality of life.

A SYSTEMS PERSPECTIVE ON PROTECTING
HUMAN PARTICIPANTS IN RESEARCH

Although many have accepted the wisdom of Henry Beecher's observation more than three decades ago that in addition to informed consent, "there is the more reliable safeguard provided by the presence of an intelligent, informed, conscientious, compassionate, responsible investigator," it would be unfair and unrealistic to expect individual clinicians and researchers, who often face multiple conflicts of interest, to both recognize and resolve by themselves the complex moral problems arising from the use of human subjects in research trials. It is not adequate to focus these ethical responsibilities only on the individual investigator who, in fact, functions within a much broader research and clinical environment.

National Bioethics Advisory Commission (NBAC, 1998, p. 15)

Clinical Research as a Complex, High-Stakes Enterprise

Clinical research today is a complex, high-stakes enterprise. A clinical trial may cost many millions of dollars, and one recent estimate put the cost of developing a new drug at nearly $900 million (including postmarketing studies) (Kaitin, 2003). The challenges of accommodating the physical, intellectual, social, and emotional characteristics and needs of infants, children, and adolescents may make pediatric research even more costly than studies that involve only adults.

For commercial sponsors, the financial rewards of positive research findings can be substantial, particularly when the population of potential users is large. Increasingly, research institutions and investigators too can reap substantial economic rewards from research. In addition, the careers of investigators and the stature of research institutions often hinge on success in the competition for research funding and the publication of findings in prestigious journals.

Nonfinancial conflicts of interest related to professional advancement or stature may be as potent as financial conflicts (see, e.g., NBAC, 2001b; Levinsky, 2002; and IOM, 2003a). An important rationale for requiring the inclusion and, indeed, increasing the proportion of nonscientists and community members on IRBs is to provide balance by involving individuals who are independent of research institutions and sponsors (IOM, 2003a). Another concern about conflicting interests arises when physician investigators recruit their own patients. In these situations, patients' decisions may be influenced by feelings of obligation, worry about antagonizing someone on whom they depend, or confusion about the goals of the physician as a researcher versus the goals of the physician as a clinician. Given the pressures on trial enrollment created by the often small numbers of eligible children, the potential for physician role conflict must be taken seriously.

Clinical research is often organizationally and socially complicated, reaching far beyond the boundaries of single institutions. In many clinical trials, investigators work in teams that must develop and negotiate topics and protocols with multiple additional participants. These participants are likely to include government or private sponsors (or both), at least one and sometimes several research review boards, and possibly legal advisers for different parties. Depending on the study, sites might include sophisticated medical centers, community hospitals, nursing homes, private physicians' offices, research participants' homes, schools, or other locations or combinations of locations. For many pediatric studies in particular, recruitment of sufficient numbers of research participants may take years and require several, even dozens, of study sites.

Value of a Systems Perspective

Given the complexity of modern clinical research and the stakes involved, an effective program for protecting human participants in research cannot focus narrowly on individuals or organizations (IOM, 2001, 2003a). Rather, a broader perspective is needed that envisions a *system of interrelated structures, policies, procedures, and resources that function successfully across institutional boundaries to protect adult and child participants in research.* Relevant *structures* include staff positions and organizational units (e.g., university offices of research administration, institutional and freestanding IRBs, and government regulatory offices). *Policies* include both public and private rules governing individual and organizational behavior (e.g., federal laws and regulations providing special protections for child participants in research, institutional policies relating to conflict-of-interest disclosures and determinations, and journal policies on conflict of interest and informed consent). *Procedures* are the mechanisms for carrying out policies (e.g., information collection and reporting arrangements and methods for collecting and analyzing data on adverse events in research). *Resources* include funding, laws, training in research ethics and methods, and leadership. The central objective of this system of interrelated elements is to protect research participants by encouraging and sustaining responsible behavior from all those involved in sponsoring, reviewing, monitoring, or regulating research and disseminating research findings.

This systems perspective can be applied to clinical research involving children by considering whether each component of the system is adequate to the specialized responsibilities of protecting child participants in research. For example, does an IRB have sufficient expertise in child health to review the kinds of pediatric research protocols that come before it? Is sufficient expertise in child health present on the safety monitoring boards that monitor injuries and other adverse events that occur during the course of a study? Are information systems organized to report separately on protocols involving children?

The recent report *Integrity in Scientific Research* observed that the research environment, like any system, includes both "variables and constants" and that "the most unpredictable and influential variable" is the individual investigator (IOM/NRC, 2002, p. 26). Each investigator's professional integrity is shaped by his or her education, culture, and ethical upbringing and is, inevitably, unique. This means that "the constants" operating in behalf of ethical conduct must come from the institutions and larger systems within which investigators work.

One advantage of considering human research protections in a systems framework of shared responsibilities is that it reduces the temptation to focus too narrowly on discrete individuals and organizations and, thereby, to underrate or ignore the diverse forces that powerfully shape their behavior. Figure 1.1 depicts, in highly simplified form, a program of human research protections operating within a larger social, economic, and political environment and a surrounding ethical culture and climate.

As shown in Figure 1.1, a significant system component is a *human research participants protection program*. A program in this sense is not a discrete IRB but, rather, a variable mix of individuals, organizational units, and organizations (see the discussions in IOM, 2001 and 2003a). The core functions of such a human research participants protection program include review of research protocols for ethical and scientific soundness, monitoring of participant safety appropriate to the risk presented by individual studies, ethical interactions between investigators and research participants, and arrangements for assessing compliance with rules and policies and improving program performance.

The specific components or modules of a human research protection program may differ depending on the characteristics of a particular study (e.g., the setting or the risks to participants), its sponsorship, and other factors. A program consists of the collection of organizational structures, policies, and procedures that apply to a particular research protocol or group of protocols. Thus, a program may include a body appointed to monitor data related to research participant safety if a study presents appreciable risk to participants, but such a body will not be part of a minimal risk study. (See discussion in Chapter 3 of data and safety monitoring boards and data monitoring committees.)

For complex multicenter clinical trials, the human research protection program may involve multiple research organizations, IRBs, research teams,

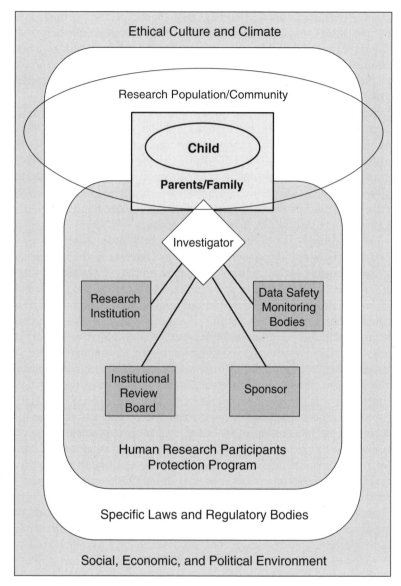

FIGURE 1.1 Simplified representation of a system for protecting human research participants (IOM/NRC, 2002; IOM, 2003).

and even research sponsors. The investigators for such trials may have to cope with different and possibly conflicting institutional policies and practices, legal frameworks (e.g., different state policies on when minors make decisions in their own right), social and economic conditions, and community cultures and ethical norms. Even within a single community, investigators, research participants, and others involved may be immersed in or influenced by more than one culture.

The government has recognized the importance of a systems perspective in its creation of a quality improvement initiative that will "work together with all components of the human research community (e.g., subjects, institutions, IRBs, investigators, sponsors, and the public)" to strengthen programs for protecting human participants in research (OHRP, 2002b, p. 1). The statement announcing the initiative noted that "public trust in our nation's human research enterprise is threatened" and that investigations have "too frequently discovered serious systemic deficiencies" in programs for protecting human participants in research (OHRP, 2002b, p. 1).

An important but underdeveloped part of a system for research protections for children is the prospective, rigorous evaluation of potential long-term benefits and harms of research and the identification of emerging or nontraditional research risks. For example, given the rapidly evolving state of knowledge of the human genome, it is important for investigators, IRBs, and sponsors of research involving children to develop methods to identify and evaluate risks that are unique to or specially evident in genetic research. Such methods should take into account the long-term nature of the potential psychological effects of such research on children who are developing cognitively, emotionally, and socially. They should also consider the risks to family members and family relationships. Although the risks of adverse drug reactions may be clear for all involved in a traditional drug study, such is not the case for the risks of learning (based on genetic investigations) that one will or may develop a debilitating or lethal disease. Long-term follow-up of child research participants and their families will help identify risks that are not now well understood and thereby provide a basis for better protecting children and families from future harm.

ETHICAL PRINCIPLES FOR A SYSTEM TO PROTECT HUMAN RESEARCH PARTICIPANTS

If a study is unethical to start with, it does not become ethical because it produces useful results.
                                        Henry Beecher, 1970, p. 122

The core ethical principles for protecting the dignity and well-being of human participants in research originate from a variety of historical and philosophical sources, some of which are discussed further in the next section of this chapter. Today, in the United States, the most widely cited statement of these ethical principles is the *Belmont Report* of the National Commission for the Protection of Human Subjects of Biomedical and Behavioral Research (hereafter referred to as the National Commission) (National Commission, 1978a).[5] The U.S. Congress created the National Commission in 1974 and charged it with, among other tasks, identifying basic principles for ethical research involving human subjects and developing ethical guidelines for applying those principles to the conduct of research. The charge also called for the National Commission to examine issues in research involving fetuses, prisoners, children, and those with mental disabilities, which it did in a series of additional reports (National Commission, 1975, 1976, 1977, and 1978b). Although the principles laid out in the Commission's reports are generally accepted, their interpretation or their application in specific cases may be unclear or contentious.

As summarized in Box 1.1, the *Belmont Report* presented three basic principles to guide ethical research involving humans: respect for persons, beneficence, and justice. In some formulations, respect for persons is labeled autonomy and beneficence is subdivided to distinguish a fourth principle, nonmaleficence (see, e.g., Beauchamp and Childress, 1994, and Jonsen et al., 1998). The latter division has ancient roots in the injunction of Hippocrates "to help or at least to do no harm" (Goold, 1923, p. 165). Although ethicists and others differ in their analyses of these principles, the following overview presents the committee's perspectives. Later chapters offer additional discussion as indicated below.

The principle of *respect for persons* underlies the emphases on the confidentiality of personal information and the provision of voluntary, informed consent for both medical treatment and participation in research. Voluntary participation in research also entails the freedom to withdraw from a study. Respect for research participants further requires that participants not be asked to expose themselves to risks or invest their time and energy in studies that are directed at unimportant questions or that are not properly designed to answer the research question.

The *Belmont Report* emphasized protection of vulnerable individuals as an element of respect for persons. A somewhat different perspective not mentioned in the report stresses respect for children's emerging autonomy (or respect for the capacities of other vulnerable individuals) as a basis for involving them in decisions, consistent with their capabilities. As discussed

---

[5]The report was issued in 1978 but was then published in the *Federal Register* in 1979. This report uses the 1978 date, but citations for the report often use the later date.

BOX 1.1
Ethical Principles for Human Research Identified in the
Belmont Report

1. Respect for Persons. Respect for persons incorporates at least two ethical convictions: first, that individuals should be treated as autonomous agents, and second, that persons with diminished autonomy are entitled to protection.

2. Beneficence. Persons are treated in an ethical manner not only by respecting their decisions and protecting them from harm, but also by making efforts to secure their well-being. Such treatment falls under the principle of beneficence. The term "beneficence" is often understood to cover acts of kindness or charity that go beyond strict obligation. In this document, beneficence is understood in a stronger sense, as an obligation. Two general rules have been formulated as complementary expressions of beneficent actions in this sense: (1) do not harm and (2) maximize possible benefits and minimize possible harms.

3. Justice. Who ought to receive the benefits of research and bear its burdens? This is a question of justice, in the sense of "fairness in distribution" or "what is deserved." An injustice occurs when some benefit to which a person is entitled is denied without good reason or when some burden is imposed unduly.

SOURCE: National Commission, 1978a.

---

in Chapters 3 and 5, the seeking (when appropriate) of children's assent to research participation demonstrates such respect, but legal permission for participation must ordinarily come from parents.

It can be argued that the *Belmont Report* weakened the argument for respecting autonomy by joining it with the argument for protecting the vulnerable from undue influence or coercion (Kopelman, in press). For individuals who are capable and competent to make their own decisions and who are not harming others, the report's formulation of the principle of respect for persons should not be interpreted to permit a balancing of autonomy against protection. For these competent individuals, respect for persons generally takes the form of noninterference within broad limits.

The *Belmont Report* observes that it is not possible to draw a precise line between justifiable persuasion and undue influence. It notes that unjustifiable pressure typically involves an individual with authority or commanding influence (e.g., a physician who could determine treatment options for a patient) over a prospective research participant. Although the report does not mention financial incentives for research participation, much attention has been devoted to payments to research participants as a potential source of undue influence (see Chapter 6 of this report).

In clinical research, particularly research that entails some risk but holds no prospect of benefiting the research participant, respect for individuals and their right to self-determination may conflict with values that focus on the potential benefits of research to the larger society. As discussed further in Chapter 4, some of the thorniest debates about research ethics involve pediatric studies that present some risk to children and that offer no prospect of direct benefit but promise to build knowledge beneficial to children in the future. Studies of the mechanisms of disease typically fall into this category.

The real-world application of the moral principle of respect for persons faces a number of practical difficulties in clinical care and research. These include imbalances in information and power between clinicians and patients and between investigators and research participants or their parents. For parents, the physical and emotional stresses associated with a child's illness or injury and, frequently, the time constraints on decision making also may compromise their ability to obtain, absorb, and evaluate information, weigh options, and then provide truly informed permission for their child to be treated or enrolled in research. How to move from the general principle of respect for persons and the abstract concept of informed consent to effective implementation and desired outcomes is a major, open question for clinicians, investigators, administrators, ethicists, regulators, and others concerned with clinical care and research. Chapter 5 returns to this question as it examines what is known about children's and parent's comprehension of research and about parent's permission and children's assent to research participation.

The principles of *beneficence* and *nonmaleficence* specifically direct attention to the potential benefits and harms of participation in research. From these principles derive the responsibilities of investigators to maximize potential or expected benefits in research, minimize risks (i.e., potential harms), and balance or weigh the potential harms to an individual of participating in research against the potential benefits of participation.[6] Also, because children usually do not have the intellectual capacity to assess and weigh the potential harms and benefits of research, parents and others have a duty to do this for them.

In the context of research, the principle of *justice* primarily involves the fair distribution of the potential harms and benefits of participating in research. Children and other vulnerable groups, including prisoners, residents of mental institutions, and the economically disadvantaged (in the United States and other countries), should not be disproportionately used in research or exploited because they are convenient, readily controlled or

---

[6]Although some research may involve no harm, much beneficial research does involve the risk of harm, sometimes serious harm. The precept to "do no harm" would, if interpreted literally, rule out such research (Kopelman, in press).

coerced, or unduly susceptible to economic or other inducements to re-search participation. Overuse of vulnerable groups is a special concern when they are unlikely to benefit from the knowledge gained from research. Research in resource-poor countries has been particularly criticized as un-just when it is not responsive to needs of those of countries, for example, when the aim is to develop medical treatments that will not be practical or affordable except in wealthier countries (see, e.g., Edejer, 1999 and NBAC, 2001a).

Underuse as well as overuse of vulnerable groups in research also raises problems of justice when it limits the extent to which a group can experi-ence the potential benefits of research. The principle of justice has been central in successful arguments for the expanded involvement in research of women (as exemplified in the congressional mandate for the Women's Health Initiative announced by NIH in 1991 [NIH, 1994; IOM, 1994b]), children (see Chapter 2), elderly adults (ASCP, 1991; FDA, 1994b), and minorities (NIH, 1994)—and, generally, for not limiting clinical studies to nonelderly white adult males.

The *Belmont Report* emphasized the societal benefits "that serve to justify research involving children—even when individual research subjects are not direct beneficiaries" (National Commission, 1978a, p. 7). It did not review the debate on this point. The earlier National Commission report on children, however, included a lengthy discussion of the arguments for and against subjecting children to research involving some risk but no prospect of direct benefit (National Commission, 1977). In particular, that report reviewed the arguments of theologian Paul Ramsey that only potentially beneficial research was ethically permissible with children or others who could not provide informed consent (Ramsey, 1970). To engage children in research that could not benefit them was to treat them as "means to others' ends" (National Commission, 1977, p. 93).

The 1977 report presented an extended analysis of Ramsey's argu-ments and those who had offered various alternative views, including Rich-ard McCormick, Stephen Toulmin, Victor Worsfold, Stanley Hauerwas, William Bartholome, Tristram Engelhardt, and others. The Commission eventually proposed that "nonbeneficial" research was acceptable but only under conditions more limited than those applicable to adults. The report pointed to the lack of alternative populations for studying certain condi-tions affecting children, the limitations of extrapolation from adult studies, and the serious consequences for children of prohibiting all child research that did not have the prospect of benefiting the participants.

The complexity and difficulty of the moral arguments about children's participation in research are reflected in the multiple statements of views from members of the Commission in the report's final chapter. In essence, the Commission (with two dissents) adopted what may be seen as a utilitarian rationale—albeit a significantly limited one—that "foreseeable benefit to an identifiable class of children may justify a minor increment of risk" to child participants in research in certain restricted situations (National Commission, 1977, p. 125). Chapter 4 of the current report discusses the complexities and controversies in (1) identifying the types, probabilities, and magnitude of potential harms and benefits to which child research participants may be exposed; (2) judging whether the potential harms to the child are reasonable in relation to potential benefits; and (3) assessing whether the potential harms have been minimized.

HISTORICAL EVOLUTION OF POLICIES FOR PROTECTING HUMAN PARTICIPANTS IN RESEARCH

There is a long history of research on children . . . but a relatively short history of legal control of this activity.
Leonard Glantz, 1994, p. 103

Systematic attention to research ethics largely postdates World War II. For much of the period since the war, policymakers, ethicists, and others have focused on the articulation and refinement of general principles, guidelines, and regulations for research involving humans. Intensive attention to the special ethical issues related to research with children developed rather slowly. Policymakers then took longer to adopt special proposals to increase protections for children than to accept proposals affecting pregnant women, fetuses, and prisoners. Nonetheless, controversies about the ethics of research involving children have frequently served as a stimulus for proposals—if not action—to adopt or strengthen human research protection policies.

Before 1947

In 1945, '50, the doctor . . . was king or queen. It never occurred to a doctor to ask for consent for anything . . . People say, oh, injection with plutonium, why didn't the doctor tell the patient? Doctors weren't in the habit of telling the patients anything. They were in charge and nobody questioned their authority. Now that seems egregious. But at the time, that's the way the world was.
Leonard Sagan (radiologist), 1994
(as cited in ACHRE, 1995, p. 83)

Broadly viewed, research involving children is not an innovation of the twentieth century. Instances of experimentation with children date back centuries. Lederer and Grodin (1994) observed that physicians often used their own children, children of their servants or slaves, and institutionalized children as subjects for early infectious disease and immunization "experiments" because the children were convenient and lacked experience with the diseases being investigated (p. 4). One widely cited example from the 1790s is Edward Jenner's experimental injection of his gardener's son and his own son with cowpox material to vaccinate them against smallpox (NLM, 2002). In the 1700s and later, physicians also used children in experiments with measles, pertussis, syphilis, gonorrhea and other infectious diseases.

The nineteenth and early twentieth centuries saw scattered or passing comments on ethical research conduct.[7] In Prussia at the turn of the last century, public controversy over research practices (including the inoculation of healthy children with syphilis serum) led to appointment of a committee that issued recommendations for ethical research practices (Grodin, 1992; Vollmann and Winau, 1996). Prussian authorities subsequently issued the first known governmental directives on research practices in 1900. They advised medical directors of hospitals and clinics that research interventions should not go forward if "the human subject was a minor or not competent for other reasons." If competent, subjects should provide "unambiguous consent" after a "proper explanation of the possible negative consequences." The consent was also to be "documented in the medical history" (quoted in Vollmann and Winau, 1996, p. 1446). It is not evident that the nonbinding directive or the ethical analysis supporting it had any effect on research practices (Vollman and Winau, 1996).

At about the same time in the United States, legislative proposals were made after controversies arose about experiments with healthy children in hospitals, orphanages, and schools.[8] As recounted by Lederer (1992, 1995) and Lederer and Grodin (1994), experiments with children in the late

---

[7]Three sources are usually cited. Thomas Percival's *Medical Ethics, Or a Code of Institutes and Precepts Adapted to the Professional Conduct of Physicians and Surgeons*, published in 1803, was the basis for the American Medical Association's first code of ethics in 1846. Percival focused mainly on physician practice, not research, but he noted the need for innovation based on sound methods and responsible investigators. William Beaumont, in his 1833 book, *Experiments and Observations on the Gastric Juice and the Physiology of Digestion*, set forth ethical principles for investigators that stressed voluntary consent. In 1865, Claude Bernard published *An Introduction to the Study of Experimental Medicine*, which did not discuss consent but did distinguish between research that might benefit the participant and research that would not. For further discussion see Grodin, 1992 and Rutkow, 1998.

[8]Proposals to regulate research came before the United States Senate as early as 1900. These proposals and several proposals at the state level would have required informed written consent and would have banned experimentation with those not competent to provide consent (Lederer and Grodin, 1994).

nineteenth and early twentieth centuries included investigations of digestive processes (including the use of stomach tubes in infants), deliberate efforts to induce various sexually transmitted diseases to identify their causes and natural history, lumbar punctures, and studies of scurvy in orphaned infants that involved withholding of orange juice. A Swedish physician's admission that he had used children provided by a foundling home rather than calves in a smallpox experiment because calves were costly prompted a U.S. pamphlet "Foundlings Cheaper than Animals" (Lederer, 1995, p. 50).

One American researcher who used institutionalized children in various studies commented in a 1914 publication that conditions in these institutions were similar to the "conditions which are insisted on in . . . [infection experiments] among laboratory animals, but which can rarely be controlled in a study of infection in man (Alfred F. Hess, quoted in Lederer and Grodin, 1994, p. 6). Despite considerable controversy, neither public action nor voluntary standards for human research won acceptance in the United States before World War II.

In 1931, the German government issued extensive new regulations protecting human participants in research after controversies over the use of healthy children in harmful studies on tuberculosis vaccines (Grodin, 1992). Among other provisions, the regulations stated that the potential adverse effects of research should be proportionate to the anticipated benefits and that disadvantaged individuals should not be exploited as research participants. The 1931 policies were both unprecedented for the era and profoundly ineffectual under the Nazi regime that took power in 1933.

Most current discussions of research ethics start with the Nuremberg Code's *Directives for Human Experimentation*, which were announced by an American military tribunal in 1947 before the verdict in the trial of several Nazi physicians and others for atrocities in medical experiments (Annas and Grodin, 1992).[9] (The tribunal convicted 16 of 23 defendants, most of them physicians, of war crimes and crimes against humanity and sentenced 7 of them to be executed.) These directives were the first internationally accepted statement of ethical principles in research. The lead principle stated that "the voluntary consent of the human subject is absolutely essential" meaning that "the person involved should have the legal capacity

---

[9]The Nuremberg Code's directives, by and large, reflect principles and advice provided in separate statements to the military prosecutors by Dr. Leo Alexander and Dr. Andrew Ivy. Ivy acted as the American Medical Association's adviser to the prosecutors (ACHRE, 1995). The statement developed by Ivy applied to research with healthy volunteers, not sick patients. His principles also provided the foundation for a 1946 statement of policies for human experimentation by the American Medical Association.

to give consent" (Nuremberg Code, 1949, p. 181–182). The directives did not mention children. Strictly construed, they would have precluded research involving children or mentally or legally incapacitated adults.[10]

Although ethicists, investigators, and policymakers have considerably refined and extended the principles of ethical research (e.g., to cover children), many of the basic tenets in current national and international statements on the conduct of research are similar to those set forth by the Nuremberg judges in 1947. In addition to voluntary, informed, and competent consent, these tenets provided that the research should be necessary and that its risks should be balanced by its social importance and potential benefits. Research should also be designed and conducted by scientifically qualified investigators to produce valid results and minimize risk to participants.

1948 to 1974

It was just that we were so ethically insensitive that it never occurred to us that you ought to level with people that they were in an experiment.
Louis Lasagna on research in 1950s, 1994
(quoted in ACHRE, 1995)

By mid-1960, NIH officials were concerned about the agency's traditional practice of relying exclusively on the moral character of investigators to safeguard humans in research. Moreover, NIH had no way to monitor the conduct of the investigators it was funding.
Irene Stith-Coleman, 1994, p. 7

As medical research accelerated in the 1950s and 1960s, the Nuremberg principles were both increasingly recognized and increasingly questioned in certain of their specifics (Faden and Beauchamp, 1986; ACHRE, 1995). Some of the questions highlighted the lack of provision for research involving children and others not competent to consent to research in their own right.

Early in the 1950s, the new Clinical Center at NIH developed explicit policies for the protection of human participants in research (which applied to studies conducted at the facility). Among other elements, the policies

---

[10]The statements by Dr. Leo Alexander and Dr. Andrew Ivy appear to have included provisions for consent by next of kin or guardians for people lacking mental competence. These provisions may have been excluded from the directives because they were not relevant in the case before the judges (ACHRE, 1995).

provided for peer review of certain kinds of research (e.g., high-risk research, nontherapeutic research involving patients, and research involving healthy volunteers). They also directed attention to ethical questions in the review of research. According to Faden and Beauchamp, "[o]fficials at the Center expected these procedures to set the standard for other institutions . . . but [this] pioneering venture was an isolated and largely ignored event" (1986, p. 202). For example, as Faden and Beauchamp reported, a survey by researchers at Boston University, which was supported by a federal grant and published in 1962, suggested that few research centers had guidelines for clinical research or even accepted the concept of committee review of protocols.

With respect to research involving children, the 1995 report of the Advisory Committee on Human Radiation Experiments stated that "in the 1940s and 1950s there were apparently no written rules of professional ethics for pediatric research in general" (ACHRE, 1995, p. 203).[11] In summarizing the discussion during a 1961 conference on Social Responsibility in Pediatric Research, the same report observed that it was not uncommon for "pediatric patients to be used as subjects of nontherapeutic research without the permission of their parents" (ACHRE, 1995, p. 202). The report also noted that some researchers, including researchers who failed to get parental permission, recognized that this was unethical (see Box 1.2).

In 1962, the U.S. Congress passed legislation that expanded the scope of FDA's authority by passing amendments to the Federal Food, Drug, and Cosmetic Act (P.L. 87-781). The legislation included provisions that required investigators to obtain a subject's consent to the use of an experimental drug unless it was not feasible or was not in the subject's best interest (at Section 501(i)(4)). Four years later, the FDA commissioner issued explicit regulations providing for consent to participation in research, "at least partially in recognition of the widespread failure of the industry to obtain [it]" (Glantz, 1992, pp. 183–200; see also the discussion in Faden and Beauchamp, 1986).

After years of debate within NIH about the balance between ethical principles and scientific inquiry, the U.S. Surgeon General issued policy statements in 1966 that significantly expanded the conceptualization and application of informed consent for external clinical research funded by

---

[11]As early as 1949, however, a Subcommittee of the Atomic Energy Commission set forth rules for evaluating proposals for medical research using radioisotopes that generally "discouraged" but did not preclude nontherapeutic research involving healthy children (ACHRE, 1995, p. 203).

BOX 1.2
Summary of Discussion of Pediatric Research in the 1950s

In the opening minutes of the meeting, this researcher reminded his colleagues that "the question for us to discuss here today is how we operate on a daily basis." He offered for discussion a provocative case from his personal experience in which he and his associates "wanted [to do] lumbar punctures on newborns." He explicitly noted that "this study [was] not of benefit to the individual; it was an attempt to learn about normal physiology." One of the other conferees asked, "Did you ask [parental] permission?" The researcher responded, "No. We were afraid we would not get volunteers." The case prompted a great deal of discussion at the conference, but perhaps most tellingly this researcher frankly acknowledged toward the end of the discussion—in a meeting that had begun with an assurance of confidentiality from the organizers—that he had "sinned" in carrying out these lumbar punctures in "normal infants" without parental permission.

SOURCE: Closed meeting on Social Responsibility in Pediatric Research, Boston University, 1961 (as described in ACHRE, 1995, p. 202).

U.S. Public Health Services grants (U.S. Surgeon General, 1966). The policy statements also required research institutions to establish committees (IRBs) to review proposed human research (Faden and Beauchamp, 1986). This institution-level review was to consider the methods for obtaining informed consent, the balance of risks and benefits in proposed research, and the welfare of the research participants.

The 1966 NIH policies were shaped in part by the 1964 Declaration of Helsinki, published 2 years previously by the World Medical Association (WMA, 1964).[12] The Declaration, which has been revised several times, set forth principles for ethical research that enlarged the Nuremberg directives and went beyond the Association's first statement in 1954 (Annas et al., 1977). The 1964 Declaration distinguished research with aims seen as "essentially therapeutic for a patient" from research with only "scientific aims." It specified looser standards of consent for the former, recommending that consent be obtained "consistent with patient psychology." The 1964 document did not specifically mention children or minors, but it did provide for

---

[12]Also in 1966, the General Assembly of the United Nations adopted the International Covenant on Civil and Political Rights, which went into effect in 1976. Article 7 of this document declares, "No one shall be subjected to torture or to cruel, inhuman or degrading treatment or punishment. In particular, no one shall be subjected without his free consent to medical or scientific experimentation" (UNCHR, 1976, online, unpaged).

the consent of legal guardians to the participation in "nontherapeutic" research of those not legally able to provide consent. Subsequent revisions to the Declaration added specific references to children and included provisions for children's agreement to participate in research (for those children who are capable of providing it). More recent revisions refer to minor's "assent" rather than "consent," recommend committee review of research, and call for journals not to accept reports of research that are inconsistent with the Declaration.

During the 1960s, criticisms of unethical research practices in research involving children gained new attention (see, e.g., ACHRE, 1995 and Lowen, 1995). In an often cited 1966 article in the *New England Journal of Medicine,* Henry Beecher reviewed 22 studies, most of which involved "experimentation on a patient not for his benefit but for that, at least in theory, of patients in general" (Beecher, 1966, p. 367). Four of the studies discussed in the article included children. As described by Beecher, one used multiple spot X-rays to study bladder filling and voiding in babies; another involved the suturing of adult skin grafts to the chest wall of a subset of children being treated for congenital heart disease to examine the effect of thymectomy on growth and development; and a third included some children with mental retardation who were given an antibiotic (for the treatment of acne) to determine whether it caused liver dysfunction (which it did) (Beecher, 1966).

The fourth study involved children at New York's Willowbrook State School. Researchers infected some of the child participants with a mild form of hepatitis during the initial stages of a study of the natural history, prevention, and treatment of viral hepatitis that extended from 1956 to 1972 and that eventually contributed to the development of a successful hepatitis vaccine. The Willowbrook research also contributed to the public debate over research ethics and the impetus for regulation (see, e.g., Goldman, 1971, 1973; President's Commission, 1981; Faden and Beauchamp, 1986; Lederer and Grodin, 1994; ACHRE, 1995; and NBAC, 1998). Among the major points of discussion were the infecting of healthy institutionalized children and the adequacy or appropriateness of the process for securing parental consent (permission) during some stages of the study. In the 1970s, controversy over the ethics of this study reached medical journals, major newspapers, and Congressional hearings (see Goldman, 1971, 1973 generally and, e.g., Ramsey, 1970; Edsall, 1971; and Goldby, 1971 who criticized the research and, e.g., Krugman and Shapiro, 1971 and Ingelfinger, 1973 who defended it).

Many of the researchers in the studies cited by Beecher were well regarded, and research oversight committees had reviewed some of the study proposals. In the Willowbrook research, parents had been asked for and had provided consent in an era when that was not uniform practice.

Beyond public controversy about particular studies, problems with the Surgeon General's 1966 policy statement became a concern. As described in a later report, site visits "to randomly selected institutions revealed a wide range of compliance . . . [and] widespread confusion about how to assess risks and benefits, refusal by some researchers to cooperate with the policy, and in many cases, indifference by those charged with administering research and its rules at local institutions" (ACHRE, 1995, pp. 100–101). The report also noted widespread complaints about overworked review committees and requests for policy clarification and guidance.

In 1971, what was then the U.S. Department of Health, Education, and Welfare (DHEW) further formalized its policies on protecting human research participants in the *Institutional Guide to DHEW Policy for the Protection of Human Subjects*. Faden and Beauchamp (1986, p. 212) describe this as a "major monograph on the subject of ethics and regulation of research." The guide set forth six basic conditions for informed consent, including the condition that the discussion of participation describes risks and discomforts, expected benefits, alternatives to research participation, and freedom to discontinue participation at any time.

The 1971 Guide also required the consent of research participants or their authorized representatives. The Guide stated that review committees "should consider the validity of consent by next of kin, legal guardians, or by other qualified third parties representative of the subjects' interests . . . [and] whether these third parties can be presumed to have the necessary depth of interest and concern with the subjects' rights and welfare . . . [and are] legally authorized to expose the subjects to the risks involved" (quoted in National Commission, 1977, p. 93).

In 1973, DHEW issued a working document on experimentation with children that proposed several special protections for children (DHEW, 1973b; see also Glantz, 1994). The draft provided that children would be excluded from participation in research under several conditions, one of which was if they were age 6 or over and had not consented to participation—unless the agency waived the requirement.[13] The draft also proposed

---

[13]The working document noted that children could not provide legally effective consent, but it nonetheless used that term in discussing children's agreement to participate in research. In rules proposed the following year, the term *assent* was used to refer to agreement by "institutionalized mentally disabled" persons (DHEW, 1974, p. 30656). The government adopted neither these proposed rules nor the 1978 recommendations by the National Commission. Rules adopted in 1983 described "the mentally disabled" as a vulnerable population in need of additional—but undefined—protections by IRBs, and they required consent to research participation by a legally authorized representative (see the discussion in NBAC, 1998).

that an "ethical review board" should review research protocols involving children and that a "protection committee" should monitor aspects of research once it was initiated. This intensity of review does not appear to have been seriously considered in later assessments or policy deliberations.

DHEW did not include special provisions for children in the general regulations that it issued in 1974 (DHEW, 1974). In July 1975, however, the NIH Clinical Center is said to have required for its intramural research program that investigators obtain a child's agreement to participate in research (National Commission, 1977).

During the 1970s, policymakers and the public were shocked to learn about the Tuskegee Syphilis Study. For more than 30 years, health researchers had followed black men diagnosed with syphilis but had neither informed them of their condition nor treated them for it (Heller, 1972; DHEW, 1973a; Jones, 1992; ACHRE, 1995). Revelations about this study contributed significantly to the passage in 1974 of the National Research Act (P.L. 93-348). That Act explicitly provided for the creation of IRBs to review biomedical and behavioral research that involved humans and was funded by DHEW. As noted earlier, it also established the National Commission and directed it to identify ethical principles for research involving humans with additional attention to research involving vulnerable individuals, including children, prisoners, and those with mental disabilities.

1975 to 1995

By the time that its mandate expired in 1978, the National Commission had produced 17 reports and supplementary documents. The best known is the *Belmont Report*, which was discussed earlier in this chapter, but other reports were also influential. DHEW revised its 1974 regulations following reports by the National Commission on research involving fetuses (National Commission, 1975) and prisoners (National Commission, 1976). In 1975, the agency added to the general regulations on human research protections (which became Subpart A of 45 CFR 46) a set of special regulations for pregnant women and fetuses and in vitro fertilization (Subpart B). In 1978, it added regulations relating to prisoners (Subpart C).

The U.S. Department of Health and Human Services (DHHS, formerly DHEW) did not adopt specific regulations on research involving children until 1983 (see below), 6 years after the National Commission produced the report, *Research Involving Children* (National Commission, 1977). That report laid out the case for involving children in research, described the extent of such research, surveyed institutional practices regarding consent for research involving children, and reviewed legal and ethical issues in pediatric research. In contrast to the *Belmont Report*, which has links from many IRB and other websites related to human research protection programs,[14] neither the 1977 report on children nor its summary appear to be available online for easy reference.[15]

Two years later, DHHS issued revised general regulations governing human research, but these still did not include special protections for children (DHHS, 1981). The new rules expanded provisions related to informed consent. For example, they included requirements that the process of securing informed consent include descriptions of the extent, if any, to which confidentiality will be maintained, explanations that refusal to participate will not result in a penalty or a loss of benefits, and information about whom to contact with questions or in the event of a research-related injury.

The 1981 regulations also allowed IRBs to exempt or expedite certain categories of minimal-risk research involving, for example, many kinds of educational and survey research. The exempted research did not have to meet the requirements for informed consent, although IRBs might still impose the requirements. These provisions for exempt and expedited research review responded to some of the concerns from the social and behavioral science research communities that the 1974 regulations inappropriately imposed on their fields regulations that had been devised for the often different circumstances and risks of biomedical research.

Finally, in 1983, 10 years after its first proposals and 6 years after the National Commission report on children, DHHS issued special regulations for research involving children (Subpart D). The recommendations of the National Commission formed the foundation for these rules. In 2000, the Children's Health Act (P.L. 106-310) required FDA to bring its regulations into conformity with the DHHS regulations providing additional protections for children participating in research (FDA, 2001b). The DHHS and FDA regulations are discussed further in Chapter 3 and subsequent chapters of this report.

In 1986, the government published proposed rules to extend the general regulations governing research conducted or supported by DHHS to all federal agencies and all federally supported research. This step followed earlier recommendations by the President's Commission for the Study of Ethical Problems in Medicine and Biomedical and Behavioral Research

---

[14]Availability does not guarantee familiarity. In a 1998 discussion with another federal commission, ethicist Albert Jonsen observed that he had recently spoken to group of IRB participants. "What they knew [were] the federal regulations. They didn't know Belmont" (Jonsen, 1998b).

[15]During the course of this IOM study, a scanned copy of the report—obtained from committee member Robert Nelson—was made available for viewing on the study's website. Chapter 8 encourages the Office for Human Research Protections (OHRP) to make the report available as a resource on its website.

(President's Commission, 1981). Not until 1991 did the government officially extend the rules to 15 other federal agencies (USDA et al., 1991).[16] This step standardized a variety of different agency policies under what is termed the Common Rule. The Common Rule does not include Subpart B, C, or D, although the Department of Education, which also funds considerable research involving children, has adopted Subpart D.

Although FDA has been part of what is now DHHS for many decades (FDA, 2002a), it has separate rules applicable to the research that it oversees based on its specific statutory authority and associated legal codification. The regulations related to protection of human participants in research are found at 21 CFR 50 and 56. The FDA has not adopted the Common Rule as such but has revised its regulations to bring them into general conformity (FDA, 1991a). Interestingly, in 1979, FDA solicited comments on a proposed rule that would apply the principles set forth in the 1973 DHEW regulations to all pediatric research that was subject to FDA jurisdiction (FDA, 1979b). The proposed rules were never adopted and were formally withdrawn in 1991 (FDA, 1991b). In 2001, following directives in the Children's Health Act of 2000, FDA brought its regulations largely into line with the provisions of Subpart D (FDA, 2001b).

Recent Years

Except for some limited revisions, the regulations issued in the 1980s still govern research conducted, supported, or regulated by DHHS, including research involving children. These regulations are discussed further in Chapter 3. Recent years have been marked by various critical reports on the performance of IRBs and DHHS in implementing these regulations. Chapter 7 reviews some of these reports as well as DHHS responses.

Arguably, the most attention-getting recent developments related to the protection of human participants in research have involved the temporary suspension or restriction of federally funded research at more than a dozen

---

[16]These agencies are: U.S. Department of Agriculture; U.S. Department of Energy; National Aeronautics and Space Administration; U.S. Department of Commerce; Consumer Product Safety Commission; International Development Cooperation Agency, Agency for International Development; U.S. Department of Housing and Urban Development; U.S. Department of Justice; U.S. Department of Defense; U.S. Department of Education; U.S. Department of Veterans Affairs; Environmental Protection Agency; National Science Foundation; and U.S. Department of Transportation. The Common Rule also covers the Social Security Administration (by legislation) and the Central Intelligence Agency (by executive order) plus the Office of Science and Technology Policy (by agency signature), which does not conduct research.

institutions (NBAC, 2001b). Problems cited by the agency included inappropriate enrollment of patients in research, poor documentation of protocol approvals and continuing review of approved proposals, and deficiencies related to the design, approval, and conduct of research, including a study in which a volunteer died (NBAC, 2001b; McNeilly, 2001). In addition, after the death of Jesse Gelsinger, FDA shut down gene transfer trials at the University of Pennsylvania. Further investigation continues.

Responding to criticisms of its own performance, DHHS has recently taken a number of steps to underscore the importance of human research protections. In 2000, it moved the lead responsibility for issues related to the protection of human participants in research out of an office within NIH and into the Office of Public Health and Science within the Secretary's Office (DHHS, 2000). To underscore program goals, the Office for Protection from Research Risks became the Office for Human Research Protections (OHRP). FDA took a similar step in March 2001 when it created the Good Clinical Practices Program within the Office of the Commissioner to take the lead on policy issues related to the protection of human participants in research. Individual centers, for example, the Center for Drug Evaluation Research still maintain research monitoring units relevant to their jurisdictions (David Lepay, M.D., Ph.D., Food and Drug Administration, personal communication, October 4, 2003). FDA and NIH have also taken steps to improve oversight and public disclosure of safety programs in gene transfer trials and, in the words of the FDA Commissioner, "restore the confidence in the trials' integrity that is essential if gene [transfer] studies are to be able to fulfill their potential" (FDA, 2000c, online, unpaged).

Another recent development involves an increasing number of referrals to DHHS of proposed research protocols involving children that IRBs have determined they cannot approve under the federal regulations (sections 404, 405, and 406 of 45 CFR 46) but which can be approved by the Secretary of DHHS under 45 CFR 46.407. For all such proposals, DHHS has created a public review and comment process, which is described further in Chapters 3 and 8. The referred protocols have, to cite a few examples, proposed to test a diluted smallpox vaccine in children, study sleep mechanisms with children, and investigate precursors to diabetes in Japanese youth (DHHS, 2002a,b; DHHS, 2003b).

As noted earlier, OHRP has created a voluntary quality improvement program that includes institutional self-assessment tools and various opportunities for obtaining guidance and counsel from agency staff or through written materials (OHRP, 2002b; see also the discussion in Chapter 7). The initiative also will promote interactions and idea sharing among research institutions and review boards.

Another major development in recent years has been the growing amount of research funded by American companies that is being conducted in other countries. Recent data indicate that approximately 25 percent of investigational new drug applications include critical data from studies conducted outside the United States (Lepay, 2003). In 2001, the DHHS Office of the Inspector General (OIG) reported that the number of foreign investigators conducting research under an FDA Investigational New Drug filing rose from 41 in 1980 to 271 in 1990 to 4,458 in 1999. The OIG concluded that FDA "receives minimal information on the performance of foreign institutional review boards . . . [and] has an inadequate database on the people and entities involved in foreign research" (OIG, 2001, p. ii). Furthermore, it "cannot necessarily depend on foreign investigators signing attestations that they will uphold human subject protections" (OIG, 2001, p. ii).

In a report that explored the ethical and practical complexities of overseeing foreign research in more depth, the National Bioethics Advisory Commission also expressed concern about current DHHS policies and procedures (NBAC, 2001a). Chapter 3 discusses federal regulations on human participants in research as they apply to research conducted in other countries.

The globalization of clinical research has encouraged international efforts to "harmonise" (to use accepted international spelling) national regulations and practices relating to human research. Examples include the *Guideline for Good Clinical Practice: E6* (ICH, 1996) and *Clinical Investigation of Medicinal Products in the Pediatric Population: E11* (ICH, 2000b) of the International Conference on Harmonisation (ICH) and the *International Ethical Guidelines for Biomedical Research Involving Human Subjects* of the Council for International Organizations of Medical Sciences (CIOMS, 2002, updating guidelines first issued in 1982).[17]

---

[17]The ICH is a collaboration involving representatives of regulatory bodies and industry in the discussion and development of common procedure and requirements for the ensuring the safety, quality, and efficacy of drugs, primarily new drugs. At the time that the collaboration was initiated in 1990, most new drugs were developed in the United States, Western Europe and Japan, but ICH activities now include observers from the World Health Organization (WHO), which provides a link to other regions. The Council for International Organizations of Medical Sciences (CIOMS) is a private, nonprofit, international organization that was created in 1949 by WHO and the United Nations Education, Social and Cultural Organization (UNESCO). It has both "national" members (including the National Academy of Sciences) and members representing international organizations. In its recent revision of guidelines for ethical biomedical research, the group noted that the changes to the guidelines "related mainly to controlled clinical trials, with external sponsors and investigators, carried out in low-resource countries (CIOMS, 2002). The guidelines include specific provisions for children. The first appendix to the guidelines provides a concise list of information to be included in a clinical protocol submitted for review under the guidelines.

The movement of clinical research overseas reflects an array of economic, social, and political forces related to such factors as the cost of doing research and the rigors of regulations governing the conduct of research (and the ease of on-site inspection of research sites). It also reflects the higher prevalence of many serious medical problems in less developed countries and, thus, the larger pool of potential research participants. This is not a trivial attraction, given that most children in developed countries are healthy, which means that recruiting sufficient numbers of children for clinical studies is often difficult.

As noted earlier in this chapter, international research can raise problems of justice, particularly when sponsors of research in resource-poor countries largely ignore the needs of those of countries; for example, when knowledge derived from research in those countries will mainly benefit wealthier countries. This may occur when diseases that are rare in wealthy nations but common in poorer countries are neglected or when the prices or costs of new preventive or therapeutic measures are beyond the resources of poorer countries.

A major impetus for the CIOMS guidelines has been concerns about ethics in international biomedical research and the challenges of applying universal ethical principles "in a multicultural world with a multiplicity of health-care systems and considerable variation in standards of health care" (CIOMS, 2002, online, unpaged). The Declaration of Helsinki, last revised in 2000 and 2002, also reflects concerns about justice in research involving resource-poor countries (WMA, 2002).

The next chapter considers many of the challenges in undertaking research involving infants, children, and adolescents. It also outlines the necessity and rationale for this research.

2

THE NECESSITY AND CHALLENGES OF CLINICAL RESEARCH INVOLVING CHILDREN

At a Congressional briefing . . . [i]t was my husband Joe and our daughter Becca who spoke. Becca was 16 and becoming a vibrant young lady looking forward to her life. The only obstacle that stood in her way was a malignant brain tumor . . . [Becca] stood at the podium next to her Dad and spoke only a few sentences. She believed it was important for her to support cancer research. It gave her hope.

Maureen Lilly, parent, 2000

As discussed in Chapter 1, children and families have benefited greatly from advances in biomedical science, medical care, and public health achieved during recent decades. For medical problems for which these advances have not resulted in prevention, cure, or improved health, the promise of future progress still gives many children and families hope in dark times.

This chapter discusses why research with adults cannot simply be generalized or extrapolated to infants, children, and adolescents and, thus, why research involving children is essential if children are to share fully in the benefits derived from advances in medical science. Most obviously, some conditions—such as prematurity and many of its sequelae—occur only in children. Similarly, certain genetic conditions such as phenylketonuria (PKU) will, if untreated, lead to severe disability or death in childhood. The diagnosis, prevention, and treatment of these conditions cannot be adequately investigated without studying children. Other conditions such as influenza and certain cancers and forms of arthritis occur in both adults and children, but their pathophysiology, severity, course, and response to treatment may differ for infants, children, and adolescents. Treatments that are safe and effective for adults may be dangerous or ineffective for children. Many of the examples cited in this report involve drugs, but clinically significant differences between children and adults extend to other areas. Radiation therapy can, for example, disrupt normal tissue development in children.

Clinical research involving infants, children, and adolescents is, in some important respects, more challenging than research involving adults. As reviewed in this chapter, these challenges include the relatively small numbers of children with serious medical problems, the need for developmentally appropriate outcome measures for children of different ages, the complexities of parental involvement and family decision making, and the adaptations required in research procedures and settings to accommodate children's physical, cognitive, and emotional development. Understanding and complying with the special ethical and regulatory protections for children constitutes another challenge. These various challenges underscore the need for those reviewing research protocols that include children to have adequate expertise in different areas of child health and research.

The next sections of this chapter provide additional historical context; discuss definitions used for the periods of infancy, childhood, and adolescence in different research arenas; and expand on the rationale and complex challenges of pediatric research. The last sections describe government policies adopted in recent years to encourage research involving children while protecting them from research risks.

CONTEXT

The ideal laboratory species for accumulating data on human functions and reactions is human, and that "animal of necessity" has been widely utilized in research in the biomedical sciences in the second half of the twentieth century.
Faden and Beauchamp, 1986, p. 152

If adult humans have been the "animal of necessity" in clinical research, then children have often been "therapeutic orphans," as characterized over 35 years ago by clinical pharmacologist Harry Shirkey (1968, p. 119). To a considerable degree, children retain this disadvantaged status, despite the recent creation of policy incentives for clinical research involving children.

As described in Chapter 1, a survey of the 1991 edition of the *Physician's Desk Reference* found that approximately 80 percent of the listed medications had labels that provided no prescribing information for children (Gilman and Gal, 1992, cited in AAP, 1995). Based on data from 1991 to 1997 involving new molecular entities with potential pediatric uses, a Food and Drug Administration (FDA) report found that 62 percent lacked labeling information for pediatric use at the time that they were initially approved for marketing (Steinbrook, 2002). The committee did not locate similar information about medical devices and biological agents.[1]

When drug labels lack pediatric prescribing information, physicians can still legally prescribe drugs for children on an "off-label" basis—and they do. According to Choonara and Conroy (2002), European studies suggest that at least one-third of hospitalized children and up to 90 percent of neonates in intensive care receive such prescriptions. A study in the United States, which used 1994 data on outpatient prescriptions, reported more than 1,600,000 off-label prescriptions of nebulized albuterol for children under age 12 years, nearly 350,000 prescriptions of the anti-depression drug fluoxetine (Prozac) for children under age 16 years, and more than 200,000 off-label prescriptions of methylphenidate (Ritalin, which is used to treat attention deficit disorder) for children under age 6 years (Pina, 1997; see also Turner et al., 1999 and Conroy et al., 2000). Altogether, the 10 identified drugs were prescribed more than five million times for children in age groups for which the drug label either had a disclaimer or lacked information for children. Since 1994, the FDA has reviewed supporting studies and approved pediatric labeling for several of these drugs (e.g., Prozac for ages 7 to 17 years, Ritalin for ages 6 to 12 years, levalbuterol down to age 7 years) (FDA, 2004).

The American Academy of Pediatrics has argued that the shortage of pediatric research creates an ethical dilemma for physicians, who "must frequently either not treat children with potentially beneficial medications or treat them with medications based on adult studies or anecdotal empirical experience in children" (AAP, 1995, p. 286). Many children undoubtedly benefit when physicians follow the second course. On occasion, however, some children will experience harm, either because the dose used was ineffective or because it was toxic. Even those children who receive some

---

[1]One provision of the Medical Device User Fee and Modernization Act of 2002 (P.L. 107-250) calls for an assessment of whether clinical studies of implanted devices continue long enough to assess the impact of children's growth and development in relation to the time that children are expected to have different kinds of implants. Another provision calls for an assessment of the adequacy of FDA's monitoring of commitments for further clinical studies of pediatric medical devices that are made by manufacturers at the time they obtain approval to market a device. The Act also directs the FDA to provide guidance on the kinds of information needed to provide reasonable assurance that medical devices intended for use in pediatric populations are safe and effective.

benefit may not receive optimal treatment because their physicians lack validated prescribing information.

Although most of the concern about expanding research involving children has focused on differences between adults and children as they relate to drugs, it is also important to consider differences in other therapeutic arenas. For example, intraocular lens replacement after cataract surgery has been a standard of care for many years in adults, and in young children it can not only treat a loss of vision but also improve visual development. Use of the procedure with children, however, presents unique developmental issues (see, e.g., Dahan, 2000; Ahmadieh and Javadi, 2001; Good, 2001; and Pandey et al., 2001). For example, children's eyes show lower scleral rigidity, greater elasticity of the anterior capsule, and higher vitreous pressure. Also, the refractive state of children's eyes changes as children grow. These characteristics make intraocular lens replacement in young children surgically and developmentally different from similar procedures for adults. In addition, the sizes of the replacement lenses developed for adults are not appropriate for young children (the mean axial length of a newborn's eye is 17 mm, whereas that of an adult is 23 to 24 mm). Surgical treatment and device placement for children present special developmental issues and requirements for pediatric studies in many other areas, including cardiology and orthopedics.

For research sponsors and investigators, the challenges of research involving children are compounded by normal developmental variability. For many conditions and interventions, separate studies are required for infants, young children, and adolescents. Several pediatric formulations of medications may ultimately be required (e.g., for acetaminophen, two strengths of chewable tablets, a low-strength "swallowable" tablet, a syrup, and drops in a different concentration for infants).

Furthermore, compared to adults, children generally represent a smaller market for commercial sponsors of research. The commercial value of various preventive, diagnostic, and therapeutic options for children, especially for rare diseases, may not be enough to offset the costs of developing them. Even for relatively common childhood conditions, the numbers of potential research participants may be small and thus require more study sites and additional costs for coordination. Development costs may also be increased because more time is often required per patient to complete study procedures and because more expensive, specialized laboratory studies may be required for small-volume biological samples. The widespread off-label prescription and use of drugs for children tend to further diminish the incentives to finance pediatric research on drugs that are already approved for use by adults. In addition, companies may be unfamiliar with the clinical, ethical, and regulatory requirements for pediatric studies, and they may be concerned about financial or public relations consequences of adverse experiences in research involving children.

As recounted in Chapter 1, reactions against abusive or questionable research practices involving both adults and children have led to an evolving set of policies and practices to protect all human participants in research, with additional protections for children and other vulnerable populations. The adoption of special protections for child research participants and the growing awareness of researchers' ethical obligations have curbed what are now regarded as unethical and harmful research practices. Notwithstanding these benefits, some of these protections have also made some research involving children more administratively burdensome in certain respects than research involving adults. Debate continues about what constitutes an appropriate balance between scientific priorities and protection of child participants in research.

Later sections of this chapter describe further the rationale and complex requirements for valid, safe pediatric research. The next section discusses the different definitions of infants, children, and adolescent used in different research contexts.

DEFINITIONS: INFANTS, CHILDREN, AND ADOLESCENTS

From birth into adulthood, children change and develop physically, cognitively, socially, and emotionally. Although these changes are fairly predictable, parents, clinicians, and others who interact regularly with children recognize that children of the same chronological age may develop at different rates. Practical and legal considerations, however, often dictate the organization of services and the definition of legal rights and other policies based primarily or entirely on chronological age.

Legal issues aside, age breakdowns are "a basis for thinking about study design in pediatric patients" (ICH, 2000b, p. 7). The age range specified for particular clinical studies will depend on the research question, for example, whether it involves a condition specific to infants or whether previous research shows relevant age-related physiological differences. The choice of age ranges may also be shaped by policy considerations, research organization missions, convenience, and other factors. Thus, in guidance on drug testing, FDA may reasonably define adolescence more narrowly than other agencies based on considerations of developmental physiology related to how drugs work in the body. A broader adolescent age range, however, is reasonable for the Centers for Disease Control and Prevention (CDC) and other agencies interested in the contribution of adolescent behavior, including risk taking, to problems such as sexually transmitted disease and motor vehicle-related deaths and injuries.

Infant

The first months of life are a period of particularly rapid development and change. Thus, in its section on growth and development, the *Nelson Textbook of Pediatrics* breaks the discussion of the first and second years of life into sections on ages 0 to 2 months, 2 to 6 months, 6 to 12 months, 12 to 18 months, and 18 to 24 months (Behrman et al., 2004). Thereafter, the textbook uses larger age ranges.

The discussion later in this chapter on pediatric pharmacokinetics underscores the significance for drug studies of developmental differences and changes during the earliest period of life. The importance of these differences and changes is reflected in FDA's guidance on pediatric drug testing, which categorizes those under age 2 years as infants (FDA, 1994a; 21 CFR 201.57(f)(9)(i)) and also distinguishes the category of neonates (infants less than 28 days of age).[2] The drug testing guidelines of the International Conference on Harmonisation (ICH) identify two additional categories—preterm infants and early neonates (infants less than 7 days of age) (ICH, 2000b; FDA, 2000b). The guidelines emphasize the unique and highly variable pathophysiology of preterm infants and their different responses to medications by stage of gestation. The guidelines stress the importance of involving neonatologists and neonatal pharmacologists in the development of research protocols for studies with neonates.

In health services research, epidemiologic studies, and public policy discussions, infants are typically defined as children under age 1 year, and early neonates and neonates are defined as described above for the FDA. These age categories, which are based on National Center for Health Statistics (NCHS) guidelines for vital statistics reporting (Kowaleski, 1997), reflect in part the interest of public health officials and epidemiologists in data to guide policies and programs to reduce infant mortality. Approximately half of all deaths among individuals under age 20 years involve infants, and the majority of these occur soon after birth (Arias and Smith, 2003).

Child

The term *child* is often used broadly—as it is in the title and, frequently, the text of this report—to refer to individuals ages 0 to 19 years (i.e., under age 20 years) or to cover all persons below the age at which a person can provide legal consent to medical treatment (usually age 18 years in the

---

[2] For FDA policies related to dietary foods, however, infant is defined as a person not more than 12 months old, child is a person more than 12 months old but less than 12 years of age, and an adult is a person age 12 years or above (see 21 CFR.105.3(e)).

United States). The definitions of child in federal regulations on human research protections are cast in legal terms and do not cite an age or age range.[3]

In guidance encouraging testing of drugs in studies involving children for the purpose of establishing safe dosing levels, the FDA categorizes those ages 2 to 11 years ("up to 12 years") as children (FDA, 1994a; 21 CFR 201.57(f)(9)(i)). The ICH guidelines cited above also use this age range. The guidelines stress the importance of investigating effects of medications on growth and development in this age group. The *Nelson Textbook of Pediatrics* uses a slightly broader age range—ages 2 to 12 years—and distinguishes early childhood (ages 2 to 5 years) and middle childhood (ages 6 to 12 years) (Behrman et al., 2004).

The National Institutes of Health (NIH) policy statement on the inclusion of children in research is expansive, defining a child as "an individual under the age of 21 years" for purposes of that policy (NIH, 1998a, unpaged).[4] The policy does not differentiate among infants, older children, and adolescents and does not present a rationale for the age range selected. The policy does, however, require research proposals to describe the rationale for including or excluding particular age groups. The NIH statement notes that its policy applies notwithstanding the different age range used by FDA. It also notes that the definition differs from the regulations of the Department of Health and Human Services governing children's participation in federally conducted, supported, or regulated research. Under NIH policy, an 18-year-old would be an adult for consent purposes (under state law) but a child for study inclusion purposes.

Adolescent

The term *adolescent* seems particularly variable in its definition, depending on the medical, public health, or psychosocial context in which it is used. NCHS observes that adolescence is "generally regarded as the period of life from puberty to maturity; [but] the meaning of 'puberty' and 'maturity' are often debated by health professionals" (NCHS, 2000, p. 19). Ado-

---

[3]The regulations state that children are "persons who have not attained the legal age for consent to treatments or procedures involved in the research, under the applicable law of the jurisdiction in which the research will be conducted" (45 CFR 46.402(a); 21 CFR 50.3(o)). Chapter 5 and Appendix B discuss these regulations and state policies that allow adolescents, under certain circumstances, to make decisions about health care in their own right.

[4]The policy statement was developed in response to language in House and Senate Appropriations Committee reports for fiscal year 1996 that noted the need for the more widespread inclusion of children in research (NIH, 1998a).

lescence is clearly a period of physical and psychosocial maturation and vulnerability related to hormonal changes, changes in appearance, and transition toward adult roles and responsibilities. The metabolic and other effects of hormonal changes associated with puberty may alter disease processes (e.g., in patients with diabetes) or contribute to the onset of medical problems (e.g., depression or polycystic ovary syndrome), with corresponding implications for disease prevention, diagnosis, and management (see, e.g., Janner et al., 1994; Travers et al., 1995; Angold et al., 1999; NRC/IOM, 1999; Schultz et al., 1999; Driscoll, 2003; and Sarnblad et al., 2003). Changes associated with puberty are an important consideration in much drug research, and the combination of physical, emotional, and social changes makes adolescence a particularly challenging period for psychosocial research.

In its regulations on pediatric drug testing, FDA uses a narrow definition of adolescence—ages 12 to 15 years ("up to 16 years") (FDA, 1994a; 21 CFR 201.57(f)(9)(i)). The ICH guidelines, however, refer to adolescents as those aged 12 to 16 or 18 years (with the observation that the upper limit "varies among regions") (ICH, 2000b, p.10). When adolescents are included in studies that also include adults, the guidelines suggest that it may appropriate "to consider studying adolescent patients . . . in centers knowledgeable and skilled in the care of this special population" (ICH, 2000b, p. 10). Recently, in draft guidance on the testing of medical devices, FDA proposed a broader age for adolescents—12 to 21 years—citing "the impact that a device could have on a growing adolescent as well as the effect growth could have on the device" as a rationale for the upper age limit (FDA, 2003b, p. 3). The agency noted that other factors—including weight, physiological development, and neuromuscular coordination—may be more relevant than chronological age for the assessment of device safety and effectiveness.

The *Nelson Textbook of Pediatrics* describes three periods of adolescence: early (ages 10 to 13 years), middle (ages 14 to 16 years), and late (ages 17 to 20 years and beyond) (Behrman et al., 2004).[5] The text observes that the first visible signs of puberty usually occur between the ages of 8 and 13 years and thus the period of early adolescence overlaps with the period of middle and late childhood. In a general statement on the age limits for pediatrics practice, the American Academy of Pediatrics (AAP)

---

[5]Some of those involved with adolescent health services identify the transition period to adulthood as extending into the third decade of life (see, e.g., SAM, 1995). The spectrum of pediatric or adolescent care may also be stretched to cover the situation of children with conditions such as congenital heart disease or cystic fibrosis who survive into adulthood but who continue to benefit from care and support provided by their pediatric care team.

noted that the responsibility of pediatrics may continue through age 21 years and even beyond under special circumstances (AAP, 1988).

Clearly, complete consensus does not exist about the age ranges that define infancy, childhood and adolescence. Definitions may reasonably vary depending upon the type of research being conducted. Given the practical challenges of recruiting adequate numbers of children for clinical research, as discussed later in this chapter, investigators may opt for as wide an age range as can be justified given the particular intervention or condition being investigated.

THE RATIONALE FOR PEDIATRIC DRUG RESEARCH

I was a brand-new fellow in pediatric hematology-oncology, in July 1963 . . . Long-term survivors of childhood leukemia were so rare that I cannot recall a single conversation on the topic during my fellowship . . . It has been a privilege to participate in studies leading to the dramatic increase in the proportion of long-term survivors.

Joseph V. Simone, 2003, p. 627-628

Much of the progress in pediatric oncology that Simone's statement acknowledges stems from a concerted effort to identify promising chemotherapeutic agents for childhood cancers, set priorities for the testing of these agents, and then design and conduct clinical trials through a national cooperative network of investigators and research institutions. This effort has been necessary because childhood cancers sometimes differ biologically from adult cancers and because other physiologic differences between children and adults may affect the ways in which chemotherapeutic agents work in the body. Agents that are effective with adults are not always effective with children.

In general, several features distinguish pharmacotherapy in children from that in adults and explain why medicines must be studied in research with children to ensure their safe and effective use (IOM, 2000b; see also, Kearns and Winter, 2003, and Reed and Gal, 2004). These features include

- requirements for age-appropriate formulations that allow the accurate, safe, and palatable administration of medicines to children of a wide range of weights and with a wide range of developmental characteristics;
- age- and development-dependent changes in how medicines are distributed in and eliminated from the body (pharmacokinetics);
- age- and development-dependent changes in the response to medicines (pharmacodynamics);

- age- and development-dependent changes in the adverse effects of medicines, both short and long term; and
- unique pediatric diseases that require development of unique pediatric medications.

Requirements for Age-Appropriate Formulations

For orally administered drugs, children of different ages often need or prefer formulations that differ from those used with adults. These formulations may include liquids, chewable tablets, rapidly dissolving tablets, and more palatable flavors. A critical impetus for the Federal Food, Drug, and Cosmetic Act of 1938, (the basis for the modern FDA) was a tragedy involving a liquid sulfonamide that cost the lives of over 100 adults and children (Ballentine, 1981; Wax, 1995; Hilts, 2003). When the sulfonamides—the first truly effective antimicrobials—were developed in the 1930s, they came in pill form, which was not suitable for very young children. For a liquid formulation, the manufacturer's chief chemist tried several solvents before devising a so-called elixir of sulfanilamide dissolved in diethylene glycol, a pleasant-tasting but toxic substance. The mixture, which also included flavoring agents, was evaluated for taste and fragrance but not safety. At least 34 children and 71 adults died of kidney failure after taking this elixir (Wax, 1995).[6]

Instances of harm to children from other unsafe drug formulations continue to occur. For example, in 1982, FDA warned that 16 premature infants had experienced "gasping syndrome" (resulting from metabolic acidosis leading to respiratory distress and other severe effects) and then died after being given intravenous medicines that contained excessive amounts of benzyl alcohol as a preservative (CDC, 1982). As recently as 2001, the warnings about this syndrome were added to labeling information for an intravenous drug—with the same preservative—that has been used on an off-label basis to treat cardiac arrhythmias in infants (de Vane, 2001). In developing countries, pediatric deaths have been associated with local formulations of acetaminophen containing diethylene glycol (Hanif et al., 1995; O'Brien et al., 1998).

---

[6]At the time, the government was able to investigate the deaths and retrieve the unconsumed amounts of the toxic drug only because the manufacturer incorrectly labeled it an elixir, which wrongly implied the presence of alcohol and thus constituted illegal misbranding under the statutes of the time. The government could not have acted if the drug had been labeled simply a solution (Ballentine, 1981; Wax, 1995). Reflecting the FDA's weakness at the time, the physician who first reported a suspicious pattern of deaths following consumption of the elixir contacted not the FDA but the American Medical Association's Council on Pharmacy and Chemistry.

Evaluations of pediatric formulations need to consider not only the safety of excipients (more or less inert substances used as vehicles or media for administering or diluting medications) but also the concentrations of the medicines being administered. For example, many adult intravenous preparations have concentrations of medicines such that the appropriate dose for a small infant is too small (e.g., less than 0.01 milliliter) to be accurately measured in a clinical syringe. Such medicines may also have low water solubility; when a nurse or doctor tries to dilute the medicine in intravenous solutions, the medicine precipitates out and may clog the intravenous line. If they reach the body, the precipitated medications may lodge in the lung and cause serious, even fatal, harm.

Not all formulations of drugs specifically for children come from pharmaceutical companies. For example, parents may be advised to give a half or a quarter of an adult tablet or to crush tablets and place them in applesauce. These strategies can produce both dosing errors and, possibly, drug instability because of uncertainty about the stability of the medicine in foods.

Professional, extemporaneous formulations (e.g., liquids based on crushed tablets) for pediatric medications may be helpful when they are produced by pharmacies with appropriate expertise. However, the validation of the stability and the absorption of the medicine from such formulations (i.e., its bioavailability) is often inadequate, particularly when compared with the standards of "good manufacturing practices" and "good clinical practices" defined by the FDA for formulation development and evaluation by pharmaceutical companies (Nahata, 1992, 1999; ICH, 1996; see also, FDA, 1997 and 21 CFR 210 and 211). In addition, many pharmacists lack the expertise to produce adequate and safe extemporaneous pediatric formulations, so their availability is limited. As discussed later in this chapter, one goal of the Best Pharmaceuticals for Children Act of 2002 is to encourage pharmaceutical companies to develop safe, effective formulations of drugs for children.

Development Affects Drug Distribution in and Excretion from the Body: Pharmacokinetics

Pharmacokinetic studies investigate the way in which medicines are absorbed (including when they are given orally, topically on the skin, or rectally), the way in which they are distributed among organs in the body, and the relationship between the dose and the concentration of a medicine in the blood. (Drug concentrations are typically measured in blood.) These studies are critical in pediatric care because they provide the basis for different formulations of drugs for children that avoid the dangers of either toxicity or underdosing based on extrapolation from studies conducted with adults. A complete description of developmental changes in pharmacokinetics cannot be included here, but a few examples demonstrate the need for proper pediatric pharmacokinetic studies before clinical trials or general clinical use of medicines with children.

One important reason for pediatric drugs studies is that the absorption of medicines after oral administration (the most common route) varies with age and differs among specific medicines. For example, the anticonvulsant phenytoin is poorly absorbed in newborns; thus, although it might theoretically be a good medicine for the treatment of seizures in newborns, unreliable absorption limits the drug's use for this purpose. A factor that can affect drug absorption is gastrointestinal transit time. The more rapid transit time of young infants can lead to poor absorption of many sustained-release formulations developed for adults.

Absorption of drugs through the skin also varies with age. Compared with adults, newborns and young children have a larger skin surface per pound of weight, and other characteristics of infants (e.g., skin thickness, blood) also affect absorption of topically applied substances such as steroid creams. The result can be a much larger dose per pound in a small child with the consequent risk of adverse effects. Examples of such adverse effects include growth inhibition from topical corticosteroids and central nervous toxicity from hexachlorophene, which is used to clean the skin of newborns.

Age and level of development are related to several pharmaco-kinetically relevant variations in the relative sizes of organs, the ways in which medicines attach to proteins in the blood plasma, and the physiologic processes that exclude chemicals from sites such as the central nervous system (e.g., processes that involve what is often called the blood-brain barrier). For example, if sulfonamides are given to premature infants, the drugs will interfere with the safe removal of bilirubin (a by-product of blood metabolism) from the blood by plasma proteins. If permitted to accumulate in the bloodstream, bilirubin can penetrate the infant's immature blood-brain barrier, which can, in turn, lead to kernicterus (yellow staining of the brain) and brain damage. The objective of pharmacokinetic studies with infants, children, and adolescents is to identify such toxic effects before rather than after a drug is used in pediatric clinical care.

Medicines are excreted from the body by metabolism in the liver and other organs. They are also filtered and excreted by the kidney. Increasingly, scientists are learning that metabolism is mediated by specific enzymes and that each of these enzymes has a different metabolic pattern depending on the child's stage of development. A specific medicine may be metabolized by one or several enzymes, each with a different pattern of action related to developmental stage. In addition, a child's stage of development will affect drug excretion and the half-life of the drug (the time it takes for half the drug to be excreted from the body, which is one of the determinants for choosing a dosing schedule, e.g., once a day versus three times a day).

For example, in newborns, the enzyme glucuronyl transferase, which metabolizes the drug chloramphenicol, has a very low level of activity. When chloramphenicol was first used in newborns in the 1950s, the dose was extrapolated from adult doses without knowledge of the drug's metabolic pathway. At the time, it was also not possible to determine concentrations of drugs in serum because of a lack of technology to measure drug concentrations in the small quantities of blood that can be safely extracted from neonates, infants, and small children. With the doses selected by individual pediatricians, the drug reached much higher concentrations in infants than in adults, resulting in death from the "gray baby syndrome" (see, e.g., Weiss et al., 1960). The technologies available today allow medicines like chloramphenicol to be more fully evaluated before they are used with pediatric patients.

The rates of maturation of drug clearance pathways after the neonatal period are highly variable and relate to the specific metabolic enzymes or kidney mechanisms that are responsible for drug excretion. (Other variables such as disease state and drug-drug interactions can also influence drug clearance.) Research shows that although neonates excrete many medicines much more slowly than adults, prepubertal children often excrete drugs much more rapidly than adults. Thus, although overdosing based on the extrapolation of doses for adults to doses for neonates is likely, underdosing of children is common.

During puberty, drug clearance and half-life move toward adult levels (Goodman et al., 2001). The changes during this period depend on the specific pathways of clearance of a given medicine (i.e., which enzymes are involved in its metabolism). This process has been studied best for cytochrome P-450 1A2 (CYP1A2), an enzyme that metabolizes caffeine and theophylline (Lambert et al., 1983, 1986; Le Guennec and Billon, 1987). The enzyme activity decreases from childhood levels at earlier pubertal stages in girls than in boys (and, thus, at an earlier age, because girls begin undergoing pubertal stages at younger ages than boys). Once adolescents have reached Tanner stage 4 (of the five stages of sexual maturity identified by Tanner [1962]), drug metabolism and clearance closely resemble adult values.

Recent studies have resulted in changes in a number of recommendations or warnings about the use (or nonuse) of specific medications by children (Meadows, 2003). These changes emphasize the importance of pharmacokinetic studies of drugs that are expected to be beneficial for children of various ages.

Development Affects Response to Medications: Pharmacodynamics

In addition to developmental changes in drug metabolizing enzymes, developmental changes can also affect the drug receptors that mediate how medicines act in the body, that is, their *pharmacodynamics*. This area has not been studied as systematically as drug metabolism.

As examples of pharmacodynamic differences between adults and children, phenobarbital and antihistamines may produce sedation in adults but excitation and hyperactivity in children. This paradoxical response is thought to be related to central nervous system receptors that have not matured. Other drugs may simply not work in children of certain ages because a receptor that permits the activity of the drug is not present or has not yet developed. Major future challenges for pediatric drug development will be to develop methods to (1) assess receptor development, (2) create clinical tools to assess the relationship between how the body processes a drug and what response the drug triggers in adults, and then (3) determine whether the same relationship holds for children of various ages.

FDA and ICH guidelines provide for minimizing the burden of full clinical trials with children if a combination of clinical information about the similarity of the disease in children and adults, pharmacokinetic and pharmacodynamic measurements, and safety and other studies provide sufficient confidence that efficacy can be extrapolated from adults or older children and that an appropriate dose can be defined (FDA, 2000b). To judge the acceptability of such extrapolations, more data are needed on changes in drug receptors by stage of development and associated pharmacodynamic outcomes.

Adverse Effects of Medicines by Developmental Stage

The very fact that children are growing and developing places them at risk of adverse effects that are not observed in adults. For example, in addition to other side effects that occur in adults, corticosteroids can alter physical growth. To cite another example, tetracyclines stain developing teeth but not teeth that are fully developed.

Not just medicines used for long periods but also those used for relatively short periods with children may have long-term consequences that are not evident for years. Although study designs for short-term clinical studies need to take potential developmental toxicity into account, long-term follow-up and surveillance are important. Such surveillance is important, for example, in tracking developmental and other outcomes for children treated for cancer with chemotherapy agents. Collaborative groups such as the Children's Oncology Group (COG) have played an important role in monitoring children for long-term outcomes, and their strategies may serve as models for those studying the developmental consequences of experimental interventions for other acute or chronic illnesses. Novel epidemiologic methods will likely be needed for long-term follow-up of otherwise healthy children treated with various medicines on a short-term basis.

Medicines for Unique Pediatric Diseases

When a medicine is being developed for both adults and children, at least some data are usually available from studies with adults before studies with children start. Even for medicines with unique pediatric indications, studies with children often follow phase 1 trials that provide an initial assessment of the drug's tolerability and pharmacokinetics in adults. As molecularly targeted therapies are developed with increasing frequency, however, it is likely that more new drugs will be developed specifically for the treatment of conditions that occur only in children. If an agent is not appropriate for initial testing with healthy adult volunteers but findings from findings from prior laboratory and animal studies are favorable, then initial testing is likely to be performed with children who have such a condition. The agent may never be administered to adults. Thus, it is inappropriate to assume or require that drugs must invariably be tested in adults before pediatric clinical trials are initiated.

IMPLICATIONS FOR PEDIATRIC INVESTIGATION

The preceding sections of this chapter emphasize the need for expanded efforts to develop appropriate and safe formulations of medicines for children. The following section outlines a safe, logical and efficient process for doing so.

Before drug studies are initiated with children, several steps should be completed to minimize the number of children required for research protocols and to maximize the quality of the data collected. Whenever possible, the first step should be the completion and evaluation of phase 1 studies with adults to investigate the tolerability, bioavailability and pharmacokinetics of the drug of interest and provide the basis for designing phase 1 and phase 2 pharmacokinetic studies involving children. When feasible, data from these studies or laboratory techniques developed during their conduct may be used to minimize the numbers and volumes of blood samples necessary for pediatric studies. For drugs such as new anticancer agents for which it is desirable to expose as few children as possible to doses too low to be therapeutic, data from phase 1 trials with adults may be used to guide the selection of a pediatric starting dose and a dose escalation scheme for early-phase testing of the drug.

In some cases, the second step should involve additional preclinical toxicology studies using animals to assess potential developmental toxicity before trials with children are started. The third step should be for investigators to assess the need and specific requirements for special formulations (e.g., liquids or chewable tablets) that are suitable for children at different ages. Taken together, the data from adult and animal studies will guide the development of a rational series of clinical studies that involve children.

For many drugs, the first pediatric study is a single-dose pharmacokinetic study that involves the age groups that are likely to use the drug. This type of study is designed to discover major age-related differences in pharmacokinetics in these groups and to generate preliminary data for the design of subsequent multidose and efficacy studies. In the United States, the majority of single-dose pediatric pharmacokinetic studies involve children with an illness likely to be treated by the drug under study. Depending on what is known in advance based on trials with adults, preclinical studies, and other information, some of these early-phase trials—unlike typical phase 1 trials involving adults—may arguably be viewed as having the prospect of providing a direct benefit to the child participants. The assessment of such research may also consider whether other treatment alternatives have been exhausted and whether the probable outcome without the experimental intervention has been assessed. As described in Chapters 3 and 4, depending on the findings from the specific assessment of potential harms and potential benefits, early-phase studies involving children may or may not be approvable under federal regulations.

After the completion of phase 1 (safety and pharmacokinetic) trials, the next step is the development of appropriate phase 2 (safety and efficacy) studies. As discussed further below, a major challenge for drug manufacturers and pediatric investigators is designing these studies to incorporate appropriate outcome criteria. For all phase 2 studies involving children, trials should be designed to minimize risks and the number of study participants (while ensuring statistically meaningful results).

Broad phase 3 trials with children may or may not be appropriate for a particular drug, depending on the agent and the condition that it is intended to treat. For some "orphan" indications (i.e., rare conditions), a phase 3 or randomized trial may not be practical. Similarly, even if there is a plan for such a trial, the timing may be significantly delayed beyond the drug's approval by the FDA for adult use. This situation applies to many anticancer agents. In such cases, safety and efficacy assessments should continue beyond marketing approval and may include postmarket surveillance or targeted cohort studies.

One of the greatest ethical challenges is assessing the optimal timing for the initiation of pediatric pharmacokinetic and efficacy trials. Most medicines entering phase 1 trials with adults are never approved because of safety concerns or a lack of efficacy (Kaitin, 2003). For this reason, one could argue that research with children should await FDA approval based on studies with to avoid children's exposure to the excessive risks of early-phase trials. As noted above, some drugs are for conditions that do not exist in adults and may be inappropriate or impossible to test in adults. Moreover, particularly for seriously ill children who have exhausted standard treatment options and who may not survive until the FDA approves an investigational drug, approval of a trial may be warranted based on initial favorable findings from preclinical studies and trials with adults. Thus, judgment is required in balancing conflicting concerns. Assessment of each proposed trial should take into account the availability of other therapies, the severity of the disease in question, the assessment of adverse event profiles for adults and other relevant data, and the availability of a suitable pediatric formulation for testing.

In sum, the overall goal for pediatric drug development should be to evaluate the safety and efficacy of drugs for children as soon as possible after adequate data for adults are generated to guide the design of safe and efficient pediatric studies. When data for adults are not available or when waiting for such data may do more harm than good, particular care must be taken to justify proceeding with pediatric trials. Likewise, if a drug will be marketed for adults without a plan in place to evaluate it with children, the rationale should be explained (e.g., no equivalent condition in children, safety concerns based on the results of studies with adult, formulation problems, or a lack of pediatric clinical end points to judge efficacy). Such an explicit rationale will help pediatricians understand the possible implications for "off-label" use of the drug.

CHALLENGES OF DESIGNING AND CONDUCTING PEDIATRIC STUDIES

Clearly, determining how children's development affects drugs in the body is both a major rationale and a significant challenge for pediatric research. In addition, researchers committed to clinical research involving infants, children, and adolescents face a number of other challenges beyond those typically encountered in research involving adults. These challenges range from practical and methodological problems to regulatory requirements and ethical concerns. Those conducting initial and continuing reviews of pediatric research should have sufficient expertise—personally or through consultation—to assess the appropriateness of the investigator's strategies for managing challenges relevant to their research topic. This section discusses these challenges.

Defining and Measuring Outcomes and Other Variables

Among the challenges facing pediatric research is defining appropriate outcome measures. This challenge has basic two dimensions. One is the determination of what outcomes are meaningful for children of different ages in the context of a specific study—and then developing reliable and valid ways of measuring these outcomes. The other is the determination of normative data for purposes of comparison, for example, for comparisons between healthy children of different ages and children known or suspected of having a medical problem.

In addition, because children are developing physiologically, anatomically, cognitively psychologically, and socially, possible developmental effects of medications and other interventions may need attention. Assessment of such effects may require lengthy follow-up studies that track children for years, even decades (see further discussion below).

Identifying Age-Appropriate Clinical Outcomes

Among meaningful outcomes, death is a relatively straightforward outcome across age groups, although the accurate identification of the cause of death is a continuing concern, particularly in studies relying on death certificates. For example, for deaths among children, health officials have made particular efforts to distinguish cases of child abuse from instances of sudden infant death syndrome. As research has led to improved therapies and prolonged survival for children with many fatal childhood illnesses (e.g., acute lymphoblastic leukemia, severe prematurity, and cystic fibrosis), death has become—as hoped—an uncommon or long-delayed outcome of these illnesses. As a result, other outcome measures become more significant in further clinical studies.

Survival after diagnosis and disease-free survival are also meaningful outcomes across age groups, but considerable caution may be needed in interpreting survival statistics and changes in survival across time. In particular, changes in diagnostic technologies or the frequency of their use can push the time of diagnosis earlier for many individuals; this can make survival statistics look better independent of any real improvement. Such changes are particularly relevant to genetic disorders that are now being diagnosed prenatally or at birth, before clinical signs develop.

To support accelerated marketing approval of new drugs and biologics aimed at serious pediatric diseases, FDA has in recent years accepted evidence from phase 3 efficacy trials that use "surrogate" physiological measures if they are "reasonably likely, based on epidemiologic, therapeutic, pathophysiologic, or other evidence, to predict clinical benefit" (21 CFR 314.510). This acceptance may be accompanied by requirements for additional postapproval follow-up studies to demonstrate long-term clinical benefit and safety in the target population. Many convenient physiological measures (e.g., blood pressure, tumor shrinkage, and the levels of different substances in the blood) do not fulfill the FDA criteria for this kind of "surrogate" outcome measure. Although the measures track changes relevant to the administered treatment, these changes may not correspond to physical or mental outcomes that directly improve the child's life. For example, a drug may shrink a tumor without affecting survival, function, or quality of life.

Pediatric investigators and FDA staff may find it difficult to agree on the best surrogate for a particular disease entity. An acceptable measurement must not only be relevant to the child's long-term well-being but also be easy to use with children and reproducible when used at multiple sites. Further, sufficient normative data should be available to permit statistical comparisons and analyses.

An example of a surrogate physiologic marker is forced expiratory volume at 1 second (FEV_1). For many lung disorders, FEV_1 is used as a measure of obstruction (blockage) of airway passages. Until the 1990s, no FDA-approved therapy had been developed for the treatment of patients with cystic fibrosis. Two new therapies were developed in the 1990s, a drug to breakdown bronchial mucus (dornase alfa [Pulmozyme]) and an inhaled antibiotic (tobramycin solution for inhalation [TOBI]). Through a series of meetings, the FDA and the cystic fibrosis community decided that FEV_1 was the optimal surrogate (in conjunction with the frequency of pulmonary infections) for this disorder because of the published data relating FEV_1 to the survival rate (Kerem et al., 1992; Corey et al., 1997; Liou et al., 2001) and the hospitalization rate (Emerson et al., 2002). As a result, FEV_1 was a key factor in FDA approval of these therapies and has become the primary outcome measure for most subsequent clinical trials (Fuchs et al., 1994; Ramsey and Boat, 1994; Ramsey et al., 1999).

Like most surrogates in pediatric research, FEV_1 is far from perfect. First, as new therapies continue to improve survival and function (CFF, 2002), FEV_1 becomes a less sensitive marker of change and of early disease. Second, measurement of FEV_1 requires a voluntary maneuver that most children under 6 years of age cannot reproducibly perform, which means it cannot serve as a surrogate outcome measure for this group. As a result, both Pulmozyme and TOBI were initially approved only for children ages 6 years and older. Newer techniques are being developed to measure lung function in infants and toddlers (Gappa et al., 2001; Castile et al., 2000). FEV_1 exemplifies the challenges of developing a surrogate outcome measure for children, especially young children.

Assessment of outcomes related to physical or cognitive functioning may be more complicated in pediatric studies than in adult studies, given normal developmental differences. The inability to walk or talk is characteristic of infants but is a serious problem for a 3-year-old. In evaluating protocols, institutional review boards (IRBs) will need to consider whether the proposed outcome measures are developmentally appropriate.

In addition to survival and functioning, outcomes related to the prevention of pain, nausea, vomiting, and other symptoms may be crucially important to children and families, depending on the child's medical condition and its treatment. Among symptoms, instruments to assess pain are the furthest advanced. For infants and young children, symptom assessment strategies commonly used with adults, for example, numerical rating scales with 10 representing severe pain and 0 no pain, need to be replaced by other more developmentally appropriate methods. Such methods in use include face scales (representing a continuum for grimaces to big smiles) and observation of infant behaviors such as crying and body movement (see, e.g., Wong and Baker, 1988; Broome et al., 1990; Krechel and Bildner, 1995; Hockenberry-Eaton et al., 1999; Gallo, 2003; Manworren and Hynan, 2003; and Naar-King et al., 2004). If child-appropriate instruments do not exist for a symptom or group of children, the development and validation of such instruments can take years.

Quality-of-life measures have become important indicators of clinical benefit and therefore important in measuring the efficacy of new treatments. Again, instruments developed for adults are usually not suited for children. Instrument development for pediatric uses is complicated and slowed by the need to create forms appropriate for children at different stages of development. Work continues to develop, test, and refine generic (for all conditions) and disease-specific instruments for both healthy and ill children of different ages.[7] For example, the PedsQL 4.0 instrument has both self-report forms and parent-proxy report forms for children ages 5 to 7, 8 to 12, and 13 to 18 years and a parent-proxy form only for children ages 2 to 4 years (Varni, 2003). This instrument has disease-specific modules for asthma, arthritis, cancer, cardiac disease, and diabetes. Other pediatric instruments are being developed or have been developed for some of the same conditions as well as for other conditions, including cystic fibrosis, cerebral palsy, atopic dermatitis, and obesity (see, e.g., Henry et al., 1997; Gee et al., 2000; Quittner et al., 2000; and Bullinger et al., 2002).

---

[7]In discussing quality of life measures for children with life-threatening conditions, Bradlyn and colleagues (2003, p. 477) observe that "[a]lthough health status, functional status, and health-related quality of life (HRQL) are terms that have often been used interchangeably, a meta-analysis suggests that health status and functional status most commonly are used to refer to the physical functioning dimensions of the broader HRQL construct, while HRQL additionally includes the psychosocial dimensions of emotional, social, and role functioning, as well as related constructs (Smith [et al.], 1999)."

Establishing Norms

Development of new treatments for children requires an assessment of both the beneficial effects and the safety of the therapy. Critical to such an analysis are comparative data about what constitutes normal values for a wide range of physiological variables. Such comparative data must be age appropriate and, frequently, disease specific. Many laboratory norms are based on easily accessible data for healthy adults. For pediatric studies, efforts must be made to ensure that laboratories processing clinical samples have age-appropriate norms. The collection of data for the development of such norms is often difficult because routine laboratory studies (e.g., chemistry profiles) are rarely performed for healthy children. The lack of normative data becomes an even greater issue for children with rare conditions. For example, to assess the potential toxicity of new drugs for premature infants or children with AIDS, it is essential to have baseline "normal-for-the-population" laboratory parameters, such as white blood cell counts and liver function test results. These children may already have abnormal white blood cell counts, which makes it more difficult to monitor the effects of drugs that may have bone marrow suppression as a toxic side effect.

An advantage of disease-specific clinical trials cooperatives or networks is their greater ability to collect age- and disease-specific normative data across multiple trials. Baseline data collected before administration of a study drug(s) are most useful for this purpose. Investigators should be encouraged to publish these data, and journals should also be encouraged to accept such publications.

Administering Interventions and Measurements

When they evaluate a pediatric protocol for potential harms and benefits and for appropriate efforts to minimize risks to child participants, IRBs should consider the qualifications and expertise of investigators and others to conduct the research, taking into account the procedures and age groups described in the protocol. They should likewise assess the appropriateness of the facilities and settings for the proposed research.

Particularly in studies involving infants and young children, the administration of interventions and measurements may lead to complications not encountered with adults. Some complications are physiological. For example, it is more difficult to draw blood from the small veins of infants or toddlers than from those of older children and adults. Furthermore, the smaller volume of blood in children sets limits on how much blood can safely be drawn. Fortunately, newer analytical methods permit accurate assays using much smaller volumes of blood than was possible in the past.

Other challenges in administering pediatric studies are behavioral. Young children may not understand instructions. If they do, they may still be too immature to cooperate consistently, for example, by staying still when asked. Certain procedures that depend on verbal feedback from the research participant (e.g., more complex or complete assessments of pain, hearing, or other sensations or sensory functions) may not be possible with very young children. Older children and adolescents may present different challenges, for example, rebellion against adult authority, including that of their parents and the investigators. Peer pressure may also be a constraint for studies that require participants to be "different" (e.g., to take medications during school hours or to miss after-school activities to go to a clinic for an assessment). Depending on the study and the ages of the children involved, providing adequate time for training and preparation of children before the initiation of study protocols may be useful. Children may be more receptive to procedures requiring cooperation if they have a good understanding in advance of what is expected of them.

Whether undertaken for therapeutic or research purposes, tests and treatments for children often require or benefit from modifications in procedures, equipment, staffing, patient and family communication, and other dimensions of care that are tailored to their special developmental needs. Thus, it may be less stressful for all involved when persons drawing blood or spinal fluid from a child have been trained to work with infants and children and their families and when they have routine access to small-gauge needles, appropriate topical anesthetics, and even colorful bandages. Indwelling catheters may be used in pediatric studies to avoid multiple needle sticks. Children should always be given the option to receive a topical anesthetic to reduce needle-stick pain.

Laboratory personnel accustomed to analyzing blood and other biological samples from children may be more accepting of small samples than personnel who mainly work with adult specimens. Furthermore, depending on expectations about possible adverse events, the safety of research protocols may be increased by the availability of personnel and facilities prepared for pediatric emergencies.

Children with chronic disorders have frequently had previous experiences (both good and bad) with medical procedures. Careful discussion of the child's perceptions and fears of any procedures before the initiation of research protocols may help correct misunderstandings and allay the child's fears. The involvement of child-life specialists and child psychologists may reduce the stress on children and families during clinical studies as well as during usual clinical care.

Undertaking Research When Study Populations Are Small

Because most children today are healthy, children suffering from serious conditions such as cancer or heart disease are relatively few in number compared with the number of adults who have such conditions. As one indicator of children's good health, children aged 0 to 19 years accounted for 29 percent of the total U.S. population of 272.7 million in 1999 but only 2 percent of all deaths—about 55,000 deaths for children compared with more than a half million deaths for adults aged 20 to 64 years and 1.8 million for those age 65 years and over (NCHS, 2000).

To cite another example, the American Cancer Society has estimated that approximately 1.3 million new cases of cancer would be diagnosed in 2003, of which an estimated 9,000 would involve children ages 0 to 14 years (ACS, 2003). For any specific cancer in children, the numbers are much smaller. For example, each year approximately 300 children are diagnosed with retinoblastoma (a tumor of the retina), 1,100 are diagnosed with astrocytoma (a brain tumor), and 2,400 are diagnosed with acute lymphoblastic leukemia (based on data from 1977 to 1995) (Ries et al, 1999). Moreover, as treatments for childhood cancer have improved and rates of cancer-free survival have increased, researchers find fewer children with relapsing disease who are potentially available for the study of new chemotherapeutic agents.

Exceptions exist to the "small-numbers" phenomenon. Each year approximately 75,000 babies are born very prematurely at 31 weeks gestation or earlier, and more than 350,000 babies have low or very low weights at birth (Martin et al., 2002). (For various reasons, however, many of these newborns will not be appropriate to include in research.) Asthma is a growing problem among children, and the increase in childhood obesity has become a major concern. A number of less serious conditions, such as otitis media, acne, and mild allergies, are quite common.

Although the numbers of children affected by some of these illnesses are greater than the numbers affected by rare genetic disorders, not all children with a disorder or condition will be eligible or able to participate in clinical trials. For any one research location, the numbers available for a study are usually quite low.

For many pediatric studies, the relative scarcity of potential study participants means that it often takes considerable effort and some creativity to enroll and retain sufficient numbers of children who meet the criteria for study participation. It may also mean that studies must extend for quite long periods just to secure enough participants. One recently published article on the prevention of fungal infections in children and adults with chronic granulomatous disease reported that it took 10 years to enroll 39 participants, most of whom were children at the time that the study started (Gallin et al, 2003).

Without a large enough number of participants, studies may not be able to generate statistically reliable estimates of differences between a study drug and a control treatment or placebo. A review of randomized controlled trials published in the *Archives of Diseases in Childhood* from 1982 to 1996 reported that about half of the studies recruited less than 40 children, with medians of 80 children for multicenter trials and 36 children for single-center studies (Campbell et al., 1998; see also Pattishall, 1990 and, generally, Freiman et al., 1986 and Moher et al., 1994). The authors comment that these small studies "have inadequate power to detect small or moderate treatment effects and result in a significant chance of reporting false-negative results" (Campbell et al., 1998, p. 196).

Children's developmental differences create further complications that often require separate subanalyses or studies with infants, older children, and adolescents to assess the safety and efficacy of an intervention. The production of reliable estimates of effects for each subgroup usually increases the total number of research participants required for a study. In some cases, depending on the condition and the question being investigated and various technical considerations, special study designs can allow the use of smaller numbers of participants. For example, in so-called crossover studies, research participants act as their own control group, typically by first receiving and being evaluated on the experimental intervention and then receiving and being evaluated on a placebo or a standard treatment. In the study by Gallin and colleagues (2003) cited above, participants were randomly assigned to receive an experimental drug or a placebo at enrollment but were then switched annually to the alternative.

As discussed further in Chapter 4, one justification for the use of placebo-controlled trials is that they may allow smaller sample sizes than may be required for studies that compare the efficacy of two standard treatments or the efficacy of an experimental and a standard intervention. Such designs may raise ethical questions, and they require particularly careful design, monitoring, and analysis. Nonetheless, they have many advantages when their use is ethically and scientifically appropriate.

Large, multisite trials have become increasingly important for studies with adults as researchers seek to understand differences in medical conditions and treatment effects among population subgroups and to demonstrate reliably treatment effects that are modest but still important. Even more often than with adults, research involving children requires multisite trials and fairly long periods of participant enrollment to generate the minimum required numbers of study participants. The relative success of pediatric oncology researchers, as described below, is based in part on the large number of institutions participating in COG, which makes state-of-the-art care more accessible to children and families. In recent years other disease-specific clinical trials (Goss et al., 2002) are beginning to follow the COG model to increase participant enrollment and improve trial efficiency.

In reviewing all protocols but especially protocols involving children, IRBs should be particularly attentive to potential problems in achieving adequate numbers and classes of study participants and to the appropriate strategies for managing such problems. Such strategies may include modifications of classic clinical trial designs and innovative approaches to recruiting children and then retaining them throughout the course of the study. At the same time, reviewers of research protocol should be alert to the appropriateness of strategies for recruiting children, including payments to children or parents. This topic is discussed further in Chapter 6.

Designing Long-Term Studies

Importance of Long-Term Studies in Pediatric Populations

As mentioned earlier in this chapter, long-term studies are a particular challenge and a particular need for many serious pediatric medical conditions. Assessing the possible developmental effects of medical treatments or interventions may require extremely lengthy follow-up, well beyond what the immediate study outcomes appear to mandate. For example, the adverse sequelae associated with the use of cranial radiation to prevent central nervous system spread of leukemia in children did not become evident until many years following the introduction of this therapeutic approach (Cousens et al., 1988; Roman and Sperduto, 1995). Despite the success of radiation in the short term, the eventual recognition of late effects, including impaired intellectual function, profound neuroendocrine abnormalities, and second central nervous system malignancies, ultimately resulted in efforts to eliminate cranial radiation from among the options for the treatment of leukemia.

Many other conditions may require long-term follow-up in order to understand the physical, psychosocial, or economic consequences of the condition and its treatment. For example, very-low-birth-weight infants must be monitored at least until they reach school age to assess in detail the sequelae of prematurity and its treatment (Fazzi et al., 1997). Likewise, if one wants to test certain kinds of preventive interventions, then the study must follow study participants for at least as long as it is expected to take the target condition to develop naturally without treatment.

Studies of the effects of certain drugs in children may also require long-term follow-up that is not necessary for adults. Because of developmental changes in hepatic and renal function, children may experience positive or negative changes in response as they receive certain drugs over a long period. For children receiving drug therapy for a chronic condition, the need for long-term follow-up for both safety and efficacy is therefore obvious.

Implementing Long-Term Studies with Children

The performance of long-term studies with children involves a number of logistical and ethical challenges. The investigator, for example, must have a clinical trial infrastructure that permits tracking and periodic evaluation of trial participants over many years. It is obvious that families may move, but so may researchers. Within research institutions, where both physicians and other study staff tend to change positions over time, the study infrastructure must have an "institutional memory" to manage ongoing data collection and interaction with research participants despite staff turnover. In addition to being a logistical challenge, long-term studies are usually extremely expensive. Study sponsors are rarely willing to provide funding for long-term follow-up, and few institutions have the wherewithal to support such studies independently.

Long-term studies with children may also raise ethical issues that are not relevant for studies with adults. The most obvious of these involves informed consent. Although federal regulations provide for investigators to seek children's assent when appropriate (as discussed in Chapter 5) and also allow their dissent under certain circumstances, it is almost always the parents who give legal permission for a child to participate in a study. For long-term studies, parents and children may be approached periodically for continued permission or assent, particularly if the nature of the research changes or when important developmental milestones are reached.

If a longitudinal study that started in childhood extends into adulthood, continuing participants will eventually become legally competent to consent to participation in their own right. For research that requires an individual's continued contribution (e.g., through periodic interviews or procedures), these participants can either consent or decline to continue participation when they become adults. In general, continued research use of data already collected would be permitted for the purposes covered by earlier permission and assent. Questions have, however, been raised about when new permission or consent must be sought for new research uses of stored biological specimens and about what to do with such specimens and related analyses when an individual withdraws from a study (see, e.g., NBAC, 1999, Weir, 2000; Botkin, 2001).[8] These are important questions with significant ethical and scientific implications, the analysis of which goes beyond the tasks for this study.

---

[8]Another question is whether it is ethical to offer individuals the option of consenting to any future research use of identifiable stored tissue samples. Some members of the National Bioethics Advisory Commission (NBAC, 1999) argue that the potential harms and benefits would be unknown for this option and so could not be evaluated, meaning that the ethical requirements for informed consent could not be met.

Working with Families

Family-centered care is increasingly being appreciated as one of the goals for the clinical services provided to children (see, e.g., Shelton et al., 1987; Johnson et al., 1992; Gerteis et al., 1993; MCHB, 2003; IOM, 2003b). It emphasizes care that respects and involves both the child and the family and that understands and accommodates their strengths, their coping strategies, and their cultural, religious, and other values. Family-centered care also promotes shared decision making.

Although family members are sometimes involved in discussions about the participation of adults in research, parents or other legally designated persons are almost always involved in discussions and decisions about children's participation in research. Discussions and decisions may also involve grandparents and other family members. As explained in Chapter 3, if research involves more than minimal risk but is not expected to benefit a child participant, federal rules usually require that both parents give permission for participation. In addition, federal rules require that, when appropriate, children must "assent" to participation in research.

The multiplication of participants in discussions and decisions about a child's involvement in research can place considerable demands on the interpersonal skills of the investigator and others involved in discussions about research participation. It may also increase the time needed for explanations and decision making and the potential for disagreement among those involved. When research involves acutely ill or injured children, investigators will usually face parents who are confronting complex and difficult decisions while under extraordinary stress. Chapter 5 examines some of the complexities of establishing the conditions for informed family decision making about children's participation in research.

The diversity of family contexts also creates challenges for investigators. Family decision making about health care in general and about research specifically is not done in a vacuum. Rather, it is affected by social and cultural factors. These factors have an important influence on families' perceptions of health, illness, and treatment and on their views of the role of patients and family members in decision making. Thus, in discussions about children's participation in research, investigators are also called upon to be culturally sensitive and competent and to negotiate between families' beliefs and the tenets of biomedicine.

Some research involving children raises highly sensitive issues for their families and, perhaps, their communities. Studies of such important issues as suicide, drug use, sexual behavior, family dysfunction, and other topics are sensitive enough when they involve adults. When studies on these topics involve children, the challenges for investigators grow. Parents may be reluctant to permit a child's participation in sensitive research. As discussed in Chapter 5, IRBs may approve federal requirements for waiver of parent permission in certain situations, and this committee encourages IRBs to consider carefully protocols that propose such waivers. In general, however, parental involvement and permission are advisable.

Meeting Ethical and Regulatory Standards for Pediatric Research

As discussed in Chapters 1 and 3, recent decades have seen the development and refinement of ethical principles to guide research with vulnerable populations, including children. These principles have been translated into government regulation, which, in turn, have directed the development of institutional structures and procedures to implement the principles and regulations.

The regulations restrict the range of research that can be undertaken with children, particularly studies that involve more than minimal risks for healthy children or children who have no prospect of directly benefiting from participation in the research. For example, traditional phase 1 clinical trials that use healthy volunteers to test the safety of a new medication face higher hurdles to approval if investigators propose to include children. Placebo-controlled trials of a drug's efficacy likewise face more scrutiny when children are involved if the trial does not hold the prospect of benefiting the children who receive the placebo but does expose them to more than a minimal amount of risk. Chapter 4 discusses in detail the criteria for approving research that includes children.

Notwithstanding the ethical rationale for the special regulations that protect child participants in research, the regulations add to the administrative burdens on investigators in preparing, justifying, and implementing research protocols. Investigators may find themselves confronting unexpected questions and criticisms from IRBs, changing procedures for obtaining parents' and children's agreement to participate in research, redesigning protocols, and delaying the enrollment of participants. When investigators have not been adequately educated about the special regulatory protections for children, they may be at a particular disadvantage in this process.

The extended time required to gain IRB approval for pediatric studies, even though it is necessary for participant safety, may frustrate both the investigators and the families of children with life-threatening disorders. In multicenter trials, some study sites are never able to enroll participants because the site does not receive IRB approval until after study enrollment is already completed at other sites. This not infrequent scenario leads to significant disappointment among researchers and potential research participants at the site. Chapter 8 discusses further these and other issues with multicenter trials.

Training and Retention of Clinical Investigators

Not only are child participants in short supply for much pediatric research, but so are properly trained and experienced pediatric investigators. Pediatricians who pursue careers in clinical research must receive specialized, post-residency training. Until recently, most subspecialty pediatric fellowship training was directed toward laboratory science rather than human-based research. To conduct the kinds of pediatric research described in this report, it is important to attract recently trained pediatricians into fellowship programs that are oriented toward clinical research and that have strong curricula that cover study design, biostatistics, the ethical conduct of trials, and similar essentials of sound clinical investigation. To ensure that new and established investigators alike are sufficiently knowledgeable about the protection of human research participants, NIH requires education on this topic for all investigators submitting new NIH grant or contract applications or receiving non-competing awards for research involving human participants (NIH, 2001).

NIH offers institutional grants, such as the K-30 clinical research curriculum awards, that are specifically intended to stimulate academic institutions to expand or improve the training of clinical investigators. Recently, NIH announced a new career development program aimed specifically at multidisciplinary clinical research (NIH, 2003b). As examples of the core components of a multidisciplinary curriculum, the program announcement listed clinical research methodology, epidemiology, biostatistics, informatics, ethical issues, safety of research participants, regulatory requirements, team leadership and management, grant writing, and interactions with industry.

In 1996, the Federation of Pediatric Organizations revised and reaffirmed its 1990 *Statement on Pediatric Fellowship Training* (FOPO, 1991), which is once again being revised. The statement stresses that fellowship training should prepare trainees to be competent in clinical care, education, and research. Such training should occur at sites that have sufficient faculty who are committed to scholarship and research excellence and who, collectively, have appropriate expertise in hypothesis-driven investigations. In addition to providing direct research experience, programs may also provide that trainees serve in some capacity on or with an IRB.

Once clinical faculty are hired, their retention depends, in part, on adequate mentoring by successful clinical investigators, sufficient protected time to conduct research, and the rapid critique of grant proposals by faculty members, including the chair and the mentor(s). Clinical investigators should be more successful if they work in an environment with a supportive research infrastructure that includes appropriate staff (including research nurses and grant administrators), adequate access to computers and data sets (if needed), and capable administration of institutional and government policies on the ethical conduct of human research.

DATA ON THE EXTENT OF CHILDREN'S PARTICIPATION IN CLINICAL RESEARCH

Data on the extent of children's participation in research are limited for most conditions. Most data located by the committee involve children with cancer. Cancer and heart disease are the leading disease-related causes of death for children, but they account for a small percentage of all childhood deaths. About half of childhood deaths occur in infancy (primarily as a result of congenital anomalies, short gestation, or complications related to pregnancy), and almost a third are the result of intentional or unintentional injuries (NCHS, 2000). As discussed elsewhere in this report, clinical trials of emergency care with both adult and pediatric populations face particular difficulties related to informed consent.

The National Cancer Institute (NCI) reports that in 1998 and 1999 some 50 percent of child cancer patients (ages 0 to 14 years) participated in clinical trials undertaken by NCI cooperative groups compared to 20 percent of patients ages 15 to 19 years and less than 3 percent of patients age 20 years or over (NCI, 2002b; data from Sateren et al., 2002; see also, Shochat et al., 2001). An earlier study based on data obtained from 1991 to 1994 reported that 70 percent of child cancer patients (ages 0 to 19 years) were enrolled in trials (Tejeda et al., 1996). A recent study calculated that about 70 percent of child cancer patients under age 15 years were registered by pediatric oncology trial groups compared to only 24 percent of patients ages 15 to 19 years (Liu et al., 2003).

The committee found no comparable data on the percentages of children with other conditions enrolled in clinical trials. A simple search of the NIH clinical trials website (http://www.clinicaltrials.gov/) generated a list of 163 leukemia studies for children from birth to age 17 years, 14 studies for cystic fibrosis, 12 studies for prematurity, and 29 studies for diabetes (all types). The search also yielded 146 studies for the terms *infant* and *infancy*, 238 for the term *neonatal*, and 159 for the terms *adolescent* and *adolescence*. The list of trials includes studies that do not test therapies. Closer examination of the listed studies suggests that some do not actually involve children. The number of studies is not a direct indicator of the total enrollment in clinical trials because trials vary greatly in size.

Some studies suggest that recruitment of children from minority populations may be particularly difficult. For example, in a longitudinal study of the risk factors for the development of cardiovascular disease during childhood, the recruitment of sufficient numbers of minority children took 2 years whereas researchers needed only 1 year to recruit the target number of nonminority children (Grunbaum et al., 1996). An analysis of enrollment in pediatric cancer treatment trials suggested, however, that minority children were proportionately represented (Bleyer et al., 1997). Some other studies report similar results (NINR, 1993; Rosella, 1994; Villarruel, 1999), whereas some show underrepresentation (Bonner and Miles, 1997; Peterson and Sterling, 1999). A recent report from the General Accounting Office suggested that FDA needed to improve its monitoring of the inclusion of minority children in research regulated by the agency (GAO, 2003).

The high referral and enrollment rates for child cancer patients in clinical trials likely reflects a number of factors, including the imminent threat posed by many types of cancer and the success of researchers in increasing survival rates for important childhood cancers, such as leukemia. Other factors appear to include the large number of institutions participating in cooperative trials, the relatively large number of therapies being tested, and the concentration of cancer treatment for children in institutions participating in cooperative trials. Care at these institutions is widely regarded by pediatricians and families as "state of the art." The committee found no other serious condition with a clinical trials cooperative group as large as COG, which includes nearly 240 member institutions in the United States, Canada, and other countries. According to its website, COG typically has approximately 100 trials open to enrollment at any time, with approximately 5,000 participants enrolled and some 35,000 being actively monitored (COG, no date).

In contrast to the number of institutions participating in COG, the National Institute of Child Health and Human Development funds 13 centers in the Pediatric Pharmacology Research Network (PPRU, no date) as well as 16 centers in the Neonatal Research Network (NICHD, 2003). As noted above, prematurity, problems associated with childbirth, and low birth weight are the leading causes of death among children.

The Cystic Fibrosis Foundation supports various research programs, including 14 centers in the Therapeutics Development Network. The National Institute of Allergy and Infectious Diseases (NIAID) and the National Institute for Child Health and Human Development (NICHD) support 18 centers of the Pediatric AIDS Clinical Trials Group (plus a data management center and a coordinating operations center) (NICHD, no date). A centralized national registry of clinical trials is clearly needed to better understand the number of children (particularly healthy children) participating in clinical research and to promote more cooperative clinical trial groups. An earlier IOM report (2003a) recommended the creation of such a central registry of all clinical trials.

INITIATIVES TO INCREASE INVOLVEMENT OF CHILDREN IN RESEARCH

Given the challenges described above, many investigators and sponsors of research have been reluctant to undertake research with children. Responding to concerns from pediatricians and family advocacy groups, policymakers have attempted, particularly in the last decade, to stimulate research that involves infants, children, and adolescents.

Legislation

Congress has long provided funding and directives to NIH and other agencies to support research on a variety of child health problems. In 1963, it established NICHD as part of NIH. This NIH unit supports a range of biomedical, epidemiologic, and other research with the goal of ensuring "that every person is born healthy and wanted, that women suffer no harmful effects from the reproductive process, and that all children have the chance to fulfill their potential for a healthy and productive life, free of disease or disability" (NICHD, 2002, unpaged). Other government agencies also focus on children's health problems, for example, the venerable Maternal and Child Health Bureau, first created early in the last century.

Legislators have also attempted to influence the behavior of pharmaceutical companies. In 1997, the U.S. Congress reinforced initiatives already underway at FDA by including incentives in the Food and Drug Administration Modernization Act of 1997 (P.L. 105-115) for these companies to conduct pediatric studies. For drugs for which FDA had requested pediatric studies, the legislation provided that a company could obtain 6 additional months of patent protection for a drug by conducting studies to provide dosing and safety information for children.

Roberts and colleagues (2003, p. 906) reported that "[b]etween July 1998 and April 2002, 53 drugs were granted pediatric exclusivity and 33 drug products have new labels with pediatric information." For seven of the drugs, pediatric studies led to "major adjustments in the dosing instructions" (p. 910). To cite an example, the new information showed that doses for midazolam hydrochloride (Versed, a sedative widely used for surgical procedures) should start at lower initial levels for children with congenital heart disease and pulmonary hypertension. Between April and January 2004, pediatric use labeling became available for another 33 drugs (FDA, 2004).

The Best Pharmaceuticals for Children Act of 2002 (P.L. 107-109) renewed the exclusivity provisions. It also called for NIH to sponsor pediatric tests of certain drugs already approved but not tested or not fully tested for their effects with children. This list, published in January 2003, identified the dozen highest-priority drugs needing pediatric testing (DHHS, 2003a). Most of the drugs are no longer under patent, and therefore, the "pediatric exclusivity" incentives are largely irrelevant. The secretary of DHHS announced that $25 million in federal funds would be allocated to support research on these drugs in 2003.

Recently, Congress passed the Pediatric Research Equity Act of 2003, (P.L. 108-155). It gives FDA the authority to require pediatric studies of certain drugs and biological products. In the future, companies submitting requests for approval to market a new drug or biologic (or a new indication, formulation, dosing regimen, or route of administration for an already approved product) will be required to submit information about the safety and effectiveness of the product in relevant pediatric populations. Testing may not be required if the agency determines that it is appropriate to extrapolate data from studies with adults (usually with some supplementary pediatric pharmacokinetic or other study data). Submission of pediatric data may be deferred under certain conditions (e.g., the adult but not the pediatric studies are completed). The requirements may also be fully or partially waived under several conditions (e.g., pediatric studies are impossible or highly impractical or existing evidence suggests that the drug would be unsafe or ineffective for children). If a waiver were granted on the basis of evidence that a drug would be unsafe or ineffective, the drug label would be required to include information to that effect.

Other agencies that are not part of FDA or NIH may also have been influenced by these initiatives. For example, in its program of Centers for Education and Research on Therapeutics (CERTs), which supports research and education on effective therapeutics (i.e., drugs, medical devices, and biologics), the Agency for Health Research and Quality has designated one center to focus specifically on medical therapies for children (UNC, 2003). The CERTs program was authorized in P.L. 105-115.

Food and Drug Administration Rules and Policies

Even though the best and brightest pediatric minds have helped us establish dosages for children, we're finding out that the dose is different than we thought in some cases. And that probably came as a surprise to most of us.

Richard Gorman, quoted by Meadows, 2003, unpaged

In 1979, FDA issued regulations on the content and format of labels for human prescription drugs (FDA, 1979a). The regulations stated that if drug companies made statements about the pediatric use of a drug for an approved indication, the statement had to be based on substantial evidence from adequate and well-controlled studies, unless FDA waived that requirement. As discussed in Chapter 1, from the early 1970s into the 1990s, the proportion of drugs with specific pediatric dosing information stayed at a low level (about 20 percent of the drugs listed in the *Physician's Desk Reference*).

In 1994, FDA required drug manufacturers to determine whether they had data sufficient to support labeling information on pediatric use. If they did, they were then to request permission from FDA to make changes in their labels based on that data (FDA, 1994a). The rules also provided that clinical trials with children might not be required to support labeling if sufficient evidence existed that the disease and the drug's effects allowed extrapolation from the results of trials with adults.

Four years later, in issuing new regulations, FDA observed that "[t]he response to the 1994 rule has not substantially addressed the lack of adequate pediatric use information for marketed drugs and biological products" (FDA, 1998e, p. 66632). Under the new regulations, FDA could, in some cases, require drug companies to conduct studies of new and existing drugs to determine their safety and efficacy in children. In October 2002, a federal court struck down this so-called pediatric rule, holding that FDA exceeded its statutory authority (Albert, 2002; ruling at *AAPS v. FDA*, 2002). In response, Congress passed the Pediatric Research Equity Act of 2003, as described earlier.

National Institutes of Health Policies

NIH has encouraged pediatric research in ways both general and specific. General strategies include support for the clinical trial cooperative groups that are intended to facilitate high-quality, multisite adult and pediatric studies and, as one consequence, reduce the number of trials with undersized study populations (i.e., "underpowered" studies in the language of statistics and research methods).

In 1998, following directives in House and Senate Appropriations Committee reports for fiscal year 1996, NIH issued specific policies and guidelines for including children as research participants (NIH, 1998a). NIH analyses suggested that 10 to 20 percent of NIH-supported studies inappropriately excluded children.

The 1998 policies focus on disorders and conditions that affect adults and that may also affect children. Children are to be included in research conducted or funded by the agency unless their exclusion is justified on scientific or ethical grounds. For some medical conditions, children's developmental characteristics might suggest the need for a separate, child-only study. Proposals to NIH for funding must include a section on the participation of children that discusses the rationale for excluding children from a study or that provides a plan for their inclusion. Such plans must describe the relevant expertise of investigators and the appropriateness of the facilities to be used. The plans are then reviewed as part of the NIH peer review process for proposals. The 1998 NIH guidelines also describe the federal rules for protecting children in research.

Congress encouraged, but did not require, NIH to establish pediatric research priorities (U.S. Congress, 1995; NIH, 1998a). Although NIH does not appear to have developed an overall set of priorities, some individual institutes have identified priorities for certain clinical problems or services, including kidney disease (NIDDK, 2001), HIV/AIDS (NIH, 2003b), and emergency medical services (NIH, 2003b).

CONCLUSION

Recent years have seen a number of actions to encourage research involving children and help investigators cope with the many methodological, practical, and ethical challenges of pediatric studies. One apparent result is an increase in the number of children participating in research. Another is an increase in the number of priority drugs that have labeling information for at least some pediatric age groups.

More can be done. Chapter 8 includes a recommendation for strengthening educational programs to develop pediatric investigators who are prepared to design and conduct valid, ethical clinical research. In addition, to ensure the continuation of well-designed and well-conducted pediatric research that will improve children's health, federal policymakers should sustain and extend other aspects of the critical financial and infrastructure for this research. They should likewise support important research that is often not attractive to commercial sponsors, including long-term studies and projects to improve outcome measures relevant to infants, children, and adolescents. Because most pediatric conditions are sufficiently uncommon that statistically sound, ethical research requires multiple study sites, the federal government should continue to establish and fund discipline-specific, age-relevant research groups or consortia with the expertise and administrative infrastructure to conduct multicenter studies.

Furthermore, as research continues to become more international, it is important for governments, investigators, industry, and international organizations to cooperate to support the conduct of ethical multinational pediatric studies, increase the pace of therapeutic development for rare pediatric conditions, and move toward greater consistency in the regulatory protections for child participants in research. The next chapter, which summarizes the regulatory framework for protecting human research participants in the United States, also briefly reviews international guidelines and efforts to develop consistent or uniform—that is, harmonize—regulations across countries.

3

REGULATORY FRAMEWORK FOR PROTECTING CHILD PARTICIPANTS IN RESEARCH

The involvement of children in research raises particular ethical concerns because of their reduced autonomy and their incompetency to give informed consent. . . . The Commission has therefore sought to answer the following two questions: under what conditions is the participation of children in research ethically acceptable, and under what conditions may such participation be authorized by the subjects and their parents.

National Commission, 1977, p. xi

The federal regulations governing research that includes infants, children, and adolescents are very closely based on the recommendations of the National Commission for the Protection of Human Subjects of Biomedical and Behavioral Research in its 1977 report on that topic. The *Belmont Report*, issued by the Commission in 1978, served as the basis for the core regulations applicable to all federally supported, conducted, or regulated research involving humans (National Commission, 1978a).

Although thoughtfully designed government regulations can guide and promote responsible behavior-related regulations, they are only one part of the U.S. system for protecting child or adult participants in research. They cannot guarantee full and competent implementation by the public and private institutions that fund, administer, and oversee research. Neither regulations nor institutional programs can substitute for well-trained, well-motivated investigators who understand their obligations and the means of fulfilling them. Chapters 7 and 8 of this report consider compliance with federal regulations and the roles and responsibilities of investigators, institutional review boards (IRBs), research institutions, research sponsors, and policymakers in implementing federal regulations and, more generally, sustaining an effective system of protections for human participants in research.

This chapter presents an overview of current federal regulations. The overview is mainly descriptive, with more analysis as well as recommendations and other guidance offered in subsequent chapters. Later sections of this chapter briefly describe other policies for protecting the safety of participants in certain clinical studies and, in addition, policies relating to research conducted in other countries.

Appendix B discusses state policies relevant to the conduct of research involving children. These policies include laws defining the age of majority (when minors become adults) and the circumstances when individuals under the age of majority can provide consent to medical care or research participation. Most states do not have specific policies and regulations on the protection of human participants in research. Appendix C summarizes conflict-of-interest and privacy policies (including the Health Insurance Portability and Accountability Act) that also contribute to the protection of research participants.

Overall, the committee concluded that the federal regulations providing special protections for child participants in research are generally appropriate for children of different ages. They reasonably defer to state laws defining the age at which individuals become entitled to make decisions about their medical care and the special circumstances under which minors may make decisions in their own right. For the most part, the problems with the regulations relate to variability in the interpretation of criteria for approving research that include inherently subjective elements that the committee doubts would be substantially and predictably clarified by the time-consuming process of revising the regulations. As discussed in Chapter 5, one change the committee does recommend is that the Food and Drug Administration (FDA) make its policies on the waiver of parental permission consistent with the U.S. Department of Health and Human Services (DHHS) regulations that permit such waivers under certain circumstances.

A number of commissions and committees have recommended that federal policymakers formally extend regulatory protections for human participants in research to all research, regardless of the source of funding or the regulatory status (see, e.g., NBAC, 2001b and IOM, 2003a). As discussed in Chapter 8, this committee agrees. It recognizes, however, that the federal government may not have the authority to do this, so it also encourages state governments to exercise their authority to regulate research in ways that are consistent with federal regulations and supportive of multistate studies.

FEDERAL REGULATIONS TO PROTECT
CHILD PARTICIPANTS IN RESEARCH

The federal regulations that govern research involving children have two basic elements. One element is the Common Rule, codified by DHHS at Subpart A of Title 45, Part 46 of the Code of Federal Regulations (45 CFR 46). The Common Rule, which applies to 17 federal agencies, sets forth the general regulations for protecting participants in federally conducted, supported, or regulated research. (The label reflects the common application of rules initially adopted by DHHS as described in Chapter 1.) The second relevant element of the regulations consists of Subpart D, additional protections for children involved in research. These regulations have been adopted by DHHS, the Central Intelligence Agency, the Social Security Administration, and the U.S. Department of Education. FDA has separate regulations (21 CFR 50 and 56) that are similar but not identical, as explained further below.

Because these regulations apply to studies conducted or supported by DHHS and to research regulated by FDA, they cover research conducted by investigators employed by the National Institutes of Health (NIH) or other DHHS agencies, outside researchers whose studies are funded by DHHS agencies, and investigators whose research must meet the requirements set forth by FDA, even if that research is privately funded. One provision of Subpart A reaches further. It requires research institutions to provide and have approved a written "assurance" that they will comply with the human research protection regulations. To have such an assurance approved, an institution must have a "statement of principles" that governs the institution in protecting human participants in research "regardless of whether the research is subject to Federal regulation" (45 CFR 46.103(b)(1)). In the spirit of this provision, many institutions require all research involving humans to go through the same basic review process, whether or not the research is explicitly covered by the regulations.

The Common Rule or Subpart A: Basic Regulations

As discussed earlier, in 1991 the federal government slightly revised and extended to 17 other federal agencies the regulations that formed Subpart A of the human research protection regulations that had been adopted in 1981 by DHHS. (The regulations that established this Common Rule also provided that each agency could adopt procedural modifications appropriate to its functions and responsibilities.) FDA did not adopt the Common Rule as such in 1991 but revised its regulations, which were already generally similar to those of DHHS, to bring them into greater conformity (FDA, 1991a).[1] Following promulgation of the requirements of the Children's Health Act of 2000, FDA issued interim rules that include additional protections found in Subpart D of the DHHS regulations (FDA, 2001b).

Although FDA is part of DHHS, for convenience, this report refers to the regulations found in 45 CFR 46 as the DHHS regulations and the regulations found in 21 CFR 50 and 56 as the FDA regulations. Also, because this report focuses on clinical research that is conducted, funded, or otherwise regulated by DHHS, the rest of this chapter usually will refer to Subpart A rather than the Common Rule. Differences in the FDA regulations will be noted as appropriate. The summary below focuses on selected elements in Subpart A that are important to understand as context for the interpretation and application of the regulations covering children.

Institutional Assurances and Responsibilities

Institutions whose members or agents (e.g., contractors) undertake research involving human subjects that is conducted or supported by one of the 17 Common Rule departments or agencies must assure the government that they comply with relevant regulations (45 CFR 46.103; see also OHRP, 2002a). DHHS can approve a "federalwide assurance" for an institution that other federal agencies can then accept for research that they conduct or support. As part of ensuring their compliance with the applicable regulations, institutions are held to a number of requirements, including:

- the development of an acceptable statement of ethical principles for the protection of human participants in research, *whether or not* the research is covered by federal regulations;
- the designation of one or more IRBs and the provision of resources to those IRBs sufficient to meet their responsibilities;
- the provision and updating of a list of IRB members that includes information sufficient to indicate their expected contributions to the IRB and their relationship (if any) to the institution;
- the development of written procedures that IRBs should follow in conducting their reviews and fulfilling their other responsibilities; and

---

[1]The FDA regulations are found in two parts of the Code of Federal Regulations, 21 CFR Parts 50 (Protection of Human Subjects) and 21 CFR 56 (Institutional Review Boards). 21 CFR 50 has two general subparts, Subpart A (scope of regulations and definitions) and Subpart B (informed consent), in addition to Subpart D, which covers children. Subpart C, which covers prisoners, has been stayed indefinitely. 21 CFR 56 has five subparts that present requirements for IRBs.

- a certification that the research projects covered have been reviewed and approved by an IRB and will be periodically reviewed as required by regulations.

General Criteria for Approving Proposed Research

Subpart A establishes several important criteria that must be met for proposed research to be approved. These criteria are listed in Box 3.1. Research involving children must meet these and additional criteria that are set forth in Subpart D.

In combination with other regulations and government guidance documents, several of these criteria have given rise to additional policies or structures. For example, as discussed in a later section of this chapter, NIH may require the creation of a board that monitors the data from and safety of clinical trials.

Requirements for Informed Consent

Subpart A sets forth a number of requirements for the process of obtaining an individual's informed consent to participate in research. These requirements, in addition to provisions of Subpart D, also apply when agreement to participate in research is being sought from a parent or other authorized representative for a person not legally competent to provide consent in his or her own right. Informed consent is not required for research that is exempt from review, and it can also be waived under certain conditions. Chapter 5 describes the general provisions for informed consent in more detail.

Institutional Review Boards (IRB)

Beyond the general institutional responsibilities of IRBs described above, the federal regulations specify additional requirements for IRBs. One set of requirements covers IRB membership (45 CFR 46.107; 21 CFR 56.107). Other requirements relate to IRB functions and operations, including both the initial review of projects and their continuing review.

At a minimum, an IRB must have at least five members. At least one member must be concerned primarily with scientific topics, and at least one member must be concerned primarily with nonscientific topics. At least one must be community based, that is, not affiliated with the institution directly or through a family member. Taken together, the members must have sufficient expertise, experience, and diversity of backgrounds to promote competent review of the usual kinds of research conducted by the institution and to promote "respect for its advice and

---

BOX 3.1
General Criteria That Research Must Meet to Be Approved
Under Federal Regulations (excluding criteria related to
special protections for children and other identified groups)

For research to be approved, all of the following requirements must be met:

• Risks to subjects are minimized: (i) by using procedures which are consistent with sound research design and which do not unnecessarily expose subjects to risk, and (ii) whenever appropriate, by using procedures already being performed on the subjects for diagnostic or treatment purposes.
• Risks to subjects are reasonable in relation to anticipated benefits, if any, to subjects, and the importance of the knowledge that may reasonably be expected to result. In evaluating risks and benefits, the IRB should consider only those risks and benefits that may result from the research (as distinguished from risks and benefits of therapies subjects would receive even if not participating in the research). The IRB should not consider possible long-range effects of applying knowledge gained in the research (for example, the possible effects of the research on public policy) as among those research risks that fall within the purview of its responsibility.
• Selection of subjects is equitable [taking into account] . . . the purposes of the research and the setting in which the research will be conducted and . . . special problems of research involving vulnerable populations, such as children, prisoners, pregnant women, mentally disabled persons, or economically or educationally disadvantaged persons.
• Informed consent will be sought from each prospective subject or the subject's legally authorized representative, in accordance with, and to the extent required by [other sections of the regulations].
• Informed consent will be appropriately documented, in accordance with, and to the extent required by [other sections of the regulations].
• When appropriate, the research plan makes adequate provision for monitoring the data collected to ensure the safety of subjects.
• When appropriate, there are adequate provisions to protect the privacy of subjects and to maintain the confidentiality of data.

SOURCE: 45 CFR 46.111.

---

counsel." Diversity of backgrounds includes not only areas of scientific or professional expertise but also culture, race, and gender.

IRBs that regularly review proposals that include children are not required to have a member or members who have expertise and experience with children, but they are advised to consider the inclusion of such individuals. The regulations provide that IRBs may seek assistance with the review of proposals from individuals who have expertise that is not represented on the IRB. (Chapter 8 of this report stresses the importance of pediatric expertise for IRBs that review research involving infants, children, and adolescents, and it recommends approaches that IRBs can use to secure this expertise.) DHHS guidance to institutions strongly recommends that institutions provide appropriate education and training for investigators, IRB members, and others to prepare them to fulfill their responsibilities to protect human subjects.

Continuing Review

IRBs are responsible not only for the initial review of research protocols but also for the continuing review of ongoing research (see, e.g., 45 CFR 46.109 and 21 CFR 56.109). The latter must occur at least annually with more frequent review required if the research protocol changes significantly or if the level of risk presented by the protocol warrants it. If the IRB detects that the research as conducted does not meet the requirements of the federal regulations and is not consistent with the IRB's initial approval or if it finds unexpected and serious harm to participants in the research, the IRB may suspend or terminate its approval of the research. The IRB must give the reasons for such action and promptly notify the investigator, the institution, and the Office for Human Research Protections.

As described by FDA, the IRB is to review the investigator's written progress report. These reports are to include "the number of subjects entered into the research study; a summary description of subject experiences (benefits, adverse reactions); numbers of withdrawals from the research; reasons for withdrawals; the research results obtained thus far; a current risk-benefit assessment based on study results; and any new information since the IRB's last review" (FDA, 1998a, unpaged). In its review, the IRB is to pay particular attention to identifying whether any unanticipated risks have emerged. (See discussion below of additional requirements for adverse event reports and data and safety monitoring bodies.)

Exempt Research and Expedited Review

Certain categories of research may be exempt from review under the provisions of Subpart A, although research institutions may independently require that research in these categories be reviewed. Exempt categories include much research that

- is conducted in educational settings (e.g., studies of educational techniques);
- involves a federally funded or approved research or demonstration project to evaluate a public benefit or service program;
- uses existing data, documents, records, pathological specimens, or

diagnostic specimens that are either publicly available or not directly or indirectly linked to individuals;

- evaluates food quality or taste or consumer acceptance; or
- employs educational tests, survey procedures, interview procedures or observation of public behavior (unless individual subjects can be identified and disclosure of the information could damage the subject's reputation, liberty, financial standing, or employability).

When research involves children, the exemption for survey and interview procedures does *not* apply unless the procedures relate to educational techniques and involve no sensitive topics. Likewise, the exemption for research that uses observations of public behavior does *not* apply when children are involved if the investigator participates in the activities under observation.

Some research, including research that involves children, may be eligible for expedited review. Eligible research is periodically identified by the Secretary of DHHS with a notice in the *Federal Register*. The most recent list of such research appeared in 1998 (DHHS, 1998). Examples of research eligible for expedited review include collection of biological specimens for research purposes by noninvasive means (e.g., by clipping fingernails or toenails or by cutting hair) or collection of data from voice or video recordings made for research purposes. A preliminary review must determine that the research presents no more than a minimal risk to participants or involves only minor changes in research approved during the preceding year. Chapter 4 discusses the concepts and interpretation of minimal risk and related terms.

Subpart D: Special Protections for Children

In 1983, DHHS adopted special protections for child participants in research, generally referred to as Subpart D because of their location in Subpart D of 45 CFR 46. In 2001, as required by the Children's Health Act of 2000, FDA issued interim regulations to bring its rules into compliance with the DHHS regulations. The interim rule incorporated most elements of Subpart D (with a few changes) into the agency's regulations at 21 CFR 50 and 56. As noted above, the U.S. Department of Education, the Central Intelligence Agency, and the Social Security Administration are the only other federal agencies to adopt these regulations. These special regulations include several important definitions, most of which have been adopted by FDA (Box 3.2).

BOX 3.2
Definitions in Subpart D That Have Also Been
Adopted by the FDA

- "Children" are persons who have not attained the legal age for consent to treatments or procedures involved in the research, under the applicable law of the jurisdiction in which the research will be conducted.
- "Assent" means a child's affirmative agreement to participate in research. Mere failure to object should not, absent affirmative agreement, be construed as assent.
- "Permission" means the agreement of parent(s) or guardian to the participation of their child or ward in research.*
- "Parent" means a child's biological or adoptive parent.
- "Guardian" means an individual who is authorized under applicable State or local law to consent on behalf of a child to general medical care.**
- "Legally authorized representative" means an individual or judicial or other body authorized under applicable law to consent on behalf of a prospective subject to the subject's participation in the procedures involved in the research.

Definition added by FDA

- A "ward" is a child who is placed in the legal custody of the State or other agency, institution, or entity, consistent with applicable Federal, State, or local law.

---

* The FDA rules clarify "that permission applies to participation in clinical investigations involving FDA-regulated products" (FDA, 2001b, p. 20592).
** The FDA rules add that "for a guardian to be able to grant permission for a child to participate in research, the guardian must either have authority to consent to a child's general medical care (where participation in clinical research falls within general medical care) or must have authority to consent to a child's participation in research" (FDA, 2001b, p. 20592).

SOURCE: 45 CFR 46.102 and 21 CFR 50.3

Assessment of Risks and (Potential) Benefits

The regulatory criteria for IRB approval of research involving children are more restrictive than those for research involving adults and focus, in considerable measure, on the assessment of risks and benefits. (As discussed in Chapter 4, because risk involves potential harms, it is more appropriate to refer to "risks and potential benefits" or "potential harms and potential benefits.") The general boundaries of research involving children that DHHS can conduct or support are laid out in four sections of Subpart D that largely correspond to the recommendations of the 1977 report on children by the National Commission for the Protection of Human Subjects of Biomedical and Behavioral Research (National Commission, 1977). The four sections are often referred to by their section numbers in the regula-

---

BOX 3.3
Research Involving Children That DHHS Is Permitted to Conduct or Support *

§46.404 Research not involving greater than minimal risk
DHHS will conduct or fund research in which the IRB finds that no greater than minimal risk to children is presented, only if the IRB finds that adequate provisions are made for soliciting the assent of the children and the permission of their parents or guardians, as set forth in §46.408.

§46.405 Research involving greater than minimal risk, but presenting the prospect of direct benefit to the individual subjects
DHHS will conduct or fund research in which the IRB finds that more than minimal risk to children is presented by an intervention or procedure that holds out the prospect of direct benefit for the individual subject, or by a monitoring procedure that is likely to contribute to the subject's well-being, only if the IRB finds that:
    (a) the risk is justified by the anticipated benefit to the subjects;
    (b) the relation of the anticipated benefit to the risk is at least as favorable to the subjects as that presented by available alternative approaches; and
    (c) adequate provisions are made for soliciting the assent of the children and permission of their parents or guardians, as set forth in §46.408.

§46.406 Research involving greater than minimal risk and no prospect of direct benefit to individual subjects, but likely to yield generalizable knowledge about the subject's disorder or condition
DHHS will conduct or fund research in which the IRB finds that more than minimal risk to children is presented by an intervention or procedure that does not hold out the prospect of direct benefit for the individual subject, or by a monitoring procedure which is not likely to contribute to the well-being of the subject, only if the IRB finds that:
    (a) the risk represents a minor increase over minimal risk;
    (b) the intervention or procedure presents experiences to subjects that are

---

tions: 404, 405, 406, and 407. Box 3.3 presents the regulatory language for each section. FDA interim regulations (21 CFR 50.51 to 50.54) include the corresponding sections, except that they refer to research involving an FDA-regulated product rather than to research funded or supported by DHHS, and they provide that the FDA commissioner rather than the secretary of DHHS can approve certain research that does not meet the criteria for IRB approval.

As discussed further in Chapter 4, the four regulatory categories involve an escalating set of assessments that need to be made and requirements that need to be met before a research proposal is approved. Several of the terms in these regulations (e.g., minimal risk and minor increase over reasonably commensurate with those inherent in their actual or expected medical, dental, psychological, social, or educational situations;

(c) the intervention or procedure is likely to yield generalizable knowledge about the subjects' disorder or condition which is of vital importance for the understanding or amelioration of the subjects' disorder or condition; and

(d) adequate provisions are made for soliciting assent of the children and permission of their parents or guardians, as set forth in §46.408.

§46.407 Research not otherwise approvable which presents an opportunity to understand, prevent, or alleviate a serious problem affecting the health or welfare of children.

DHHS will conduct or fund research that the IRB does not believe meets the requirements of §46.404, §46.405, or §46.406 only if:

(a) the IRB finds that the research presents a reasonable opportunity to further the understanding, prevention, or alleviation of a serious problem affecting the health or welfare of children; and

(b) the Secretary, after consultation with a panel of experts in pertinent disciplines (for example: science, medicine, education, ethics, law) and following opportunity for public review and comment, has determined either:

(1) that the research in fact satisfies the conditions of §46.404, §46.405, or §46.406, as applicable, or (2) the following:

(i) the research presents a reasonable opportunity to further the understanding, prevention, or alleviation of a serious problem affecting the health or welfare of children;

(ii) the research will be conducted in accordance with sound ethical principles;

(iii) adequate provisions are made for soliciting the assent of children and the permission of their parents or guardians, as set forth in §46.408.

---

*The corresponding, slightly modified, FDA regulations are at 21 CFR 50.51 to 54.

SOURCE: 45 CFR 46.

---

minimal risk) involve subjective or ambiguous concepts that have caused and that continue to cause considerable uncertainty, confusion, and disagreement among IRB members, investigators, and others who encounter them.

Agreement to Participate in Research

Parental Permission Because children are not legally able to provide consent in their own right, the federal regulations generally require that parents or guardians provide permission before children can be enrolled in research. If the IRB determines that the research involves more than minimal risk but is not expected to benefit the child participant, the regulations require that investigators secure permission from both parents. If the IRB determines that research involves no more than minimal risk or that it holds out the prospect of direct benefit to the child, the IRB may decide that the permission of one parent is sufficient. Permission from one parent is also sufficient if that parent is legally responsible for the care and custody of the child or when the other parent has died or is unknown, incompetent, or not reasonably available. Chapter 5 describes circumstances in which the DHHS but not the FDA regulations provide for exceptions to the parental permission requirement.

Child Assent Although children cannot legally consent to participation in research, the regulations provide for children's agreement or assent to research participation. The regulations do not describe the information that must be provided to children but rely on IRBs to use their discretion in judging assent provisions. Researchers must seek a child's assent unless the IRB determines that

  •   the children to be involved (as a group or individually) are not capable of providing assent, given their age, maturity, or mental state;
  •   the research has a prospect of an important direct benefit for the child that is possible only in the research context; or
  •   the research involves circumstances that would allow waiver of consent for adults.

As noted previously in Box 3.2, federal regulations on human research protections define children in terms of state laws defining the legal age at which an individual can consent to the treatments or procedures involved in the research. The legal age of majority is now 18 in all states except Mississippi (age 21) and Nebraska and Alabama (both age 19).[2] Chapter 5 and Appendix B discuss when those below the age of majority may agree to participate in research without permission from a parent or other authorized adults, for example, when they are accorded the status of emancipated or mature minors. They also consider special requirements related to research participation by children who are wards of the state.

---

[2]In Mississippi, a person age 18 or over can consent to medical or surgical care. In Alabama, a statute permits minors to consent to medical or surgical treatment at age 14. See Appendix B.

ADDITIONAL FEDERAL POLICIES FOR MONITORING SAFETY OF PARTICIPANTS IN CLINICAL RESEARCH

Beyond the policies summarized above, both NIH and FDA have established additional policies and procedures for monitoring the safety of participants in clinical research. As discussed below, one set of policies relates generally to the reporting of adverse events, and another involves the creation of committees to monitor data on such events in certain clinical trials.

An earlier IOM report included a constructive recommendation that "[f]ederal oversight agencies should harmonize their safety monitoring guidance for research organizations, including the development of standard practices for reporting adverse events" (IOM, 2003a, p. 148). The report also recommended that NIH provide additional guidance about the elements that should be included in data and safety monitoring plans for clinical trials and that NIH-funded clinical trials be monitored "with the same rigor and scrutiny as trials carried out" for products subject to FDA approval (IOM, 2003a, p. 151). Further, "any monitoring report for studies under a [research ethics review] board's purview [should] be shared with that board" (p. 145). This recommendation extended to reports for studies that a sponsor ended without seeking FDA approval of a drug or other product. This committee supports these recommendations.

The summary below focuses on the identification of unexpected and serious research-related problems and the monitoring of participant safety during clinical trials. Because most clinical trials are relatively limited in duration and in the size and diversity of study populations (e.g., by age, severity of illness, and diagnosis), they may fail to identify adverse events that are relatively uncommon, that are late effects that do not emerge for years after an intervention, or that occur as a result of long-term use of a drug or other intervention.[3] For example, genetic studies, particularly those

---

[3]As one response to concerns about patient or consumer safety problems that arise after drugs, devices, and other medical products have been approved for marketing, FDA has created various programs and procedures—under the rubric of postmarketing surveillance—that attempt to identify such problems. Surveillance may take several forms, including mandatory reporting of serious adverse events by manufacturers and health care providers, voluntary reporting by consumers and professionals, patient registries, surveys, and ad hoc investigations (e.g., laboratory or epidemiologic investigations). In addition, FDA may require further clinical studies as a condition of marketing approval. These studies—like other clinical research—require IRB review. In general, the postmarketing surveillance tools are limited in their ability to detect problems that arise after marketing begins. Also, the FDA requirements only cover FDA-regulated products and do not apply to certain kinds of surgical procedures or behavioral interventions. Reporting and analysis of adverse events are also important elements of voluntary efforts to improve the quality and safety of patient care (see, e.g.,

that identify inheritable genetic defects, may have consequences for research participants, family members, and family relationships that emerge or intensify after the study ends. Long-term consequences are also an important concern for many cancer treatments (see, e.g., the recent report on long-term survivors of childhood leukemia [Pui et al., 2003]). The identification of studies that warrant long-term follow-up and the design and sponsorship of such studies should be recognized as elements of a comprehensive system for protecting human participants in research.

Adverse Event Reporting

In a general sense, an *adverse event* is an occurrence that causes harm to a patient or research participant or that has the potential to do so. The focus is usually on serious, unexpected problems (e.g., not described in the research protocol) that appear to be associated with the research. The reporting of adverse events in clinical studies is a complex topic, and the role of IRBs in relation to adverse events is not well-defined, which causes considerable frustration and uncertainty. As observed in a popular handbook for IRB members, "guidance [to IRBs] from federal authorities has been both confusing and contradictory" (Amdur and Bankert, 2003, p. 64).

Without mentioning adverse events as such, both DHHS and FDA regulations require that IRBs have written procedures for the prompt reporting to the IRB, appropriate institutional officials, and the relevant Department or Agency head of "any unanticipated problems involving risks" to human research participants or others (e.g., investigators) (45 CFR 46.103(b)(5); 21 CFR 56.108(b)(1)). The regulations also require prompt reporting to the investigator, appropriate institutional officials, and the Department or Agency head of any suspension or termination of an individual research protocol related to "unexpected serious harm" (45 CFR 46.113; 21 CFR 56.113). In separate regulations relating to investigational new drugs, FDA specifies additional requirements for investigators or research sponsors to report unanticipated or unexpected adverse experiences,

---

JCAHO, 2003). In the Best Pharmaceuticals Act of 2002 (P.L. 107-109), FDA was directed to review adverse events reports for the year after a drug was granted pediatric exclusivity (as described in Chapter 2). FDA staff have reported to the FDA Pediatric Advisory Subcommittee on several products. For some of the products, staff asked the subcommittee whether an additional year of follow-up was advisable, given the small number of reports (Iyasu, 2003). Staff also reported on the limitations of the current monitoring system. The limitations include the questionable quality of individual reports, biased or selective reporting and underreporting, and an inability to calculate problem rates because the system lacks denominator data (i.e., data identifying the number of individuals who are, for example, taking a particular drug).

events, effects or problems (the terminology varies) associated with the use of the drug (21 CFR 312.32; 21 CFR 312.53; 21 CFR 312.64; 21 CFR 312.66). Sponsors are required to report to FDA and participating investigators adverse experiences that are "both serious and unexpected" (21 CFR 312.32). The FDA regulations also include requirements for reporting of adverse experiences or effects for medical devices and biological products. Since 1999, NIH has required that summary reports of adverse events be provided to the IRB at each trial site for multisite studies that have a data safety and monitoring board as described below.

Serious adverse events or experiences include deaths (which usually must be reported even if mortality is an identified risk in a study), hospitalizations, persistent or significant disabilities, and birth defects. Unanticipated problems are those not described or foreseen as risks in the study protocol. They include harms that are more serious or frequent than expected.

DHHS and FDA regulations require IRBs to have written procedures for ensuring effective communication regarding problems with or changes to research activity (45 CFR 46.103; 21 CFR 56.103). The regulations do not provide further direction, and the committee found no comprehensive overview of actual IRB procedures related to adverse event reports. Information from individual institutions and committee experience make it clear, however, that IRB policies and practices vary with respect to what, when, and how investigators should report problems and how the IRB should evaluate the reports received. For example, adverse event reporting forms created by institutions vary in the information required, the guidance provided, and the extent to which the form highlights a report involving a serious, unanticipated, research-related event.

Some IRB policies specify that the chair or other qualified individual will do an initial screening of adverse event reports submitted to the IRB; others use a group. In certain emergency situations, the individual or group may act to suspend or modify a study subject to later review by the full IRB membership. Depending on the information received, the IRB may require modifications in the study (e.g., changes in the consent form and process), increase the frequency of continuing review, reconsider the approval of the study, halt the study, or decide that no action is needed. IRBs are required to notify investigators of any decisions in writing (45 CFR 46.109(d)).

Data and Safety Monitoring Boards and Data Monitoring Committees

The discussion below focuses primarily on federal policies for data and safety monitoring during clinical trials designed to test the safety and efficacy of drugs and other products. In addition, during their review of a research protocol, IRBs may determine that a data safety and monitoring board or committee should be established if not already provided for or required.

Building on guidelines dating back to the 1970s, NIH has issued rules requiring the creation of data and safety monitoring boards (DSMBs) for multisite clinical trials that are supported or conducted by NIH and that involve potentially risky interventions (NIH, 1998b). The National Cancer Institute (NCI) has issued more detailed policies and guidance about the level and kind of monitoring appropriate for the phase 1, 2, and 3 clinical trials that it supports or conducts (NCI, 1999). The NCI policy provides that phase 1 and 2 trials may be monitored by the principal investigator or project manager or by NCI staff (or some other designated person) or jointly. Phase 3 randomized clinical trials must have a DSMB. As noted above, NIH requires that summary reports of adverse events be provided to relevant IRBs for multisite trials.

Commercially sponsored research regulated by FDA is covered by draft guidance on the establishment and operation of what the agency calls data monitoring committees (FDA, 2001c). Except for certain research conducted in emergency situations, FDA does not require such committees. It does, however, have additional requirements for the reporting of adverse events both before and after the approval of products over which it has jurisdiction (see below). As discussed further in chapter 7, FDA has an extensive monitoring system that also includes inspections of investigators and IRBs (and sometimes research sponsors) to assess compliance with guidelines. Large trials are more likely to prompt inspections than smaller trials (IOM, 2003a).

Institutions that routinely engage in clinical trials may establish a standing monitoring committee, unless a trial has an externally appointed body. Many clinical trials testing drugs for the treatment for cancer operate under the umbrella of some kind of cooperative research group and have their own DSMB. For example, protocols sponsored by the Children's Oncology Group are monitored under the procedures established by that group. The NCI website has links to several examples of approved data monitoring plans (NCI, 2002a). Box 3.4 summarizes the general responsibilities of monitoring boards or committees, however they are appointed and wherever they are located.

DSMBs have the power to stop studies early when the results reveal a clear benefit or a clear harm. For example, the 076-AZT trial, which tested a drug regimen to prevent mother-to-fetus transmission of HIV, was stopped early by the DSMB because of the obvious efficacy of the regimen (Mofenson, 2000). Recently, a placebo-controlled randomized trial of inhaled tobramycin in young children with cystic fibrosis was stopped early based on the basis of evidence that the drug had a significant effect on

---

BOX 3.4
General Responsibilities of Data and Safety Monitoring Boards and Data Monitoring Committees

- Reviewing research protocols (initial and major revisions), including the descriptions of potential harms and benefits and the plans for data and safety monitoring.
- Evaluating the progress of trials and periodically assessing the quality and timeliness of the reported data, the recruitment and retention of participants, the performances at the various trial sites, and other factors.
- Identifying external factors (e.g., publication of results from other studies involving the same condition) relevant to the safety of participants or the ethical status of studies.
- Recommending revisions in protocols when indicated by the review of data and procedures.
- Determining when circumstances warrant suspension or early conclusion of a trial.

Pseudomonas aeruginosa infection, a common cause of morbidity and mortality in these children (Gibson et al., 2003).

The primary responsibility of data and safety monitoring bodies, whatever their label, is to protect the safety of human participants in research (Ellenberg and Braun, 2002). A second major responsibility is to help protect the integrity of clinical trials so that the results will be trustworthy and useful. To that end, monitoring committees should be independent of the studies being monitored. Independence from the institutions involved may also be desirable.

The appropriate composition of a monitoring group depends on the nature of the study or studies being monitored. Usually, the membership will include individuals who are experts on the medical condition or intervention under study and statisticians who are familiar with the kinds of data that a trial will generate. Depending on the trial, the monitoring group may also include experts in clinical trials methodology, ethicists, epidemiologists, representatives of the patient community being studied, and others. When the research in question involves infants, children, or adolescents, then the monitoring group should also include pediatric expertise appropriate for the condition and population under study. For long-term genetic studies involving children or family members, monitoring boards may include individuals familiar with the short- and long-term impact of genetic information on the psychological status of children.

In general, even if it is not required by sponsors, IRBs should require that some form of data and safety monitoring be incorporated into pediatric research protocols that involve more than minimal risk and that this plan be reviewed by the IRB as part of the approval process. The type of data and safety monitoring plan will depend on specifics such as the degree and the nature of the risks associated with the trials. IRBs should examine the plan to assess the independence of the strategy from individuals and organizations with conflicting interests. IRBs should then be provided with periodic reports regarding data and safety monitoring activities and findings. IRBs should also have the opportunity to refer concerns for data and safety monitoring.

FEDERAL RULES FOR RESEARCH CONDUCTED
IN OTHER COUNTRIES

As discussed in Chapter 1, research and protections for participants in research must increasingly be viewed in an international context. Many multicenter studies involving adults or children include sites in both the United States and foreign countries, and some research that is submitted to FDA as part of the process of securing approval to market drugs, devices, or other products may be conducted entirely outside the United States. About one-quarter of the new drug applications submitted to FDA include important data from foreign sites, and almost all of these submissions involve commercial sponsors (Lepay, 2003). Examples include applications for the drugs lamivudine and didanosine.

Both DHHS and FDA rules include provisions on foreign research. The DHHS rules note that procedures for protecting human research participants may differ in other countries and that these procedures may be substituted if the department or agency head determines that the procedures provide protections equivalent to those provided for under DHHS rules (45 CFR 46.101(h)). When such a substitution is approved, the agency is usually supposed to publish a notice of the action.

For foreign institutions, the DHHS requirements for an assurance of compliance provide that institutions will be guided by ethical principles, such as the World Medical Association's Declaration of Helsinki (WMA, 2002 [see Chapter 1]) or the *Belmont Report* (National Commission, 1978a). They must also comply with the guidelines outlined in 45 CFR 46 or other recognized guidelines and procedures for research involving human subjects.[4] Recognized guidelines include the *Guideline for Good Clini-*

---

[4]In addition to requiring that institutions provide adequate resources and written policies for the review of research, the terms of an assurance for a foreign institution include agreement to requirements that informed consent be obtained and documented consistent with 45 CFR 46.116 and 117.

cal Practice: E6 (ICH, 1996) from the International Conference on Harmonisation (ICH) and the *International Ethical Guidelines for Biomedical Research Involving Human Subjects* (CIOMS, 2002).

The 1996 ICH guideline, which was also published as guidance by the FDA, does not provide explicit special protections for children (except as part of provisions related to informed consent). Children are, however, discussed in a separate ICH statement, *Clinical Investigation of Medicinal Products in the Pediatric Population: E11* (ICH, 2000b). This ICH guideline was also published as guidance by FDA, which described it as not binding but as representing the agency's "current thinking" (FDA, 2000b, p. 1). This guidance covers a variety of technical and practical issues in pediatric research in addition to ethical issues. In addition to the ICH efforts, FDA has also been working with the European Agency for the Evaluation of Medicinal Products on issues related to international pediatric oncology research (Stephen Hirschfeld, M.D., Center for Biologics Evaluation and Research, Food and Drug Administration, personal communication, November 21, 2003).

For drug companies or other firms seeking to have foreign studies considered in FDA decisions, FDA provides two options (FDA, 2001a; OIG, 2001). The first (applicable to all U.S. studies) requires the submission of an Investigational New Drug Application, under which studies are to be conducted consistent with the research protections described earlier in this chapter. The second option does not require prior approval or explicit conformity with the rules applicable to U.S. research. Rather, the conduct of foreign research must be consistent with international guidelines, such as the Declaration of Helsinki, or the host country's laws and regulations.[5]

---

[5]FDA regulations (21 CFR 312.120 (c)) require that sponsors of studies using the second option "explain how the research conformed to the ethical principles contained in the Declaration of Helsinki or the foreign country's standards, whichever were used. If the foreign country's standards were used, the sponsor shall explain in detail how those standards differ from the Declaration of Helsinki and how they offer greater protection." In addition, sponsors must provide information that allows the FDA to judge whether the studies are scientifically sound. The regulations governing approval of drug applications specify the 1989 version of the Declaration of Helsinki, whereas the regulations governing medical devices specify the 1983 version. Unlike the 1989 document, the 1983 version does not require that review be independent of the investigator or sponsor of the research. The most recent update of the Declaration of Helsinki occurred in 2000, with a clarification in 2001 (WMA, 2002). In March 2001, FDA issued guidance to industry under the title "Acceptance of Foreign Clinical Studies." This guidance notes that FDA did not incorporate the 2000 amendments to the Declaration. The guidance also indicated that the agency was reviewing the regulations related to foreign studies.

CONCLUSION

This largely descriptive chapter has provided an overview of federal regulations intended to protect adults and children involved in research. It has noted several issues that are considered further in the remainder of the report. These issues include the uncertainty and confusion over the interpretation of key concepts in the regulations; the adequacy of pediatric expertise in IRB review of research involving children; and the lack of regulatory protections for adults and children participating in research that is not federally conducted, funded, or regulated.

The following chapters highlight a number of additional concerns, including the lack of data on the performance of the system of research protections for children. Without such data, it is impossible to judge how effectively and efficiently the system is working overall and where it may be failing those whom it is supposed to protect.

4

DEFINING, INTERPRETING, AND APPLYING CONCEPTS OF RISK AND BENEFIT IN CLINICAL RESEARCH INVOLVING CHILDREN

In research involving human subjects, risk is a central organizing principle, a filter through which protocols must pass.
National Bioethics Advisory Commission (NBAC), 1998, p. 89

If risk is an important filter for research protocols involving adults, it is an even finer filter for research that involves children. Federal regulations and international guidelines have established criteria for approving and conducting research involving children that are generally more stringent than those that apply to research involving mentally competent adults. This stringency is most notable as it relates to the level of risk to which child research participants can be exposed, particularly when the research does not offer the prospect of direct benefit.

The committee was specifically asked to consider the regulatory definition of "minimal risk." Because this concept is closely related to several other concepts in the federal regulations on research involving children, the committee also examined certain of these concepts, including "minor increase over minimal risk," "disorder or condition," "commensurate experience," and "vital importance." In addition, the chapter discusses the regulatory requirements that risks to research participants be minimized and that the risks be reasonable in relation to the anticipated benefits. In this chapter, as elsewhere in the report, when the text mentions requirements for the approval of research, it is referring to research covered by federal regulations because it is federally supported, conducted, or regulated or because an individual institution has extended the regulations to all of its research.

Although the interpretation and application of risk criteria to research protocols are sometimes straightforward, disagreements between investigators and reviewers of proposed research and disagreements among reviewers are not uncommon. The analysis and recommendations presented in this chapter are intended to encourage greater consistency in regulatory interpretation and promote explicit attention to all the criteria for approving research protocols that include children.

It is important to note at the outset that much research—whether having a prospect of benefit or not—cannot be known to be entirely free of risk. If applied to studies without prospect of benefit, a "no risk" standard for approving research would make impossible much research that can advance the health and well-being of children. The risk categories analyzed in this chapter—involving minimal risk or a minor increase over minimal risk—are intended to allow important research to go forward by permitting children who do not have the potential to benefit directly from research to be exposed to only a small risk of harm. Still, a clear tension can exist between the goal of advancing clinical research that may benefit future children and the goal of limiting the risks to individual children who participate in clinical studies. That tension underscores the importance—as discussed further in chapter 5—of a sound process for explaining to parents and, as appropriate, children the purposes of a study, its potential harms and benefits, and the rights of prospective research participants to refuse participation.

BASIC CONCEPTS OF RISK, HARM, AND BENEFIT

Risk is a complex concept that has different meanings in different contexts. Broadly, risk refers to a potential harm or the potential of an action or event to cause harm. Specific risks can be characterized along several dimensions, including the probability of a given harm as well as its likely severity and duration.

A *harm* is a hurtful or adverse outcome of an action or event. It makes one's situation worse, temporarily or permanently. Research harms can occur or be evident close in time to the research intervention, but they also may occur or become apparent long after the research has been completed.

Harms resulting from research participation may be physical (e.g., pain, disability, discomfort, or death), psychological (e.g., fear, anxiety, depression, or embarrassment), or social (e.g., peer disapproval, economic loss, or legal jeopardy). For research that includes children, investigators and reviewers of research must consider potential harms such as fear and separation from parents that are usually not considered in studies involving adults (AAP, 1995). Discussions of research ethics also identify harms related to the violation of privacy or confidentiality and, more abstractly, to the lack of respect for individuals that occurs if research participants are treated as objects or means to an end (see, e.g., NBAC, 2001a and NHRPAC, 2002).

One difference between the federal regulations and the 1977 report of the National Commission for the Protection of Human Subjects of Biomedical and Behavioral Research (National Commission) is that the regulatory definition of minimal risk refers to harms or *discomfort*, whereas the latter report's definition mentions only harm (National Commission, 1977). This could be seen as unimportant because a discomfort is, by definition, a kind of harm, in that it makes a person's situation worse. A certain amount of discomfort could also be viewed as unimportant in assessments of overall risks of harm to a child. For example, the supplementary discussion in the National Commission report refers to "unusual discomfort" as a harm. The regulatory language, nonetheless, calls the attention of investigators and reviewers of research to harms that children may experience but that are less dramatic than, for example, death, disability, prolonged pain, or other lasting physical, psychological, or social harm. Such discomfort-as-harm covers a range of transitory but unpleasant physical and psychosocial experiences (e.g., pain, nausea, embarrassment, and fear).

A *benefit* is a positive or valued outcome of an action or event. A *potential benefit* is a positive but uncertain outcome, for example, the desired result of an experimental intervention. Discussions—and federal regulations as well—often refer to "risks and benefits" when it is appropriate to use the parallel language of "potential harms and potential benefits."

Potential benefits, like risks or potential harms, have the dimensions of probability, magnitude, and duration. They likewise may be physical (e.g., cure of a disease, slowing of the progression of a disease, or relief from pain), psychological (e.g., relief from depression or improved quality of life), or social (e.g., removal or lessening of a condition that is stigmatizing or that interferes with employment).

Most discussions of risk, harm, and benefit focus on potential harms or potential benefits to the individual research participant. For certain studies involving children, however, federal regulations require consideration of possible benefits to other children. Specifically, as discussed below, when proposed research involves a minor increase over minimal risk and does not offer the prospect of direct benefit, the research must be limited to children with a disorder or condition *and* must be expected (among other criteria) to generate vital knowledge about the disorder or condition (45 CFR 46.406; 21 CFR 50.53). That is, the child participating in the research is not expected to benefit directly from the study, but future children may. In addition, studies that are otherwise not approvable under the regulations may be approved by the Secretary of the U.S. Department of Health and Human Services (DHHS) or the Commissioner of the Food and Drug Administration (FDA) if the studies, among other things, present "a reasonable opportunity to further understanding, prevention or alleviation of a serious problem" with children's health or welfare (45 CFR 46.407; 21 CFR 50.54). Again, any potential benefit is not directly to the child research participant but to other children in the future.

Although federal regulations include, as one element of informed consent, "a description of any benefits to the subject or to others which may reasonably be expected," the corresponding description of risks cites only risk to the research participant (45 CFR 46.116(a)(3); 21 CFR 50.25(a)(3)) from the research. The regulations require research protocols to include written procedures for promptly reporting of "problems involving risks to subjects or others" (45 CFR 46.103(b)(5); 21 CFR 56.108(b)(1)), but overall, the emphasis in the regulations is on risks to research participants.

Some research clearly presents risks to others. For example, participants in a smallpox vaccine trial may pose a risk of disease transmission to individuals in close contact with them. Certain genetic studies have the potential to cause serious emotional distress to family members and impair family relationships in the short- and long-term. If confidentiality is breached, such studies may present the additional risks of stigmatization or economic harm to the family. Investigators and reviewers of research should normally consider such risks as part of their broader moral responsibility to minimize or prevent harm.

In addition, certain research involving children may pose risks to members of ethnic, cultural, religious, or other communities. Studies may, for example, focus attention on the prevalence of a medical condition or problem (e.g., diabetes or teen alcohol abuse) in certain ethnic or other groups (see, e.g., Arrillaga, 2001 and Stiffman et al., 2002). Such attention may reinforce prejudices about minority groups, stigmatize their members, and promote discrimination (Fisher et al., 2002). Reflecting concerns about stereotyping, discrimination in jobs or insurance, and other short- or long-term negative effects of research, some Indian tribes such as the Navaho Nation and the Cherokee Nation have organized formal institutional review boards (IRBs) to review research protocols (Hillabrant, 2002; see also IHS, 2002). (Whether or not they have organized their own IRBs, tribes must approve research conducted on tribal lands, unless the tribe has delegated review to another entity, such as the Indian Health Service.)

ASSESSING THE LEVEL OF RISK POSED BY A RESEARCH PROTOCOL

Categorizing, evaluating, and weighing the potential harms of proposed research are among the most challenging and subjective tasks for those charged with reviewing pediatric research. In 1998, the National Bioethics Advisory Commission observed that "relatively little progress has been made in describing the *criteria for assessing risk* by IRBs" (NBAC, 1998, p. 89, emphasis in the original).

Required Determinations

Box 4.1 summarizes the determinations about possible research harms and benefits that must be made before federally funded, sponsored, or regulated research involving children may be approved. As described in Chapter 3, some of these requirements must be met for all covered human research; other provisions are specific to children.

The provisions specific to children establish four basic categories of approvable research involving children (see Box 3.3 in Chapter 3). Figure 4.1 presents an algorithm for using the assessed level of risk, the possibility for direct benefit, and other criteria to determine whether research fits one of these categories. For research that involves a control group of healthy children without a disorder or condition and without prospect of direct benefit from the research, the research procedures for that group would have to involve no more than minimal risk.

Defining Minimal Risk

Subpart A of the DHHS regulations defines *minimal risk* as meaning "that the probability and magnitude of harm or discomfort anticipated in the research are not greater in and of themselves than those ordinarily encountered in daily life or during the performance of routine physical or psychological examinations or tests" (45 CFR 46.102(i); 21 CFR 50.3(k)). Subpart D of the regulations then explicitly applies this definition to research involving children.

The interpretation of what constitutes minimal risk is important to investigators because several practical consequences may flow from a judgment that a proposal does not exceed that risk threshold. For example, under certain circumstances, as described in Chapter 3, such a proposal may be eligible for expedited IRB review.

BOX 4.1
Determinations Related to Research Risks and Potential Benefits Required by Regulation for Federally Supported, Conducted, or Regulated Research Involving Children

Are risks to participants minimized by using procedures that are consistent with sound research design and that do not unnecessarily expose subjects to risk and, whenever appropriate, by using procedures already being performed on the subjects for diagnostic or treatment purposes? 45 CFR 46.111(a)(1); 21 CFR 56.111(a)(1)

Are risks to participants reasonable in relation to anticipated benefits to subjects and to the importance of the knowledge reasonably anticipated from the research? 45 CFR 46.111(a)(2); 21 CFR 56.5111(a)(2)

Is the selection of participants equitable, taking into account the purposes of the research, its setting, and the special problems of research involving vulnerable populations, such as children? 45 CFR 46.111(a)(3); 21 CFR 56.111(a)(3)

Are safeguards included to protect participants who are likely to be vulnerable to coercion or undue influence, such as children? 45 CFR 46.111(b); 21 CFR 56.111(b)

Does research meet the regulatory criteria for research involving children? 45 CFR 46.404-407; 21 CFR 50.51-54 (see Figure 4.1)

Are appropriate provisions made for monitoring participant safety? 45 CFR 46.111(a)(6); 21 CFR 56.111(a)(6)

Are appropriate provisions made for protecting privacy and confidentiality? 45 CFR 46.111(a)(7); 21 CFR 56.111(a)(7)

How Investigators and IRBs Interpret Minimal Risk

The committee found few systematic studies documenting how clinical investigators or reviewers of research interpret minimal risk in general or with reference to the risks of either "daily life" or "routine medical or psychological examinations." The first comparison (daily life) covers a very large array of possible experiences involving a sizeable range of risks, even for people not engaged in clearly high-risk activities such as skydiving. As described by Kopelman, this part of the definition may try "to explain the obscure (what studies have an appropriately low risk to allow participation by child-subjects) with the more obscure (what is the probability and magnitude of risk people normally encounter in daily life) (Kopelman, 2000, p. 751). The concept of "minor increase over minimal risk" builds on the

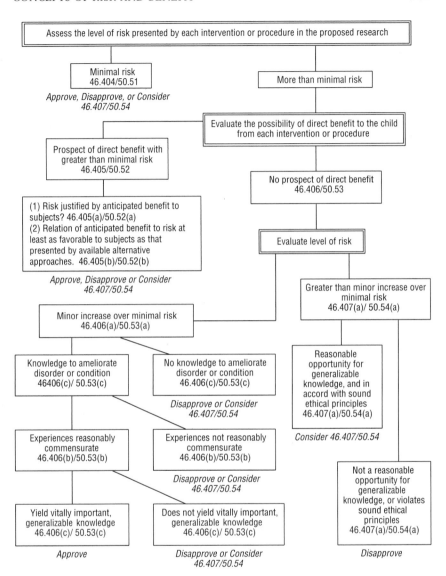

FIGURE 4.1 Algorithm for making assessments of research protocols as required by 45 CFR 46.404-407 and 21 CFR 50.51-54 (Nelson, 2003).

interpretation of minimal risk and, therefore, shares in its uncertainty or confusion.

That the "minimal risk" standard invites variable interpretation has long been clear. A 1981 article reported on a survey of pediatric researchers and department chairs that found variations in how they applied the risk categories in proposed federal regulations to several procedures used in pediatric studies (Janofsky and Starfield, 1981). For example, when asked to assess tympanocentesis (puncturing of the ear drum) in children up to 1 year of age, 46 percent of respondents classified the procedure as involving a minor increment over minimal risk, 40 percent thought that it involved more than a minor increase, but 14 percent thought that it posed minimal risk or less. The level of agreement on a risk category typically was less than 70 percent. An accompanying editorial called for better standards of risk assessment in children's research and suggested (without results) that a task force of the American Academy of Pediatrics develop consensus opinions about the risks of different procedures (Lascari, 1981).

Some 20 years after the study by Janofsky and Starfield was published, a survey of chairs of IRBs again found variation in the assessments of risk that a variety of research procedures presented to children (Wendler, 2003; Shah et al., 2004). For example, when asked to assess the risk presented by a confidential survey of sexual activity, 29 percent of respondents classified it as presenting more than a minor increase over minimal risk, whereas 44 percent thought that it presented minimal risk. Fifteen percent of respondents classified a blood draw once a week for 6 weeks as minimal risk, but 32 percent classified it as more than a minor increase over minimal risk. Eighty-one percent judged a single blood draw as minimal risk, but 17 percent labeled it as a minor increase over minimal risk. For research involving lumbar puncture without conscious sedation, 32 percent of respondents classified the research as involving a minor increase over minimal risk when it involved ill children and 6 percent classified it as minimal risk; for healthy children, the corresponding figures were 16 and 2 percent. The respondents might have shown greater agreement if they had been reviewing real protocols, and it is not clear whether respondents were giving their own views or the views that they thought others held. Also, the study did not determine the nature and extent of the experience of the IRB chairs with protocols involving children. Nonetheless, the results still point to the considerable subjectivity of risk assessments.

Chapter 8 cites analyses of actual IRB determinations that show similar variability in risk categorization. Most involve determinations reached by multiple IRBs reviewing the same protocol for multicenter trials. This variability in risk categorization raises ethical concerns about whether children are being appropriately protected from research risks. It also presents practical problems for those involved in designing and implementing important and often complex pediatric studies. The next sections of this chapter offer interpretations of minimal risk and minor increase over minimal risk that the committee believes will reduce the confusion and disagreement surrounding these concepts. Nonetheless, given the lack of relevant data and the subjective aspects of risk assessments, differences in judgments will certainly continue. For that reason, it is important that those designing and developing research explain the evidence and rationales behind their judgments. Likewise, those reviewing a research protocol should explain the bases for their determinations about its approval or disapproval.

Indexing Assessments of Minimal Risk to the Experience of Healthy Children in Daily Life

The regulatory definition of minimal risk, which was first adopted in 1981, departs in some respects from the definitions offered by the National Commission in its 1977 report, *Research Involving Children* (see Chapter 1). That report defined minimal risk as "the probability and magnitude of physical or psychological harm that is normally encountered in the daily lives, or in the routine medical or psychological examination, of *healthy children*" (National Commission, 1977, p. xix, emphasis added). In contrast, the definition presented in Subpart A and cited in Subpart D of the federal regulations has no modifying phrase referring to healthy individuals. When what is now Subpart A was first published in the *Federal Register* in 1981, the preamble—but not the actual language of the regulations—described minimal risk in terms of "those risks encountered in the daily life of the *subjects of the research*" (DHHS, 1981, online, unpaged, emphasis added). This use of the research participants' experiences as the point of reference has come to be called the "relativistic interpretation" of the minimal-risk standard.

A relative interpretation theoretically allows high-risk studies to be approved as "minimal-risk" studies if members of target research populations experience high risks in their daily lives, including in their homes, schools, sports activities, or neighborhoods. In addition to such environmental risks, some potential target research populations may, by virtue of their medical condition or its treatment, experience substantial everyday risks, distress, and uncomfortable medical examinations that are, for them, routine but *not* minimal in burden or discomfort. A relative interpretation of minimal risk would permit comparably high risks in research for these already high-risk children. In contrast, more fortunate research populations that experience low levels of risk in daily life would have a correspondingly low risk threshold for assessing whether a study presented minimal risk.

Consistent with the conclusions of a number of other groups (see, e.g., the National Commission, 1977; NBAC, 2001a; and NHRPAC, 2001), the committee rejected a relative interpretation of minimal risk, that is, an interpretation that allows the application of different standards or thresholds of minimal risk for different children and permits greater risk for those already disadvantaged by illness, poverty, and other burdens. The relative interpretation of the minimal-risk standard is inconsistent both with an ordinary or commonsense understanding of the concept of minimal risk and with the objective of providing special protections to child participants in research. It misinterprets and undercuts the moral and social purpose behind the minimal-risk standard; namely, to guide judgments about when risks are low enough to safely and ethically enroll children in studies that are not designed to benefit them (Kopelman, 1989, 2000).

Furthermore, allowing a relative interpretation of minimal risk would violate the ethical principle of justice, which requires that the burdens and benefits of research be distributed equitably. As a political and practical matter, it could also create social dissension if those in disadvantaged communities or populations understood that their children could be exposed to a higher risk in research than better-off children (Kopelman, 1989, 2000). Thus, the standard for interpreting risk has moral and social as well as legal and scientific implications.

In rejecting a relative interpretation of minimal risk, the committee agreed with the National Human Research Protections Advisory Committee (NHRPAC) that the interpretation of the concept should be "indexed" to the experiences of the "normal, healthy, average child" (NHRPAC, 2002, p. 3).[1] The threshold of minimal risk should thus be the same for healthy and ill children.[2] Furthermore, the interpretation should not change for groups of healthy children whose daily experiences involve risks greater than those that most other children experience as part of daily life. Thus, children who live in dangerous environments (e.g., with abusive parents or in unsafe housing) would not be exposed to more research risk than children who live in safer environments.

Interpretations of risk may, however, take into account children's developmental status or age because the physical or psychological risk of a research procedure can vary for younger and older children. That is, what is minimal risk for an 8-year-old may be high risk for an infant. Also, in some cases, a procedure that is judged to involve minimal risk to healthy children

---

[1]NHRPAC was an advisory committee to the Secretary of DHHS. Its charter expired in July 2002 and it was replaced in October 2002 with a new group, the Secretary's Advisory Committee on Human Research Protections.

[2]In the earlier cited survey of IRB chairs by Shah et al. (2004), respondents asked to categorize risk level for research involving a lumbar puncture and conscious rated such research differed were more likely to categorize the research as presenting minimal risk when the example involved healthy children than when it involved ill children.

may present more than minimal risk to children with certain medical conditions. For example, intramuscular injections that are safe for healthy children would be risky for children with hemophilia. The eligibility and screening criteria described in research protocols should be sufficient to exclude such vulnerable children from studies that otherwise present minimal risk.

Determinations about risk should consider the duration and cumulative characteristics of research interventions or procedures, for example, the number of procedures included in a protocol or the number of times that an individual procedure is repeated in a given period of time. Certain studies may include several different procedures that involve minimal risk or burden individually but that taken together present more than minimal risk. Similarly, although a single blood draw by needle stick normally involves minimal harm or discomfort, multiple needle sticks for blood draws in a short period could, depending on the child's age and other circumstances, present more than minimal risk of harm or discomfort. In other words, risk can be cumulative.

The committee agreed with NHRPAC's basic argument about the meaning of minimal risk, but it had some concerns about a further statement that interpreted minimal risk as "the socially allowable risks which parents generally permit their children to be exposed to in nonresearch situations" (NHRPAC, 2002, p. 1). The terms *socially allowable* and *generally permit* were presumably intended to exclude comparisons with risky actions or situations (e.g., failing to place infants and small children in car seats during automobile trips) that might be permitted in children's daily lives by irresponsible or ignorant parents. The committee agrees that it is appropriate to discourage comparisons of minimal-risk research to such dangerous situations as "what a child might encounter . . . while playing in traffic."[3]

Nonetheless, that an action has majority social approval and is legal does not necessarily make it an appropriate basis of comparison for the assessment of risks to child participants in research. For example, researchers could conceivably claim that an experiment that involved hitting a child presented only "minimal risk" if state laws or school board policies expressly permitted spanking (see, e.g., AAP, 2001) and public opinion polls in the state showed majority support for the practice as part of school life.

---

[3]This is quoted from IRB minutes in connection with the approval as minimal risk of a study that involved an overnight inpatient hospital stay for healthy 6- to 10-year-olds and extensive testing that required several hours of intravenous infusions and placement of two intravenous lines (Carome, 2000, p. 3). The study was subsequently reclassified as involving a minor increase over minimal risk.

Comparisons with Risks of Routine Examinations for Healthy Children

In addition to the risks of daily life, the federal regulations provide a second standard for assessing minimal risk in research, specifically, the risks "ordinarily encountered . . . during the performance of routine physical or psychological examinations or tests." Just as the committee concluded that the assessment of "risks of daily life" standard should be indexed to the experiences of normal, healthy, average children, it likewise concluded that the "routine examination" standard be interpreted with reference to the experiences of normal, healthy, average children. Ill children may routinely undergo much more burdensome and risky examinations. Again, assessments can appropriately take age into account because routine examinations differ for infants, children, and adolescents.

The components of "routine medical examinations" have no precise, universally accepted definition but what is sometimes called a well-child physician visit offers a reasonable basis for comparisons. In addition to a history, such a visit typically includes several routine, age-appropriate physical and psychological examinations or tests, guidance and education (for the child, the parents, or both), and immunizations.

Recommended elements of the physical examination component of a well-child visit are not entirely uniform (see, e.g., USPSTF, 1995; Schuster, 2000; and Behrman et al., 2004), in part because those making recommendations must often rely on clinical experience and judgment rather than solid scientific evidence about the potential benefits and risks of specific assessments or tests. Depending on the child's age, the physical examination may include measurements of height, weight, and head circumference; assessment of obesity with skin-fold calipers (pincher-like devices used to determine levels of subcutaneous fat); collection of blood; measurement of heart rate and blood pressure; collection of voided urine; testing of fine and gross motor development; and hearing and vision tests. The recommended elements are most extensive for neonates and older infants and most limited for school-age, preadolescent children.

A central objective of the history component of a well-child visit is to identify health risks (e.g., poor diet or a lack of seat belt or car seat use). Because many health risks vary by age, so does the history component of an examination. For an adolescent's routine medical examination, a full history includes exploration of sexual, smoking, and other behaviors that have health consequences.

Notwithstanding some disagreement about the specifics, the components of a well-child visit appear to be fairly modest in number and, taken individually, are reasonably well-characterized in content. They clearly include a far smaller set of activities than the activities of daily life. They also present a more limited range of risk of harm.

In addition to psychological assessments that may be part of a well-child visit, psychological tests considered routine for healthy children include standardized measures of infant functioning and standardized intelligence tests for children and adolescents. For example, to assess infant behavior, including responses to stress, the Brazelton Neonatal Behavioral Assessment Scale exposes infants to both pleasant stimuli and unpleasant stimuli, such as pinpricks (Brazelton et al., 1987). If the Brazelton assessment is used as a benchmark for determining acceptable research risk, researchers would clearly be able to expose infants to mildly unpleasant stimuli. As another example, the Bayley Scales of Infant Development, which are used for children from age 1 month to 3 1/2 years, include both mental scales and motor scales (Bayley, 1993). In the administration of the Bayley scales, the child is asked to display gross motor skills, such as standing, walking, and jumping, and fine motor skills, such as grasping an object. The child may also be asked to point to pictures, imitate words spoken by the examiner, or imitate the examiner's actions. The examiner tests a child's reaction to actions such as shaking a rattle behind the child's head and placing a mirror in front of the child. The Denver Developmental Screening Test II is used with children from birth to age 6 years (Frankenburg et al., 1992). This test also assesses gross motor and fine motor skills. It also assesses language skills and social skills, for example, by having the child play ball with the examiner and by having the child wash and dry his or her hands.

Intelligence tests, such as the widely-known Stanford-Binet Intelligence Scale, the Wechsler Preschool and Primary Scale of Intelligence, and the Wechsler Intelligence Scale for Children, include questions designed to assess knowledge and reasoning (Thorndike et al., 1986; Wechsler, 1989, 1991). The Wechsler scales also include performance items that require children to perform tasks such as assemble puzzles, arrange pictures in a sequence, and reproduce a design.

For a research procedure or intervention that is not normally part of routine medical or psychological examinations for children, the question is whether it presents a risk that is "equivalent" to that encountered in such examinations (NHRPAC, 2002). In its discussion of procedures involving minimal risk, the National Commission mentioned—in addition to physical examinations and psychological tests—"immunization, modest changes in diet or schedule, . . . and noninvasive physiological monitoring" (National Commission, 1977, pp. xix-xx). For the most part, assessments of equivalence are likely to be more straightforward for comparisons to routine medical and psychological examinations than for comparisons involving the larger range of risks encountered in daily life.

Recommended Interpretation of Minimal Risk

To recapitulate, the committee appreciated the subjective dimensions involved in interpreting the concept of minimal risk and the frequent lack of data to guide assessments of the risk presented by a particular procedure in the context of a particular study. It recognized that variability in assessments will continue, which makes it important that those designing and reviewing research explain the bases for their judgments of risk. Recommendations later in this chapter call for federal agencies or advisory groups to provide additional guidance for investigators and reviewers about procedures that normally involve minimal risk or a minor increase over minimal risk.

On ethical grounds, the committee rejected a "relative" interpretation of minimal risk; that is, an interpretation that allows the application of higher thresholds of minimal risk for children who experience higher risk in their daily lives as a result of their place of residence, family situations, medical condition, or other burdensome circumstances. Instead, the assessment of risk should be indexed to the experiences of average, normal, healthy children. It may take age into account and should consider the duration of potential harms or discomfort.

> **Recommendation 4.1: In evaluating the potential harms or discomfort posed by a research protocol that includes children, investigators, and reviewers of research protocols should**
>
> • interpret *minimal risk* in relation to the normal experiences of average, healthy, normal children;
> • focus on the equivalence of potential harms or discomfort anticipated in research with the harms or discomfort that average, healthy, normal children may encounter in their daily lives or experience in routine physical or psychological examinations or tests;
> • consider the risk of harms or discomfort in relation to the ages of the children to be studied; and
> • assess the duration as well as the probability and magnitude of potential harms or discomfort in determining the level of risk.

Defining Minor Increase over Minimal Risk and Associated Terms

Minor Increase over Minimal Risk

In its 1977 report on research involving children, the National Commission recommended that children with a disorder or condition be allowed to participate in research that does not hold the prospect of directly benefiting them *if* the research involves no more than a minor increase over minimal risk *and* has the prospect of providing knowledge vital for understanding or ameliorating the disorder or condition. The Commission argued (with dissents by 2 of 11 members) that "foreseeable benefit to an identifiable class of children may justify a minor increment of risk to research subjects" (National Commission, 1977, p. 125).

In Section 406 of 45 CFR 46 and Section 53 of 21 CFR 50, federal regulations follow the Commission's advice. The section thus permits children with disorders or conditions to be exposed to slightly more than minimal risk—without prospect of direct benefit—to gain important knowledge about those disorders or conditions. For research involving adults, federal regulations provide no equivalent risk category. The assumption is that adults can decide for themselves if they wish to consent to research, including research that involves greater than minimal risk absent any prospect of direct benefit.

Whatever disputes exist about the interpretation of the "minimal risk" threshold are compounded in interpreting the "minor increase over minimal risk" threshold. Neither the regulations nor the National Commission's report provides a definition of "minor increase over minimal risk." The Council for International Medical Organizations noted that there is no precise, internationally accepted definition of a "slight or minor increase" above the risks encountered in routine medical or psychological examinations (CIOMS, 2002, Guideline 9). In commentary, the National Commission mentioned research that "goes beyond, but only slightly beyond, the minimal risk" (National Commission, 1977, p. 130). NHRPAC referred to risks that are "just a bit more" or "a little more than minimal" (NHRPAC, 2002, p. 3). The committee endorses these interpretations that stress that the increase over minimal risk should be "only slightly beyond" or "just a bit more" than that level.

In its report, NHRPAC concluded that just because children may experience invasive procedures with considerable risk and discomfort while they are being treated for a disease, this "does not justify risks greater than a minor increase over minimal in a research study that provides no prospect of direct benefit to the individual subjects" (NHRPAC, 2002, p. 3). The committee agrees. That is, consistent with the interpretation of minimal risk, what constitutes "a bit more" risk in research involving children is not relative and does not allow a higher threshold for children with high-risk or high-burden conditions than for children with less serious conditions.

Recommendation 4.2: In evaluating the potential harms or discomfort posed by a research protocol that includes children who have a disorder or condition but no prospect of benefiting from participation, investigators and reviewers of research protocols should

- interpret *minor increase over minimal risk* to mean a slight increase in the potential for harms or discomfort beyond minimal risk (as defined in relation to the normal experiences of average, healthy, normal children);
- assess whether the research procedures or interventions present experiences that are commensurate with, that is, reasonably comparable to experiences already familiar to the children being studied on the basis of their past tests or treatments or their knowledge and understanding of the treatments that they might undergo in the future;
- consider risks of harms or discomfort in relation to the ages of the children to be studied; and
- assess the duration as well as the probability and magnitude of potential harms or discomfort in determining the level of risk.

Disorder or Condition

Just as federal regulations at 45 CFR 46.406 and 21 CFR 50.53 offer no definition of a minor increase over minimal risk, they likewise offer no definitions of "disorder" or "condition." Again, this section of the regulations, among other provisions, allows children to be enrolled in studies that involve a minor increase over minimal risk but no prospect of direct benefit. Thus, the approval of much research that may ultimately benefit various groups of children hinges on the definition and interpretation of these terms.

The meaning of the term *condition* has, in particular, been variably interpreted. Some of this variability, however, probably stems from problems with the interpretation of minimal risk. For example, when IRBs narrowly interpret "minimal risk" and routinely classify research that involves potentially controversial topics (e.g., surveys of adolescent sexual activity or drug use) as involving a minor increase over minimal risk (rather than no more than minimal risk), approval may then depend on whether the target research group is determined to have a condition (e.g., "being an adolescent").

Stedman's Medical Dictionary defines *disorder* as "a disturbance of function, structure, or both, resulting from a genetic or embryonic failure in development or from exogenous factors such poison, trauma, or disease" (Stedman, 2000). This definition encompasses physical and mental health problems arising from such common sources as disease, trauma, congenital anomalies, neurodevelopmental problems, and genetic abnormalities.

The term *condition* presents more difficulties. Standard medical dictionaries do not define it (except as a verb), and other dictionaries are not helpful in the context of clinical research. In recommending that research involving children be conducted to promote children's health and well-being, the National Commission stated in its 1977 report that "it is necessary to learn more about normal development as well as disease states in order to develop methods of diagnosis, treatment and prevention of conditions that jeopardize the health of children, interfere with optimal development, or adversely affect well-being in later years" (National Commission, 1977, p. 1). The National Commission did not, however, explicitly define "condition."[4]

Views on the meaning of "condition or disorder" cover a wide spectrum. At one end of the spectrum is the view that "disorder or condition" refers only to an illness, disease, injury, or defect. The committee rejected this view as too narrow, noting that it would reduce flexibility in studying children who are currently healthy but at risk of serious illnesses that could potentially be prevented or mitigated through early interventions.

Others interpret condition so broadly that almost any social, developmental, or other characteristic would qualify as a condition and, thereby, justify exposing a child to a higher level of research risk. This would make virtually meaningless the distinction between research approvable under Section 404 and research approvable under Section 406 of the DHHS regulations. Use of such broad interpretations could also unjustly single out groups of children already burdened by poverty and other social disadvantages for research that would not necessarily benefit them.

Thus, although the committee agreed with NHRPAC that a condition "can be understood more broadly than simply a specific disease or diagnostic category" (NHRPAC, 2002, p. 3), the committee did not fully accept that group's description of condition as "relating to [1] a specific characteristic which describes a group of children, [2] a physical, social, psychological, or neurodevelopmental condition affecting children, or [3] the risk of certain children developing a disease in the future based on diagnostic testing or physical examination" (NHRPAC, 2002, p. 3, bracketed numbers added for clarity). As examples of conditions, the NHRPAC report cited two periods of childhood (infancy and adolescence) and socioeconomic circumstances, for example, poverty and institutionalization.

The committee recognized that it is important to understand the correlates of health and disease and to identify specific circumstances or conditions—not just correlates—that contribute to children's poor or good health. For example, what about poverty—for example, persistent poor nutrition—contributes to specific health problems? Nonetheless, children's social, economic, racial, ethnic, and environmental characteristics or circumstances

---

[4]The Commission generally used "condition" in ways that seem synonymous with a diagnosable, treatable, or preventable illness or medical problem rather than a social characteristic or circumstance (see, e.g., Chapter 9 of the report).

do not, in themselves, necessarily justify exposing a child to a higher level of risk in research that is not expected to benefit them directly. Issues of justice must be considered.

If a characteristic of a group of children is to be designated as a condition that allows children to be exposed to a higher level of risk without prospect of benefit, the link between the characteristic and a deficit in health or well-being should be supported by scientific evidence or clinical knowledge. Thus, for this kind of research, investigators who define a research population on the basis of social characteristics or "conditions"— such as ethnicity, family circumstances, or economic status—must present a case that the condition has a negative effect on children's health and well-being that is relevant to the research question. They must also make the case that the research can be expected to generate vital knowledge about the condition.

> Recommendation 4.3: In determining whether proposed research involving a minor increase over minimal risk and no direct benefit can be approved, the term *condition* should be interpreted as referring to a specific (or a set of specific) physical, psychological, neurodevelopmental, or social characteristic(s) that an established body of scientific evidence or clinical knowledge has shown to negatively affect children's health and well-being or to increase their risk of developing a health problem in the future.

In the committee's experience, investigators and reviewers of research sometimes ignore the "disorder" or "condition" criterion in assessing whether research is approvable under 45 CFR 46.406 or 21 CFR 50.53. Investigators and IRBs should be explicit about how this and other criteria are met for research approved under this section.

> Recommendation 4.4: For purposes of determining whether proposed research involving a minor increase over minimal risk and no direct benefit can be approved, institutional review boards should make a determination that
>
> • the children to be included in the research have a disorder or condition;
> • the research is likely to generate vital knowledge about the children's disorder or condition;
> • the research procedures or interventions present experiences that are commensurate with, that is, reasonably comparable to, experiences already familiar to the children being studied on the basis of their past tests or treatments or on their knowledge and understanding of the treatments that they might undergo in the future; and

- the research does not unjustly single out or burden any group of children for increased exposure to research risk on the basis of their social circumstances.

Commensurate

In approving research that involves a minor increase over minimal risk, investigators and reviewers of research must also determine that "the intervention or procedure presents experiences to subjects that are reasonably commensurate with those inherent in their actual or expected medical, dental, psychological, social, or educational situations" (45 CFR 46.406(b); 21 CFR 50.53(b)).[5] This provision is based on another recommendation in the 1977 report of the National Commission. The Commission suggested that this requirement would help children who have the capacity to agree or assent to research participation "make a knowledgeable decision . . . based on some familiarity with the intervention or procedure and its effects" (National Commission, 1977, p. 5). NHRPAC observed that the requirement could also help parents make thoughtful judgments about permitting a child's participation in research.

As a synonym for commensurate, the National Commission referred to research activity that was "reasonably similar" to procedures that prospective research participants ordinarily experience. Dictionary definitions of commensurate or commensurable also emphasize the concepts of sameness, as well as proportionality or correspondence (American Heritage, 1992; Merriam-Webster, 2003). Thus, a child might not have experienced a particular research procedure, but the procedure could still be described to the child as potentially presenting levels of pain, immobility, anxiety, time away from home, or other effects that would be similar to those produced by procedures that they have experienced. In any case, even if a procedure is commensurate with a child's experiences, it cannot be approved under this category of research if it involves more than a minor increase over minimal risk.

Familiarity with a procedure may make further experiences with that or a similar procedure less frightening or burdensome to an ill child than it would be to a healthy child. In some cases, however, past experience with a procedure could make a child more fearful or anxious. The National

---

[5]The committee noted that the federal regulations involving prisoners refer to determinations about the "*risks* involved in the research" being "commensurate with *risks* that would be accepted by nonprisoner volunteers" (45 CFR 46.305 (a)(3), emphasis added). In contrast to prisoners, the regulatory comparison for children involves "*experiences*" not "risks."

Commission's explanation of this provision indicates that investigators and reviewers of protocols should not assume that familiarity with a procedure reduces the burden on a child research participant. Rather, investigators should plan to assess the views and concerns of the child and the parents when children's assent and parent's permission for a child's participation in research are discussed. That advice remains appropriate.

Direct Benefit

Under 45 CFR 46.405 and 21 CFR 50.52, child participants in research can be exposed to more than a minor increase over minimal risk if—among other conditions—the research presents the prospect of direct benefit. A *direct benefit* is a tangible positive outcome (e.g., cure of disease, relief of pain, and increased mobility) that may be experienced by an individual. When a research procedure or intervention has the prospect of directly benefiting child research participants, it can be approved even if it presents more than a minor increase over minimal risk. In addition, the relationship between the anticipated direct benefit and the risk or potential harm should be at least as favorable for the proposed research procedure as for the alternatives available to the children. This follows the recommendation of the National Commission (1977) that a child should not be disadvantaged by being enrolled in a research study (see the discussion below of clinical equipoise).

Research participants may also anticipate collateral, indirect, or side benefits that are not related to the research objectives as such (Churchill et al., 2003). For example, those participating in research may appreciate the opportunity to learn more about their condition or develop social relationships with others in similar circumstances (Churchill et al., 2003). Collateral or indirect benefits should *not*, however, be considered in assessing a research procedure's potential benefits in relation to its potential harms or be allowed to make up for shortfalls in the prospect of direct benefit from the research procedure (NBAC, 2001b). Similarly, although research participants may view gifts or payments for research participation as benefits, federal guidance makes clear that such payments should not be included by investigators or IRBs in their risk-benefit assessments (OPRR, 1993; see also Chapter 6).

Ordinarily, research that holds out the prospect of direct benefit evaluates an intervention intended to prevent, diagnose, or treat illness or injury. In addition, the regulations mention monitoring procedures that might contribute to a child's well-being (45 CFR 46.405; 21 CFR 50.52). For example, a study testing a new method for monitoring blood sugar levels might have the prospect of reducing discomfort or inconvenience for the children involved in the study.

Environmental circumstances can affect assessments of whether research has the potential for direct benefit. For example, in recent discussions of a proposed test of dilute smallpox vaccine in young children, one issue was whether the threat of a terrorist attack involving smallpox was, in the words of one reviewer, "a fantastically remote possibility or a real threat" (Hammerschmidt, 2002, p. 2). That reviewer judged that the prospect of direct benefit was highly speculative and that the arguments for direct benefit were not conclusive. Another reviewer noted, in contrast, that most vaccine research involving common childhood illnesses did have the prospect of directly benefiting children participating in the research and that the risks were low (Halsey, 2002).

As discussed in Chapter 2, the usual phase 1 trial with healthy adult volunteers seeks to determine the maximum tolerated dose and pharmacokinetic characteristics of a drug intended for a condition that these volunteers do not have. Such a trial does not hold out the prospect of direct benefit. In contrast, clinical trials involving children usually follow studies with adults (and possibly special laboratory and animal studies) that have provided information about safety and pharmacokinetics and that have given at least preliminary indications of efficacy. This information can help shape the design of an early-phase pediatric trial, for example, by guiding the selection of a drug dose that will maximize the potential for benefit and reduce the associated potential for harm as much as possible, although the trial may still involve more than a minor increase over minimal risk. Particularly when standard treatment alternatives have been exhausted and the probable outcome for the child without the trial intervention is grim, the prospect of benefit may arguably be considered reasonable in relation to the risks, even when further testing of efficacy is continuing in adult studies (see, e.g., Kodish, 2003c).

Vital Importance and Research Approvable Under Section 407 or Section 54

When proposed pediatric studies involve more than minimal risk and no direct benefit, approval of the research requires that IRBs determine not only that the children included in the study have a disorder or condition but also that the proposed research may produce vitally important scientific knowledge about the disorder or condition. The committee stressed earlier that all these determinations should be an explicit part of the review and approval process.

Although the standard of "vital importance" is required for research to be approved under 45 CFR 46.406 or 21 CFR 50.53, different language is used in 45 CFR 46.407 or 21 CFR 50.54, which allows research that cannot otherwise be approved to be referred to and approved by the Secretary of DHHS or the Commissioner of FDA. Section 407 requires a determination that the research offers "a reasonable opportunity to further the understanding, prevention, or alleviation of a serious problem affecting the health or welfare of children." Arguably, the latter is a less stringent standard than the standard of vital importance. That is, proposed research might more easily be justified on the ground that it "furthers" knowledge than on the grounds that it is "vital."

As described in the 1977 report of the National Commission, the referral of proposed research for "national" review should be reserved for "exceptional situations" and research of "major significance." Given this context, the committee believed that *the criterion for judging the potential contribution of research must, ethically, be as stringent for reviews conducted under Section 407 as for those conducted under Section 406.* Thus, although it is not required by the regulations, the standard of "vital importance" should be applied by the panels involved in the review of proposals referred to the Secretary of DHHS or the Commissioner of FDA for approval. The Secretary's Advisory Committee on Human Research Protections (SACHRP) should incorporate this criterion when it considers adjustments in the process for Section 407 reviews (see Chapter 8).

Recommendation for Additional Government Guidance

Ideally, investigators and reviewers would have some data on which to base assessments of the risk presented by common research procedures, whether or not the procedures are part of routine physical examinations. For many routine medical and psychosocial interventions, however, risks may at best have been characterized (e.g., as involving bruising, pain, or anxiety) but not assessed in terms of the frequency, intensity, or duration of harms or discomfort. Although it is reasonable for reviewers of research proposals to seek information on the risks of research procedures or interventions, they may find that no evidence is available. Even when some data are available about the risk of harm, judgments about what is "minimal" or "minor" often have a significant subjective component.

The committee concluded that IRBs should be encouraged to develop written rationales (e.g., in IRB minutes) to explain the basis for their judgments about the risks presented by procedures included in a research protocol. Such a practice should help reviewers of research identify more clearly the evidence or other bases for their judgments.

In addition, the committee concluded that useful guidance can be provided to pediatric investigators and reviewers of pediatric research if continued efforts are made to develop consensus identifications of procedures that present minimal risk or no more than a minor increase over minimal risk to children participating in research (NBAC, 1998; Kopelman, 2000).

The NHRPAC work group engaged in such an effort and produced a table in which they categorized a number of common research procedures according to the level of risk presented by a single use of the procedure. That table is reproduced in Table 4.1.

Although NHRPAC has been disbanded, the successor SACHRP should be encouraged to continue its predecessor's work to develop consensus assessments about the risk of common research procedures. To provide further guidance for investigators and reviewers of research, these consensus assessments should be accompanied by examples, citations of any relevant data, and explanations of the rationales for the categorization of procedures as involving either minimal risk or a minor increase over minimal risk.

The Office for Human Research Protections (OHRP) can also assist

TABLE 4.1 Common Research Procedures by Category of Risk

| | Category of Risk | | |
Procedure	Minimal	Minor Increase over Minimal	More Than a Minor Increase over Minimal
Routine history taking	X		
Venipuncture/fingerstick/heelstick	X		
Urine collection via bag	X		
Urine collection via catheter		X	
Urine collection via suprapubic tap			X
Chest X-ray	X		
Bone density test	X		
Wrist X-ray for bone age	X		
Lumbar puncture		X	
Collection of saliva	X		
Collection of small sample of hair	X		
Vision testing	X		
Hearing testing	X		
Complete neurological exam	X		
Oral glucose tolerance test	X		
Skin punch biopsy with topical pain relief			X
Bone marrow aspirate with topical pain relief			X
Organ biopsy			X
Standard psychological tests	X		
Classroom observation	X		

NOTE: The category of risk is for a single procedure. Multiple or repetitive procedures are likely to affect the level of risk.
SOURCE: NHRPAC, 2002.

investigators and IRBs by developing explicit guidance based on the information and recommendations presented in this report and the work of NHRPAC and, eventually, SACHRP. Such official guidance is essential to direct the attention of IRBs to these resources. In addition to providing guidance about the interpretation of the terms discussed in this chapter, OHRP should provide examples of studies and procedures to clarify the limits of minimal risk and a minor increase over minimal risk. The examples should indicate qualifying factors that may affect research risk; for example, the expertise of those performing a procedure and the adequacy of the facilities (e.g., in case of a research emergency). Although FDA has provided much more detailed guidance on many aspects of research conduct and the interpretation of regulations than OHRP, it should work with OHRP on the development of this guidance.

> Recommendation 4.5: The Secretary's Advisory Committee on Human Research Protections (U.S. Department of Health and Human Services) should continue the work of its predecessor committee by developing additional consensus descriptions of procedures or interventions that present minimal risk or no more than a minor increase over minimal risk. In addition, the Office for Human Research Protections and the Food and Drug Administration should cooperate to develop and disseminate guidance and examples for investigators and institutional review boards to clarify important regulatory concepts and definitions (including definitions of minimal risk, minor increase over minimal risk, condition, and prospect of direct benefit).

OTHER ISSUES RELATED TO THE ASSESSMENT OF RISK

In addition to the issues discussed in the preceding sections, other questions about the assessment of research risks warrant consideration. The following discussion considers three questions. First, should determinations about potential harms and benefits be made individually for each research procedure or intervention included in a study, or is it appropriate to judge the research as a whole or as a package? Second, how should research risks be assessed in relation to the anticipated or hypothesized benefits, given other alternatives available to research participants? Third, how should a research protocol be examined to assess whether it minimizes risks to participants.

Assessing Level of Risk by Protocol Components or as a Whole

Most complex clinical research involves several research procedures or interventions. Certain procedures may hold out the prospect of direct benefit to the research participant; others may not. A 2001 report from NBAC pointed out that all research involves some procedures or methods that are used "*solely* for the purpose of answering the research question(s)" (NBAC, 2001b, p. 77). Such procedures may be medical (e.g., collection of blood by venipuncture or via a catheter), statistical (e.g., random assignment of subjects to different arms of a clinical trial), or administrative (e.g., review of medical charts).

For example, to gain additional knowledge about an experimental intervention, a research protocol might include an aspiration of bone marrow that would not offer the prospect of direct benefit to the child participant. To be considered for approval, such a "research-only" procedure must present no more than a minor increase over minimal risk. To meet this requirement and also minimize risk, procedural sedation for the aspiration of bone marrow might be restricted to local anesthesia and intravenous medications (e.g., a narcotic and a benzodiazepine). The purpose of the restriction would be to ensure that the level of sedation was moderate, thus preserving protective airway reflexes.

When a research protocol involves multiple procedures, including some without prospect of direct benefit to the research participant, how should the protocol be assessed to determine whether it meets the regulatory criteria for approval? (For discussions related to this question, see, e.g., National Commission, 1977; Freedman, 1987; NBAC, 2001b; Weijer, 2001; and Nelson, 2003.) One answer is that a research protocol should be assessed and approved as a whole—even if some components do not individually meet the criteria for approval—as long as the level of risk overall is reasonable in relation to the anticipated benefit.[6]

An alternative view—which the committee adopted—is that not only must the research be considered as a whole, but each intervention or procedure must also be assessed independently against the regulatory criteria for approval. Thus, for pediatric studies, the presence of an intervention or procedure that offers the prospect of direct benefit cannot be used to justify the exposure of a child to other procedures that present more than a minor increase over minimal risk but no prospect of direct benefit. Furthermore, as noted earlier, the cumulative risk or burden of a protocol should be assessed. This is important because research may involve several different

---

[6]For example, in clarifying the analysis that recently led one IRB to refer a protocol to the Secretary of DHHS for consideration, the IRB stated that federal regulations imply that the IRB should make "a risk determination regarding the collective nature of the research procedures" and argued that making "determinations for individual procedures seems of little help in determining an overall risk assessment" (see questions and answers at http://ohrp.osophs.dhhs.gov/panels/407-04pnl/response.htm).

procedures that may involve minimal risk or burden individually but that may present more than minimal risk when considered collectively.

In the DHHS regulations, Section 405 (concerning approval of studies presenting more than minimal risk and the prospect of direct benefit) and Section 406 (concerning approval of studies presenting more than minimal risk without the prospect of direct benefit) both refer to the risk presented by *an intervention or procedure* (rather, referring generally to the risk presented by the research). This regulatory language is consistent with a "component" assessment of risk. If elements are evaluated individually, then one component of a protocol might be approved under Section 405 of the regulations, whereas another might either be approved under Sections 404 or 406 *or* be judged to be not approvable under any of the three primary regulatory categories. (The corresponding FDA regulations are at 21 CFR 50.51 to 53.)

In its 1977 report, the National Commission stated that in assessing the "overall acceptability" of proposed research, "the risk and anticipated benefit of activities described in a protocol must be evaluated individually as well as collectively, as is done in clinical practice" (National Commission, 1977, p. 4). NBAC likewise recommended that "[i]n general, each component of a study should be evaluated separately" and, further, "[p]otential benefits from one component of a study should not be used to justify risks posed by a separate component of a study" (NBAC, 2001b, p. 77). This committee agrees.

> Recommendation 4.6: Institutional review boards should assess the potential harms and benefits of each intervention or procedure in a pediatric protocol to determine whether each conforms to the regulatory criteria for approving research involving children. When some procedures present the prospect of direct benefit and others do not, the potential benefits from one component of the research should not be held to offset or justify the risks presented by another.

Assessing Whether Risks Are Reasonable in Relation to Anticipated Benefits: Clinical Trials and Clinical Equipoise

Current regulations provide that a child should not be exposed to more than a minor increase over minimal risk unless the research intervention or procedure offers a prospect of direct benefit. In its report on children, the National Commission argued further that a child should not be disadvantaged by being enrolled in a research study (National Commission, 1977). Two requirements follow from this argument. First, if more than a minor increase over minimal risk is involved, the risk of harm associated with an intervention must be justified by the prospect of direct benefit to the child.

No similar justification is required for research with adults (45 CFR 46.111; 21 CFR 56.111). Second, the balance of anticipated benefits and the risk of harm must be comparable to that for the alternatives available to the child outside of the research. When these other alternatives are taken into account, a child's health or welfare should not be placed in jeopardy by the decision to enter the child into a research protocol.

The argument of the National Commission bears some resemblance to the concept of "clinical equipoise" (or "research equipoise"), which, in turn, is related to the notion of a null hypothesis (i.e., that there is no difference between two alternatives). The concept of equipoise has emerged as an important criterion in evaluating the ethical acceptability of a clinical trial and determining the appropriate comparison groups—or arms—for a trial (see, e.g., Freedman, 1987; Weijer et al., 2000; and NBAC, 2001b; see also Sackett, 2000 and Shrier, 2001). As originally defined by Freedman, clinical equipoise exists when "there is genuine uncertainty within the expert medical community—not necessarily on the part of the individual investigator—about the preferred treatment" for a condition (Freedman, 1987, p. 141; see also Tri-Council, 1998).

Thus, at the beginning of a clinical trial with an intervention arm and a control arm, no participant would be assigned to receive care known to be inferior to an alternative. Reflecting their assessment of findings from laboratory, animal, or other human research, some experts might view one option as inferior; but both options should be endorsed by "at least a respectable minority of expert practitioners" (Weijer et al., 2000, p. 757) based on "reasoned" uncertainty about the evidence (Mann and Djulbegovic, 2003). The case that such uncertainty exists can be presented by investigators and assessed by reviewers of research protocols.[7]

Freedman and colleagues (1996), among others, have argued that the principle of clinical equipoise is founded in part on a physician investigator's therapeutic obligation to patients and that one situation that can violate this obligation involves the use of placebo controls when an effective, active treatment can serve as a control (Rothman and Michels, 1994). A counterview distinguishes the obligation of clinicians to act in an individual patient's best interest from the obligations of researchers to create knowledge using ethical, scientifically valid methods, which may—under carefully defined

---

[7]Others have argued that the views of the broader community, including patients and prospective research participants, be considered as part of decisions about the desirability of trials (see, e.g., Karlawish and Lantos, 1997). Although the underlying point may be worthy, extending the term *equipoise* to these types of ethical judgments may detract from the term's usefulness in focusing on the medical community's uncertainty about the effectiveness of diagnostic, preventive, or therapeutic options.

and limited conditions—include a placebo-controlled trial when an effective treatment exists (see, e.g., Emanuel and Miller, 2001 and Miller and Brody, 2002; see also, Ellenberg and Temple, 2000 and Truog et al., 1999).[8] One such condition is an especially meticulous informed consent process that carefully explains what a placebo is and makes clear to prospective research participants that they could be assigned to the placebo arm of the trial.

The use of placebo control groups has long been controversial (see, e.g., Ellenberg and Temple, 2000; NBAC, 2001b; and Emanuel and Miller, 2001). This controversy flared in October 2000 when the World Medical Association (WMA) revised the Declaration of Helsinki (WMA, 2002). One revision (paragraph 29) stated that any new preventive, diagnostic, or therapeutic method should be tested against the best current method and that the use of a placebo (or no treatment) control group should be limited to situations in which there is no proven alternative method. After considerable controversy over the revision, WMA qualified its opposition to state (in a footnote) that a placebo control may be ethical if a compelling scientific case supports the use of a placebo control rather than an active control *or* if the condition being studied is minor and the risk to the group receiving the placebo is minor (WMA, 2002).

In 2000, the International Conference on Harmonisation adopted a guideline that would allow a placebo control when there is no serious harm of withholding effective therapy (ICH, 2000a; see also FDA, 2001d). A placebo-controlled could also be ethical when the proven effective treatment has such severe toxicity that many patients would refuse treatment or when comparison with an active control treatment would not yield scientifically valid results. Similarly, the recent revision of the Guidelines of the Council of International Medical Organizations stated that placebo controls can be ethical (1) when there is no established effective intervention, (2) when withholding and established effective intervention would result in only temporary discomfort or a delay in the relief of symptoms, and (3) when an active control trial would not yield scientifically reliable results

---

[8]FDA is perceived by many as conditioning the approval of drugs, in most instances, on the provision of information from placebo-controlled trials (see, e.g., Cowdry, 1997). FDA rules and guidelines do not explicitly require such trials. FDA policies require "adequate and well-controlled studies" and identify five types of studies that may be acceptable under some circumstances: placebo concurrent control, dose-comparison concurrent control (in which at least two different doses of the same drug are compared), no treatment concurrent control, active treatment concurrent control, and historical control (21 CFR 314.26(b)(2)). In responding to comments on the so-called pediatric rule (see Chapter 2), FDA stated that alternatives to placebo-controlled trials should be used *if* such trials can provide adequate information about the effectiveness of a therapy (FDA, 1998e).

and the use of placebo would not pose any risk of serious or irreversible harm to the research participants (CIOMS, 2002).

The Committee on Drugs of the American Academy of Pediatrics (AAP) also has a statement on the use of placebo controls. Such use should be limited to situations

1. when there is no commonly accepted therapy for the condition and the agent under study is the first one that may modify the course of the disease process;

2. when the commonly used therapy for the condition is of questionable efficacy;

3. when the commonly used therapy for the condition carries with it a high frequency of undesirable side effects and the risks may be significantly greater than the benefits;

4. when the placebo is used to identify incidence and severity of undesirable side effects produced by adding a new treatment to an established regimen; or

5. when the disease process is characterized by frequent, spontaneous exacerbations and remissions and the efficacy of the therapy has not been demonstrated (AAP, 1995, p. 294).

The AAP statement does not mention the withholding of commonly accepted therapy when that would only result in minor discomfort. Such research would likely be approvable under federal regulations.

Whatever the criteria outlined by national and international organizations, they may still not justify the inclusion of children in a placebo-controlled trial. For research involving children and a placebo control group to be approved by an IRB under federal regulations, either (1) the balance of potential harms and benefits for children in the placebo control arm must be as favorable as those for children receiving the active, standard treatment or (2) the potential harms to which children in the placebo control arm would be exposed are no more than minimal or involve only a minor increase over minimal risk. Although ethical and regulatory principles allow adults to give their informed consent to participate in research involving more risk, they do not allow parents or children to agree to accept such research risk for a child.

Other requirements also apply. As for all research, risks must be minimized (see further discussion below). In addition, the creation of a data and safety monitoring board is typically required for clinical trials (see Chapter 3).

For a placebo-controlled trial, the process of requesting parental permission should make clear that the proposed research could involve foregoing or delaying a known effective therapy and that the child could be assigned to *either* a placebo-control group (with no benefit expected) *or* a group receiving an experimental intervention (with a prospect of benefit). (The same kind of explanation is also necessary when active treatment control groups are employed.) Parents should also be informed if children in the placebo-control group will eventually "cross over" to the experimental intervention. They should likewise be provided clear explanations about why a placebo arm is necessary to answer the research question and what measures that will be taken to ensure the child's safety and well-being. As discussed in the next chapter, studies indicate that research participants and parents of research participants may not understand these and other aspects of research.

Given the controversy over placebo-controlled trials, more published data are needed on health outcomes for research participants receiving placebos. A common misperception among patients (and even some clinicians) is that research participants assigned to placebo arms are necessarily at greater risk than those assigned to treatment arms. Particularly in early-phase studies, however, the participants in placebo arms may have fewer adverse events. As discussed above, if the condition of research equipoise is indeed met, then no research participants should be exposed to treatment (including administration of a placebo) known to be inferior to an alternative.

Assessing Whether Risk Is Minimized

One ethical and regulatory responsibility of investigators is to minimize the risk that research presents to participants. In assessing whether risks are being minimized, attention often focuses on the risk presented by the procedures or interventions that are being tested for safety or efficacy. Investigators and reviewers must, however, also consider whether risks are minimized for interventions or procedures intended solely to collect information (e.g., blood draws and lumbar punctures). One advantage of separately evaluating each intervention or procedure in a research protocol, as recommended above, is that it encourages attention to risk minimization for all the procedures.

As observed in Chapter 1, poorly designed research will usually fail to answer the research question. One example is research that is designed without adequate attention to the sample size needed to detect a meaningful difference between an experimental intervention and a placebo or control treatment. At a minimum, such research wastes the time of research participants. Depending on its particular faults, poorly designed research can also expose research participants to avoidable harm and can dissipate potential benefits. An important emphasis of specialized education for clinical researchers is techniques of modern research design and data analysis that help minimize the exposure of research participants to such avoidable risks.

Depending on the procedures or interventions involved in a research protocol and the characteristics of the research population, investigators and reviewers of research may consider several questions in determining whether the protocol proposes appropriate steps to minimize risk. Box 4.2 lists a number of these questions. Some—for example, whether the research design is sound—apply to any research, whereas others—for example, whether the research setting is equipped to meet children's developmental requirements—focus on particular concerns in studies that include infants, children, or adolescents.

The guidelines listed in Box 4.2 include several items related to the qualifications of the research team and the characteristics of the research site that may affect the risk associated with a particular clinical study. The creation of pediatrics as a specialty and the founding of children's hospitals as institutions were motivated, in part, by perceptions that excellent physical and psychosocial care for children requires specialization. Similarly, the creation of regional pediatric trauma and neonatal intensive care centers reflects a judgment that the concentration of care for patients with complex conditions in designated units will improve outcomes.

Many interventions or procedures would clearly involve unacceptable risks if they were undertaken by generalist physicians in ordinary community hospitals. Even within pediatric centers, research involving high-risk procedures, for example, gross surgical resections and stem cell transplants may involve higher risks if they are performed by staff and institutions that are less experienced with those highly specialized procedures or the management of their side effects in children with specific cancers. Thus, reviewers of research protocols may consider the relevance of specialization in facilities and personnel when making their determinations about risk. In addition, the IRB may determine that information about staff and institution experience should be included in discussions with parents about a child's research participation.

IRB members may sometimes find it appropriate to examine specific data about the performance of the investigators and the research setting to help them assess the level of risk posed by a research procedure and the extent to which risks have been minimized. Most data available to IRBs are likely to involve serious adverse outcomes (e.g., death, disability, hospital admission or extension of the hospital stay, or the need for a "rescue" procedure). No data may be available to judge outcomes such as pain, fear, or other forms of distress. Ideally, comparative data could be used to assess performance history.

BOX 4.2
Guidelines for Considering Risk and Risk Minimization in Research That Includes Children

- Is inclusion of children necessary to answer the scientific question posed by the research? What are the ages of the children to be included? Are any of the potential research harms age dependent?
- Will potential child participants be screened for known vulnerability to the risks associated with specific elements of the research?
- What does the research require of children and their families? Is adherence to the research protocol a concern? If so, what are the risks of nonadherence?
- Are all the procedures or interventions necessary to answer the research question? Can the investigators collect the required information using procedures that the child participants will undergo as part of normal therapy or monitoring?
- Have prior laboratory studies, animal research, studies with adults, or other data provided a sufficient basis for proceeding with research involving children?
- Does the study follow principles of sound research design?
- What are the theoretical risks involved with the research as proposed? Are data available to estimate the probability and magnitude of each risk as they relate to the categories of children to be included?
- For the sites where the research procedures will be performed, have the investigators provided data on the site-specific frequency of adverse events for those procedures (e.g., sedation for research procedures)?
- Are the investigators and other members of the research team qualified to perform each of the procedures or assessments specified in the protocol and recognize potential risks and adverse outcomes? Does the research team have appropriate skills and expertise in caring for children of the ages included in the study?
- Will research be performed in a setting that is "friendly" to children of the ages included in the study? Is the setting appropriate for the physical, clinical, psychological, and emotional needs of these age groups?
- For research having more than a minimal risk, does the research protocol have an adequate plan for monitoring the safety of the child participants? Does the monitoring plan provide for the inclusion of professionals with the appropriate expertise in pediatrics?
- If the protocol presents the risk of a physical or psychological emergency, is the research setting equipped to respond? Are plans for responding to an emergency specified in the protocol?
- What are the "stopping rules" or "end points" for early discontinuation of the research on the basis of strong findings about harms or benefits? Are they specific and appropriate?
- What happens to the data once they are collected? Where are research records stored, and who has access to them? What are the practices and procedures for maintaining the short-term and long-term confidentiality of the data?

CONCLUSION

Under federal regulations, some research that would be approvable for adults involves more risk than is allowable for children. The regulations recognize children's greater vulnerability and need for protection. Unfortunately, the concepts of risk on which decisions about approvable research hinge have significant subjective elements. The same applies to several other key concepts in the regulations. Reasonable people may disagree when interpreting these concepts, especially when little or no evidence is available to inform judgments. Nonetheless, if investigators and IRB members apply the definitions presented here, judgments about similar protocols should be more consistent. They should also conform more to the ethical principles underlying the regulations.

In addition, the consistency and quality of evaluations can be improved if investigators and IRB members pay more systematic attention to all the requirements (not just the provisions related to risk) included in the four sections of the DHHS and FDA regulations that set criteria for permissible research involving children. Applications for IRB approval and IRB records should include rationales related to each of the key concepts. The last chapter of this report recommends that IRBs and federal agencies provide clear, easily located guidance that will help both investigators and IRB members understand and fulfill their responsibilities.

5

UNDERSTANDING AND AGREEING TO CHILDREN'S PARTICIPATION IN CLINICAL RESEARCH

> *My daughter will be nine years old and she needs some kind of input in what's going on with her. . . . She's presently in a study and I need for her to be able to understand what she's getting herself into. . . . She's at the point where she asks a lot of questions . . . which is good.*
>
> Andrell Vaughn, parent, 2003

The quote above shows a mother's concise, personal appreciation of the values underlying requirements that children be involved, when appropriate, in discussions and decisions about their participation in research. This mother recognizes her daughter's growing maturity, increasing curiosity, and developing moral right to be involved in choices about "what's going on" in the context of a close parent-child relationship.

When research involves children such as this 9-year-old, investigators and institutional review boards (IRBs) cannot rely on the conventional concept of *informed consent*, which applies to decisions about research participation made by those with the legal and intellectual capacity to make such choices in their own right. Children usually lack such capacity. Instead, legal authority to allow a child's participation in research rests with parents or guardians, who must provide their *permission*. In addition, with respect for children's emerging maturity and independence and consistent with federal regulations, investigators—when appropriate—seek to

146

involve children in discussions about research and obtain their *assent* to participation.

Although debate continues about the ethical dimensions and boundaries of parental permission and child assent, especially when adolescents are involved, much attention today focuses on more practical questions about how to interpret and implement these concepts and honor their underlying ethical principles in research practice. For example, at what age should investigators, as a general rule, begin seeking a child's assent? What information and what role in decision making are appropriate for children at different stages of development? How should relationships between children and parents be approached?

This chapter considers two elements in the charge to the committee. The first relates to the written and oral process for obtaining assent and permission for research participation from children and their parents, guardians, or other legally authorized representatives.[1] The second involves an examination of children's and parent's expectations and comprehension of the direct benefits and risks associated with a child's participation in research and, in particular, their understanding of the distinction between research and treatment. The discussion begins with an overview of the ethical principles and legal requirements for obtaining parents' and children's agreement to a child's participation in research, including circumstances in which minors can make decisions on their own behalf. Next is a review of the literature relevant to parents' and children's understanding of research participation, which also covers the general research literature on the development of children's cognitive and decisional capacities. The last sections of the chapter offer recommendations.

ETHICAL PRINCIPLES AND LEGAL REQUIREMENTS

The Ethics of Informed Consent, Permission, and Assent

For pediatric ethics, informed consent is more properly understood as a combination of informed parental permission and (when appropriate) the assent of the child.

Kodish, 2003b, p. 90

As described in Chapter 1, the ethical principle of respect for persons underlies the obligation of investigators to treat individuals as autonomous actors who must provide their informed and voluntary consent to partici-

---

[1]For simplicity, the rest of this chapter will refer only to parents.

pate in research. Requirements for parental permission serve the ethical obligation of investigators to respect and protect vulnerable individuals. Provisions for involving children in discussions about research participation and seeking their assent, when appropriate, attest to respect for children's developing autonomy. Permission and assent are thus the intertwined foundations of ethical research involving children.

Much of the ethical analysis that underlies the principles and processes of informed consent in research derives from or is similar to the analysis of informed consent to receive medical treatment. Nonetheless, agreement to participation in research differs from agreement to receive clinical care. As discussed in this chapter, patients—and investigators—may sometimes not clearly understand that research has purposes distinct from clinical care. Such a lack of understanding can compromise the objectives of informed agreement to participation in research.

General Conditions for Informed Consent

In the classic analysis by Faden and Beauchamp (1986), the conditions for autonomous decisions or actions include intentional action, understanding of the action, and voluntary or uncontrolled action. Informed consent may be viewed as one type of autonomous choice, but a choice that must also be considered within "the web of cultural and policy rules and requirements . . . that collectively form the social practice of informed consent in institutional contexts" (Faden and Beauchamp, 1986, p. 277).

The conditions of understanding and voluntariness are central to requirements that investigators provide relevant information to prospective research participants, evaluate their understanding of this information, and assess situations for possible coercion or undue influence on the decision to participate in research. Voluntary choice extends beyond the initial, explicit agreement to participate in research to the sometimes implicit and sometimes explicit agreement to continue participation on the basis of an understanding of one's right to withdraw.

Parental permission is ethically distinct from consent, but the conditions of understanding and voluntariness and freedom from coercion or undue influence still apply to assessments of the procedures for obtaining permission. With appropriate regard for a child's or an adolescent's maturity, they also apply to procedures for seeking assent.

Although parental permission is sometimes described as "consent" or "proxy consent" and children's agreement is also sometimes labeled as "consent," such labels are misleading. They do not properly reflect the ethical differences between permission or assent and informed consent. Again, as the concept has developed, only those who are held competent to make autonomous decisions on their own behalf can provide informed consent. Thus, parents can provide informed consent only for themselves. Minors cannot provide informed consent unless they have been judged to be able to act as adults for that purpose (see the discussion below of emancipated and mature minors).

Within the limits of parental discretion described in Chapters 3 and 4, the ethical and legal provisions for parental permission assume that parents will make decisions about research participation that protect their child's interests.[2] In exceptional circumstances, for example, in certain situations involving child abuse and neglect, that assumption fails. Alternative mechanisms (e.g., appointment of a guardian) may be necessary to protect the child. In less exceptional situations, investigators who engage parents in careful discussions of research participation may still occasionally conclude that parents are not adequately considering their child's well-being. They may then judge that the ethical standards for the child's participation are not met, even though the parents are willing to give permission.

Consent, Permission, and Assent as Processes

As familiarity with the practical realities of obtaining informed consent to medical care or research participation developed, ethicists, investigators, and policymakers recognized that creating understanding is more than a simple matter of providing information or preparing clear consent forms. Rather, a careful *process* of communication is necessary, one that includes the opportunity for parents and children to ask questions and investigators to make assessments of the extent to which a decision about participation in research (and about continued participation, once it has started) is made freely and with understanding (Faden and Beauchamp, 1986).

The inclination to concentrate on physical consent forms is, however, strong. Forms are fairly easy to review, and their use is relatively straightforward to document. Two recent reports on research ethics still found it necessary to stress in their recommendations that informed consent should be understood as a process and not merely a form (NBAC, 2001b; IOM, 2003a). A third report, which focused on social and behavioral research, concluded that IRBs focus too much on the consent form and also fail to calibrate their attention to the level of risk posed by the research (NRC,

---

[2]Although parents are often expected to make decisions in their child's *best* interests given the available alternatives, some arguments allow a role for other considerations or, at least, reasonable freedom from intrusive second-guessing by others (see, e.g., Brock, 1994 and Ross, 1998). One argument is that having assigned parents the main responsibility for raising children, society should grant them reasonable discretion in doing so according to their own values. For example, under this argument, parents may consider peripheral benefits of research participation (e.g., socialization of the child in the values of altruism).

2003). That is, they do not match the intensity and specificity of their review of consent documents and processes to the risk presented by the research. The recommendations at the end of this chapter suggest some ways to direct investigator and IRB attention to the *process* of seeking parents' and children's agreement to research participation.

The focus on forms also reflects, in part, the concerns of research institutions and sponsors about litigation that might cite omitted information or other alleged deficiencies in consent forms. This concern is evident in the legal tone of many consent, permission, and assent forms, which include terminology that is unfamiliar and potentially intimidating to many. Such language may satisfy the "informed" aspect of consent but limit a prospective research participant's true understanding of the proposed research. Again, the focus should be on the process, and the forms should support that process.

Although failures of comprehension about any major element of research participation raise ethical concerns, a particular concern is whether prospective research participants understand that they will be participating in research and that the purpose of research differs from the purpose of normal clinical care. The purpose of research is to generate knowledge, usually for the benefit of patients or individuals in the future. The belief that the purpose of research is treatment is termed the *therapeutic misconception* (Appelbaum et al., 1982).[3]

In some cases, the description of an area of research may encourage this misconception. For example, Churchill and colleagues (1998) and Lysaught (1998) have made this argument about the labeling of gene transfer research as "gene therapy." As discussed in Chapter 1, references to "therapeutic" and "nontherapeutic" research may likewise contribute to misperceptions that the purpose of clinical trials is individual clinical care. Referring instead to research interventions or procedures as having or not having the prospect of direct benefit may help reduce misunderstandings.

King (2000) has argued that the threat that participants will misunder-

---

[3]Research participants may also expect that being in a clinical trial may provide them benefits in the form of more information about their condition and closer monitoring than they would otherwise receive. A recent analysis of studies that compared the outcomes of patients participating or not participating in cancer clinical trials reported that "there are insufficient data to conclude" that enrollment in clinical trials leads to improved outcomes (a "trial effect") (Peppercorn et al., 2004, p. 263). Although the results were more favorable for pediatric cancer trials than for adult cancer trials, the article emphasized the significant limitations in the quality of the data; it did not single out these trials as an exception to the general conclusion. That is, until better data are available to support a trial effect, "patients with cancer should be encouraged to enroll in clinical trials on the basis of trials' unquestioned role in improving treatment of future patients" (p. 263).

stand the purpose of research is large enough that IRBs should devote more attention to the description of potential benefits in the consent process. King argues, for example, that IRBs should require a statement in consent forms that benefit is not expected in early-stage studies, unless the investigators can make a good case for a reasonable prospect of direct benefit. King also argues that in consent forms the introductory discussion of what a study hopes to prove may mislead participants who are eager to receive treatment that will improve their lives. In addition, one of the anonymous reviewers of this report observed that in his long experience, protocols for clinical trials do not always clearly distinguish between the potential benefits or harms generally associated for treatment of a disease and the potential benefits and harms specific to the intervention being tested.

In an analysis of the therapeutic misconception, Dresser observed that patient advocacy groups "often portray study participation as the way to obtain cutting-edge therapy" (Dresser, 2003, p. 240; see also, Dresser, 2001). Dresser suggested that exaggerated expectations about research benefits not only can undermine informed decision making by individuals but also can diminish social activism that promotes better access to existing beneficial care (also see, more generally, Callahan, 2003).

When research includes medical procedures or interventions, clinical investigators have the obligation to provide them as carefully and as competently as they would in usual care situations. Nonetheless, to protect the validity of the research and its potential to create knowledge that will benefit future patients, certain elements in a research protocol (e.g., random assignment to an experimental or control group and blinding of investigators to the experimental or control group) typically limit how much a particular patient's care may be individualized to better meet that patient's best interest. "The opportunities for [clinical] choice disappear when neither the health care professional nor the subject plays a role in deciding on treatment" (Lidz and Appelbaum, 2002, p. V-57). This underscores the importance of helping prospective research participants understand what participation in the research will and will not involve and what limitations the research protocol will impose on practitioner and participant decisions about treatment.

Legal Requirements for Permission and Assent

General

The concept and practice of informed consent have evolved as much through the judicial route as through the ethical route. For the most part, however, courts have focused on informed consent to clinical care, not research participation. The term *informed consent* itself gained currency

BOX 5.1
Selected Regulatory Provisions for Informed Consent That Also Apply Generally to Parental Permission for a Child's Participation in Research

Except as provided elsewhere in this policy, no investigator may involve a human being as a subject in research covered by this policy unless the investigator has obtained the legally effective informed consent of the subject or the subject's legally authorized representative. An investigator shall seek such consent only under circumstances that provide the prospective subject or the representative sufficient opportunity to consider whether or not to participate and that minimize the possibility of coercion or undue influence. The information that is given to the subject or the representative shall be in language understandable to the subject or the representative. No informed consent, whether oral or written, may include any exculpatory language through which the subject or the representative is made to waive or appear to waive any of the subject's legal rights, or releases or appears to release the investigator, the sponsor, the institution or its agents from liability for negligence.

(a) Basic elements of informed consent. Except as provided in paragraph (c) or (d) of this section, in seeking informed consent the following information shall be provided to each subject:

(1) a statement that the study involves research, an explanation of the purposes of the research and the expected duration of the subject's participation, a description of the procedures to be followed, and identification of any procedures which are experimental;
(2) a description of any reasonably foreseeable risks or discomforts to the subject;
(3) a description of any benefits to the subject or to others which may reasonably be expected from the research;
(4) a disclosure of appropriate alternative procedures or courses of treatment, if any, that might be advantageous to the subject;

following a 1957 court case in which the court held that physicians had the duty to disclose "any facts which are necessary to form the basis of an intelligent consent by the patient to proposed treatment" (*Salgo v. Stanford Jr.*, 1957).

Aside from the direction provided by the Nuremberg tribunal, legislators and regulators, rather than judges, have been the major source of requirements for consent to research participation. As described in Chapter 1, the 1962 amendments to the Federal Food, Drug, and Cosmetic Act (P.L. 87-781) included requirements for informed consent from those participating in research involving investigational new drugs "except where it is not feasible or it is contrary to the best interests of such human beings" (21 USC 355(i)(4)). In 1966, the U.S. Surgeon General significantly expanded

(5) a statement describing the extent, if any, to which confidentiality of records identifying the subject will be maintained;

(6) for research involving more than minimal risk, an explanation as to whether any compensation and an explanation as to whether any medical treatments are available if injury occurs and, if so, what they consist of, or where further information may be obtained;

(7) an explanation of whom to contact for answers to pertinent questions about the research and research subjects' rights, and whom to contact in the event of a research-related injury to the subject; and

(8) a statement that participation is voluntary, refusal to participate will involve no penalty or loss of benefits to which the subject is otherwise entitled, and the subject may discontinue participation at any time without penalty or loss of benefits to which the subject is otherwise entitled.

(b) Additional elements of informed consent. When appropriate, one or more of the following elements of information shall also be provided to each subject:

(1) a statement that the particular treatment or procedure may involve risks to the subject (or to the embryo or fetus, if the subject is or may become pregnant) which are currently unforeseeable;

(2) anticipated circumstances under which the subject's participation may be terminated by the investigator without regard to the subject's consent;

(3) any additional costs to the subject that may result from participation in the research;

(4) the consequences of a subject's decision to withdraw from the research and procedures for orderly termination of participation by the subject;

(5) statement that significant new findings developed during the course of the research which may relate to the subject's willingness to continue participation will be provided to the subject; and

(6) the approximate number of subjects involved in the study.

SOURCES: 45 CFR 46.116 and 46.408. FDA regulations are at 21 CFR 50.25 and 50.55

requirements for informed consent in clinical research funded by U.S. Public Health Service grants. Government officials provided more explicit guidance and direction in subsequent years, notably, in 1981 U.S. Department of Health and Human Services (DHHS) regulations that remain in place today.

The regulatory language concerning informed consent is fairly detailed. Box 5.1 includes the main provisions that apply by reference to parental permission for a child's participation in research. Statements from the regulations often appear verbatim in instructions to clinical investigators and in consent forms (see, e.g., NIH, 2000a). Some studies have, however, documented discrepancies between the elements required and the elements actually found in consent forms (White et al., 1996; Silverman et al., 2001).

Parental Permission

Federal regulations usually require that parents provide permission for a child's participation in research (45 CFR 46.408; 21 CFR 50.55). (Consistent with earlier chapters, the text refers to the regulations that apply to federally conducted or supported research as DHHS regulations to distinguish them from the similar but not identical FDA regulations.) As discussed further below, the regulations define children with reference to state laws establishing the legal age for consent to the treatments or procedures involved in the research. In general, the rules for informed consent listed in Box 5.1 also apply to permission. That is, parents or guardians are to be provided the same kinds of information and disclosures that would be provided to adults consenting to research in their own right. The regulations define parents as biological or adoptive. A guardian is someone who is appointed by a court and who can authorize medical care for a child.

Both parents must provide permission for the child to be included in research when research involves greater than minimal risk and does not hold out the prospect of direct benefit to the child. The regulations allow exceptions when one parent is dead, incompetent, not reasonably available, or not legally responsible for the child's care. In these situations, permission from one parent will suffice.

Waiver of Parental Permission

Under certain circumstances when parental permission is not a reasonable requirement to protect a child, the DHHS regulations allow an IRB to waive parental permission—provided that an appropriate mechanism for protecting the child is substituted and the action is consistent with federal, state, and local laws (45 CFR 46.408(c)). As an example of a situation in which a waiver might be appropriate, the regulations cite only situations involving neglected or abused children. The National Commission for the Protection of Human Subjects of Biomedical and Behavioral Research (hereafter, the National Commission) mentioned several other circumstances in which parental or guardian permission might be waived, including when parents are incompetent to provide permission, when the research involves conditions for which state laws allow adolescents to be treated without parental consent, or when the research involves mature adolescents and only minimal risk (National Commission, 1977).

The DHHS regulations do not describe what additional protective procedures might be appropriate if parental permission is waived but only state that the choice will "depend upon the nature and purpose of the activities described in the protocol, the risk and anticipated benefit to the research subjects, and their age, maturity, status, and condition" (45 CFR 26.408(c)). One option is to appoint an independent research monitor or participant advocate. His or her role would be to verify the adolescent's understanding of the research and the assent process, determine that the agreement to participate is voluntary, and document the basis for the waiver of parental permission. If another adult (e.g., a grandparent) is knowledgeable and involved with the minor, the advocate might also seek that person's views. Other protective strategies are described later in this chapter.

In a departure from DHHS regulations, the regulations of the Food and Drug Administration (FDA) do not allow the waiver of parental permission, even when it is not a reasonable requirement to protect the child (FDA, 2001b). FDA has argued that its statute does not permit such a waiver. As noted earlier, the statute governing FDA requires the consent of those to whom investigational drugs are being administered (or their representatives) except when it is not feasible or is contrary an individual's best interests. In the committee's view, this language allows for waivers consistent with DHHS regulations.

A recommendation presented later in this chapter urges that FDA bring its policies on waiver of parental permission into agreement with those governing research conducted or supported by DHHS. It also urges FDA, the National Institutes of Health (NIH), and the Office for Human Research Protections (OHRP) to cooperate to define more explicitly the factors that should be considered in waiver decisions and the safeguards that are appropriate for different situations when parental permission is waived.

Although not limited to research involving children, OHRP (then called the Office for Protection from Research Risks) and FDA have since 1996 provided for waivers of consent or permission when research involves certain emergency situations (Ellis and Lin, 1996; 45 CFR 46.116(c) and (d); FDA, 1996b; 21 CFR 50.24). A detailed set of requirements must be met and documented before a waiver can be approved. For example, "the subjects are in a life-threatening situation, available treatments are unproven or unsatisfactory, and the collection of valid scientific evidence, which may include evidence obtained through randomized placebo-controlled investigations, is necessary to determine the safety and effectiveness of particular interventions" (21 CFR 50.24(a)(1)); "[t]here is no reasonable way to identify prospectively the individuals likely to become eligible for participation in the clinical investigation" (21 CFR 50.24(a)(2)(iii)); and "participation in the research holds out the prospect of direct benefit to the subjects" (21 CFR 50.24(a)(3)). In addition to IRB review, draft regulatory guidance from FDA specifies a process of community consultation and public disclosure (FDA, 2000a). The committee learned that at least one proposal for FDA approval of research under these regulations was being prepared under the auspices of the Pediatric Emergency Care Applied Research Network (James Chamberlain, M.D., Children's National Medical Center, personal communication, October 13, 2003).

Children's Assent

Although decisional capacity develops through childhood and even into adulthood, practical and policy considerations have led policymakers to require, in most cases, that individuals achieve a specified age (the "age of majority") before they can enter into contracts, consent to medical care, and make other crucial decisions in their own right. State policies are important for clinical research because federal regulations on human research protections define children as "persons who have not attained the legal age for consent to treatments or procedures involved in the research, under the applicable law of the jurisdiction in which the research will be conducted" (45 CFR 46.402; 21 CFR 50.3(o)). As described below, minors (those who have not achieved the age of majority) can still be held competent to consent to medical treatments under certain circumstances.

Consistent with recommendations in the National Commission's 1977 report, federal regulations generally require assent to research participation from children judged capable of providing it. They define *assent* as "a child's affirmative agreement to participate in research" and also state that "[m]ere failure to object should not, absent affirmative agreement, be construed as assent" (45 CFR 46.402(b); 21 CFR 50.3(n)). Assent is not, however, required if an IRB concludes that the research has the prospect of directly benefiting the child and that potential benefit is available only in the research context (45 CFR 46.405; 21 CFR 50.52). Assent may also be waived under the same conditions in which adult's informed consent may be waived.

The federal regulations do not specify an age at which IRBs should expect investigators to begin to seek assent from children. Rather, IRBs are to consider the ages, maturity, and psychological state of the prospective research participants. In the committee's experience, most IRBs require investigators to seek assent from children over the age of 6 or 7 years. The judgment about assent may apply to all the children who are to participate in a study or to each child individually. As discussed later in this chapter, the assent process for older adolescents may differ little from the process for seeking informed consent if that consent process is suitably structured. Thus, investigators would provide the same kinds of information as is required for adults.

The regulations permit oral presentation of assent information and allow discretion on the part of the IRB about the way assent is documented (45 CFR 46.117 (c)(2) and 45 CFR 46.408 (e); 21 CFR 50.55(g)). FDA guidance on pediatric drug research (developed by the International Conference on Harmonisation [ICH]) provides that "[p]articipants of *appropriate intellectual maturity* should personally sign and date either a separately designed, written assent form or the written informed consent" (FDA, 2000b, p. 19781, emphasis added). Although the ICH guidance puts more stress on getting a signature than do the federal regulations, the guidance also allows discretion.

The regulations do not describe what information is to be presented as part of the assent process. In general, the type and amount of information presented should be adapted to the child's cognitive and emotional status and experiences.

The process of involving children in research typically involves a progression of assessments that combine acknowledgement of the child's vulnerability with respect for the child's developing maturity (Fisher, 2003; Kodish, 2003a). IRBs must first decide whether the research is approvable under federal regulations and that it includes appropriate processes for requesting parental permission and child assent. For approved protocols, parents usually then decide whether participation in the research is appropriate given their child's characteristics and experiences. If parents agree, the child decides whether the research, *as he or she understands it*, is an activity in which he or she wishes to participate. Particularly with young children, whose decisional capacities may fluctuate with fatigue and irritability, it may be reasonable—as part of a respectful and noncoercive assent process and with parental agreement—for investigators to come back to a child who says "no" to see whether he or she may feel differently later. Depending on the child's age, the nature of the research, and the investigator's perspectives on involving children, the discussion about research participation may start with the parents or may include the child from the outset.

Emancipated and Mature Minors

Even when individuals have not reached the age of majority, states provide, under certain circumstances, that they may consent to medical treatment without parental agreement. Appendix B describes state policies (including court decisions) in more detail. It makes clear that most states have no explicit provisions about a minor's agreement to participation in research without parental consent. (See also, English and Kenney, 2003.)

In most states, minors can become *emancipated* and attain legal majority through certain actions, which usually include marriage, enlistment in the military, or being self-supporting and living independently. Although the terminology or label used in different states varies, emancipated minors can make decisions as if they had reached the age of majority. They thus can provide informed consent to medical treatment in their own right. Emancipation sometimes requires a court order.

In addition, states permit minors to consent to treatment for certain problems (e.g., drug or substance abuse or sexually transmitted disease) without parental permission. In many states, the statutes allowing such treatment also forbid the health care provider from billing the parent, lest confidentiality be breached. A number of states have general consent statutes that permit minors to consent to medical or surgical treatment at a specified age; usually it is age 16 years but in some states it is as young as 14 years. Furthermore, the jurisprudence in many other states has accepted the "mature minor" rule, in which a minor who is subjectively assessed as capable of giving the same degree of informed consent as an adult may be treated without a parent's involvement. In some states, minors who are parents may be in the paradoxical position of being able to permit treatment on behalf of their child but not on their own behalf.

Again, as Appendix B explains, statutes and case law rarely refer specifically to decisions by minors about participation in research. Because state laws are so variable and often vague, investigators and IRBs must be knowledgeable about federal, state, and local laws related to consent, confidentiality, and related matters when they consider research that involves waiver of parental permission. Differences among state policies could complicate certain studies involving sites in more than one state and might preclude the inclusion of certain sites. In addition to seeking legal counsel, investigators and IRBs may find it prudent to consult representatives from communities that might be affected by the proposed research and to consider the climate in the state regarding parental prerogatives. As emphasized earlier, federal regulations require that appropriate protective procedures be in place if parental permission for research participation is to be waived.

Wards of the State

Responding in part to some of the abuses and controversies described in Chapter 1, federal regulations impose special conditions for research participation by children who are wards of the state. Although the DHHS regulations do not define the term *ward*, the interim regulations issued by FDA define a *ward* as "a child who is placed in the legal custody of the State or other agency, institution, or entity, consistent with applicable, Federal, State, or local law" (21 CFR 50.3(q)). When the state assumes the role of parent for these children, it may still defer to the child's biological parent(s) if the custody is temporary.

For research that involves more than minimal risk and that does not hold the prospect of direct benefit to the child participant, IRBs can approve research involving a ward of the state only under specific circumstances. These are when the proposed study (1) is related to the child's status as a ward or (2) is conducted in settings such as schools or hospitals where the majority of children participating in the study are not wards. When such research is approved, each child must have an independent, competent appointed advocate (in addition to any other appointed guardian). If a minor is under detention by the state, the provisions of Subpart C of the DHHS regulations, which govern research involving prisoners, may also apply.

As discussed in Appendix B, state policies on research participation by wards of the state rarely appear to be codified in statute or clear case law. Rather, state agencies responsible for these children often appear to have little formal, written guidance for making decisions. As a consequence, investigators likewise may have little guidance beyond the federal regulations. Some states appear to be much more restrictive than others in permitting wards to be included in research and may thereby discourage research that might increase understanding of this population of vulnerable children.

RESEARCH RELEVANT TO PARENTS' COMPREHENSION OF CHILDREN'S PARTICIPATION IN RESEARCH

It's a lot easier to make a decision for yourself rather than for somebody else . . . you just don't know if you've done the right thing.

Parent (quoted in Caldwell et al., 2003, p. 557)

The literature on adults' understanding of and decisions about their own participation in research is considerably more extensive than the corresponding literature on parents making decisions about their child's participation in research. The committee believes that findings about the reasoning that adults use and the decisions that adults make on their own behalf are generally relevant to an understanding of decisions that adults make on behalf of children. It recognizes, however, that the anxieties associated with making decisions on behalf of one's child, especially one's sick child, may put particular stress on an adult's comprehension, reasoning, and decision-making capacities (Ruccione et al., 1991; Levi et al., 2000; McGrath, 2002). Some research findings about informed consent for clinical care are also relevant to the research context, although the ethical and informational requirements are usually more stringent for informed consent in the context of research.

What should parents be able to understand to make an informed decision about their child's participation in research? In general, parents of prospective research participants should have a basic understanding of

- the purposes of the research and what procedures (medical and otherwise) that the child will undergo (or may undergo, if random assignment to treatment and control groups is planned);

- the potential consequences of the child's research participation, including the likelihood, significance, and duration of possible harms and benefits;
- their right to accept or refuse research participation and to withdraw the child from a study once it has started;
- their responsibilities as the parents of a child participating in research and the child's responsibilities (if any); and
- the responsibilities of investigators to parents and children, including answering questions, maintaining the confidentiality of data, minimizing the risks of participation, and providing information about study findings.

If the child has a medical condition, certain additional areas of understanding are also important when participation in a clinical trial is proposed. Parents considering an ill or "at-risk" child's participation in a clinical trial should understand

- their child's medical condition and prognosis;
- the difference between receiving usual clinical care and participating in a trial;
- their child's options for care (e.g., standard treatment, monitoring, or hospice care) outside the trial;
- the research methods, including, if applicable, methods for assigning research participants to intervention or control groups; and
- the potential harms and benefits for the child of participating or not participating in the trial, given the child's medical status and prognosis.

The following discussion looks first at the general literature relevant to adult's comprehension of research participation. It then considers some research specific to parents' decision making on behalf of their child. The research literature supports increased attention to the *process* of seeking parental permission. It also supports a recognition that decision making about research participation—whether on one's own behalf or that of another—is an imperfect process.

General

Reading Levels, Readability, and Informed Consent and Permission Forms

Consent and permission forms are only one element of a meaningful process of parental decision making about a child's participation in research. Nonetheless, to the extent that the forms fail to assist parents in making decisions because they are not easily comprehended, this failure constitutes an important deficit in the informed consent and permission process. In principle, investigators can compensate for some shortcomings in consent forms as they talk with people and explore their understanding of research participation. In reality, little is known about these conversations, including whether they can compensate for deficient consent forms. Although forms should not be the main focus of the consent and permission process, the exercise of developing a clear, readable, and informative consent document can contribute to the design and implementation of a clear, understandable, and constructive process for seeking informed consent or permission.

Research institutions and IRBs typically provide the same forms and related guidance for studies that involve adults making decisions about their own participation in research and for studies that have parents making decisions about their child's participation. Study after study has found that the consent forms for medical treatment or research participation typically require high levels of education or, at least, levels of education higher than the average for key patient or study populations (e.g., low-income patients) (see, e.g., Ogloff and Otto, 1991; Rivera et al., 1992: Grossman et al., 1994; Hopper et al, 1995, 1998; Goldstein et al., 1996; and Paasche-Orlow et al., 2003). This is a serious problem given, that surveys suggest that more than one-fifth of adults in the United States have very limited literacy skills and that another quarter have seriously limited skills (Kirsch et al., 1993).

Consistent with other studies of consent forms for adults, one analysis of forms for the parents of prospective child participants in an array of biomedical research studies at a single hospital found that forms were written at the college-graduate level (Tarnowski et al., 1990). The researchers also found that forms had gotten longer but not more readable over a 10-year period.

Another study of institutional consent forms (for clinical care) and vaccine information pamphlets intended for parents reported that the forms generally required a reading level of 12th grade or above and the pamphlets required an 11th-grade reading level or higher (Davis et al., 1990). In reality, the inner-city parents at the investigators' institution had a median reading level just below the seventh grade. A second study with the same lead author assessed educational materials from the American Academy of Pediatrics, the Centers for Disease Control and Prevention, and other sources. It found that parents at the outpatient pediatric clinic tested at a seventh- to eighth-grade reading level but that 80 percent of the educational materials required at least a 10th-grade reading level (Davis et al., 1994).

Unfortunately, efforts to make consent forms more readable have their limitations. The authors of one recent analysis of consent forms concluded,

"IRBs commonly provide text for informed-consent forms that falls short of their own readability standards" (Passche-Orlow et al., 2003, p. 721). Nonetheless, the authors concluded that the sample text provided by some IRBs indicated that forms could be written clearly and simply at a fourth-grade level and still provide essential information.

An earlier analysis by Hammerschmidt and Keane (1992) reported that IRB review of consent forms usually did not improve their readability levels. Furthermore, after a simplified consent form was compared with the standard consent form for a clinical oncology trials group, researchers found that participant comprehension was essentially the same for the two forms, although nearly all participants found the simplified form more readable (Davis et al., 1990; 1994; 1998; see also Duffy and Kabance, 1982; Charrow, 1988; and Taylor et al., 1998).

A recent randomized clinical trial of an easy-to-read consent statement for several cancer treatment trials concluded that documents could be simplified without omitting important information (Coyne et al., 2003). Such documents could increase patient satisfaction and reduce the anxiety associated with the consent process. (The authors noted that participants in their study tested at an average literacy level at or above ninth grade, higher than might be found in many research contexts.)

Evaluations of consent forms often focus on quantitative "grade-level" measures of readability, but other aspects of written forms should also be considered.[4] These include the logical flow of ideas, the organization of headings and subheadings, type style and size, page layout, the helpful use of graphics, and cultural and linguistic appropriateness or adaptations. Actual comprehension of the text may depend not only on the characteristics of the text and the level of literacy of the individual, but also on other individual characteristics, such as motivation to learn, interest in the material, and experience with the subject matter.

The National Cancer Institute has developed guidelines for researcher design and use of consent forms and has also provided a template to serve as the basis for devising forms for specific protocols (NCI, 2001). In general, the development of templates (informed by evidence about adult learning and comprehension of information about research participation) is a useful step, especially for studies conducted at multiple sites. As discussed elsewhere in this report, local IRBs may modify consent forms in ways that

---

[4]Assessments of readability typically rely on formulas that are convenient but that may have a number of limitations (see, e.g., Duffy, 1985; and Baker et al., 1988). The simplest formulas usually involve counts of the numbers of letters or syllables used in words and the number of words used in sentences, on the basis of the assumption that longer means more complex. For texts about medical topics, however, even short words (e.g., shunt and lesion) may be unfamiliar. Some formulas take familiarity into account.

compromise the research and the practical purposes of having a common form for multicenter studies. Local modifications may sometimes be appropriate for local study populations, however.

Presentation of Quantitative Information

Just as the readability of research consent and permission forms may affect parent's comprehension, so may the way in which information about the probability of potential harms and potential benefits of research participation is presented. The committee found no studies that assessed the quantitative information provided to prospective research participants or to the parents of prospective research participants. Some studies in other areas, including medical decision making, are generally relevant.

A number of studies indicate that adults often have considerable difficulties accurately understanding and using quantitative information (see, e.g., the review by Stanovich and West, 2000). Several studies also indicate that the manner in which quantitative and other information is presented can affect accurate understanding of the likelihood of harms and can also influence an individual's choices (Edwards et al., 2001). For example, studies of people's understanding of quantitative information about the outcomes of medical screening (e.g., mammograms) suggest that they find frequency information (e.g., a 4 in 1,000 chance of an event) more understandable than probabilities (e.g., a 0.04 percent chance) (Gigerenzer, 1996). Information presented in relative terms (e.g., a 50 percent increase or decrease in some outcome) tends to be more "persuasive" than information presented in absolute terms (e.g., decrease from 2 in 10,000 to 1 in 10,000) (Forrow et al., 1992; Malenka et al., 1993; Ransohoff and Harris, 1997).

Other research suggests that framing quantitative information about possible outcomes in positive terms (e.g., a 3-in-4 chance of improvement or survival) rather than negative terms (e.g., a 1-in-4 chance of deterioration or death) may encourage individuals to choose less risky options (see, e.g., Rothman et al., 1993, Rothman and Salovey, 1997; see also, Llewellyn-Thomas et al., 1995; McGettigan et al., 1999). Increasing the number of options or the number of negative outcomes discussed can produce unexpected shifts in people's choices, at least, in hypothetical situations (Ubel, 2002). Finally, although it is tempting and common to substitute verbal descriptions for numerical descriptions, research indicates that people vary in their interpretation of qualitative expressions such as "rare" or "most" (see, e.g., Sutherland et al., 1991; Mazur and Merz, 1994; Cohn et al., 1995; Man-Son-Hing et al., 2002; Mazur and Hickam, 1991). Providing quantitative descriptions of probabilities (e.g., a 1-in-4 chance) rather than or in addition to verbal descriptions (e.g., a moderately low chance) may reduce inconsistency in the interpretation of risk information and encourage more deliberative thinking.

A considerable body of research considers people's reasoning and decision-making capacities more generally. Much of this research describes deficiencies in people's reasoning capacities, for example, selectively focusing on information that supports one's views (Stanovich and West, 2000). This underscores the importance of a careful process for helping prospective research participants reach decisions.

Comprehension of Research Purposes

> *In the end, it is only the benefit of furthering knowledge that can be honestly guaranteed to a potential research subject.*
> Advisory Committee on Human Radiation Experiments,
> 1995, p. 476

Most research evaluating people's understanding of the difference between research and usual clinical care has involved adults consenting to research participation in their own right. It generally indicates that avoiding or overcoming the therapeutic misconception can be a formidable challenge. As Appelbaum and colleagues (1982) observed many years ago about participants in psychiatric research, "subjects' ability to distort small aspects of the study design often had the effect of maintaining their therapeutic misconceptions, while they gave the appearance of having a good general understanding of the study" (p. 328).

Other studies also suggest that research participants may have difficulty understanding the purpose of research (see, e.g., Yuval et al., 2000 and Daugherty et al., 1995). When Edwards and colleagues (1998) reviewed 61 studies about attitudes toward clinical trials, they found that people mentioned self-interest more often than altruism as the reason for participating in trials. (Often, however, the specific questions and methods were not fully enough described to provide a clear picture of the results.) They also cited three studies from the 1990s that reported a near majority or majority of physicians believed that research participants did not understand the information given them or realize that they were participating in research.

Several studies suggest that research participants frequently have expectations of benefit, even in clinical trials that test safety but not efficacy (see, e.g., Daugherty et al., 1995; Schutta and Burnett, 2000; Meropol et al., 2003; and Weinfurt et al., 2003). Likewise, although they may understand and approve the knowledge-generating purpose of research in general, participants may view their own participation in research primarily in terms of benefit to themselves (Cassileth et al., 1982; Bevan et al., 1993; Wilcox and Schroer, 1994; Aby et al., 1996; Hutchison, 1998; Yoder et al., 1997; Cheng et al., 2000; Madsen et al., 2000). Individual reactions to randomization and placebo-controlled trials suggest a tendency to view the intervention arm of a trial as desirable or beneficial (see, e.g., Snowdon et al., 1997; Fallowfield et al., 1998; and Welton et al., 1999).

A survey and interviews conducted by the Advisory Committee on Human Radiation Experiments (ACHRE) produced a number of interesting findings about people's understanding of research participation (ACHRE, 1995).[5] The survey involved more than 1800 patients at 19 health care institutions across the country. A third of those surveyed believed that patients who participated in medical research usually or always benefited medically compared with those who did not. About two-thirds of the patients who had participated in research indicated that they had done so to obtain better treatment; a similar percentage reported that being in research gave them hope. Results from 103 in-depth interviews were generally consistent with the survey findings. The researchers, however, reported that patients who had been in diagnostic, epidemiologic, or survey research were more likely to differentiate between research and treatment than those who had participated in studies testing a potentially therapeutic intervention.

About three-quarters of those surveyed for ACHRE indicated a desire to help others or advance scientific knowledge. Suggesting that this altruistic motivation should be "tapped explicitly" when investigators are recruiting research participants, the ACHRE report explains that such an emphasis might reduce the potential for research to be misunderstood by underscoring "for patients that the primary objective of research is to create generalizable scientific knowledge" (ACHRE, 1995, p. 476).

Patients considering research participation may not necessarily anticipate improvement in their condition from the intervention being tested, but they may expect to receive better diagnostic evaluation, closer medical monitoring and follow-up, and more information about their condition (Mattson et al., 1985; ACHRE, 1995; Yoder et al., 1997; Madsen et al., 2000). For example, for Danish patients in a trial of interventions for inflammatory bowel disease, an important reason for participating in the research was "the expectation of being 'a special patient' during the trial" (Madsen et al., 2000, p. 463).

---

[5]The survey also had some interesting findings on patient interpretations of terms used to describe research, specifically, medical research, clinical trial, clinical investigation, medical study, and medical experiment. The last term, medical experiment, produced the strongest negative associations. Respondents thought patients in medical experiments were at higher risk and were likely to fare worse than patients in medical research. Although patients in medical research were viewed as being at greater risk and more likely to get unproven treatments than those in clinical investigations or clinical trials, they were thought to be more likely to benefit medically. The term medical study was viewed more positively than medical research, perhaps because it seemed to suggest research involving records and not patients.

Implications

Although more studies of ways to present qualitative and quantitative information about research are needed, the research summarized above provides some guidance to investigators on how they can prepare to discuss a child's research participation with parents. It suggests that documents to support the permission process can often be written at a simpler level than is customary, although investigators and IRBs should still be aware that more readable information and forms do not guarantee better understanding of research participation. A number of research institutions and IRBs set an eighth-grade reading level as the target for written materials, but as discussed earlier, a target of a sixth-grade reading level may benefit many parents and other adults as long as essential information can still be accurately presented.

Research about the comprehension of quantitative information suggests that investigators should present estimates of potential harms and benefits using frequencies rather than (or in addition to) probabilities and using absolute terms rather than (or in addition to) relative terms. They should not rely on qualitative descriptions of potential harms and benefits but should include quantitative descriptions or estimates to the extent possible. Strategies for communicating about potential harms and benefits of research should consider characteristics of study populations as well as individual variability in education levels, experiences, and other characteristics.

The general findings summarized above underscore, again, the importance of focusing on consent and permission as a process. That process should include discussion and time for questions. It should also, depending on the study, provide for a tactful assessment of the prospective participant's understanding of research purposes, potential harms and benefits, voluntary participation, and other key information.

Research on Parents' Decisions About a Child's Participation in Research

> *We didn't have time to think.*
> Mother of child with cancer (quoted by Pletsch and Stevens, 2001, p. 57)

> *Most parents . . . don't know anything beyond their current crisis, and they are trusting in the physician to carry them through.*
> Nancy Sander, family advocate, 2003

Several studies have explored factors associated with parents' decisions to involve their child in research. Many involved small numbers of parents of limited sociodemographic diversity. Some studies involved validated survey or interview instruments; others apparently did not. Publications did not always report quantitative information on parents' responses, and some relied on quotes from parents that conveyed views vividly without providing a clear sense of how representative those views were.

A few studies included both parents who permitted their child's enrollment in research and parents who did not, but most included only parents who had agreed to participation. A number of studies included at least some parents of children with serious illnesses or at risk of such illnesses. Several studies were conducted in other countries, mainly in Canada, Australia, and Western European nations. Differences in cultures, research practices, and health care norms could limit the relevance of these studies to the United States.

Reasons for Permitting or Not Permitting a Child's Participation in Research

Some studies suggest that many parents (like many adults making decisions in their own right) view research as an opportunity to gain additional access to care and information about their child's condition and treatment. In a Washington State study, 44 parents who had agreed to their child's participation in an asthma study completed a questionnaire about their motives (Rothmier et al., 2003). The authors concluded that "[a]lthough altruistic motives are present in pediatric asthma research, most parents/ guardians gave consent for their child to learn more about their child's asthma" (p. 1037). Access to the newest drugs and relationships with staff were also positive factors. Parents with lower family incomes were more likely to respond that access to free medications was a factor in their decision.

Of 181 Dutch parents who agreed to their child's participation in a study of ibuprofen for the prevention of seizures, approximately one-third reported an expected benefit to their child as the reason for agreeing (van Stuijvenberg et al., 1998). Slightly more than half cited a desire to contribute to science as a motivation for agreeing to their child's participation. Two-thirds of the parents reported that they saw no disadvantages to their child's participation in the research.

Hayman and colleagues (2001) surveyed 94 New Zealand parents who agreed (69 percent response rate) and 103 who declined (47 percent response rate) to enroll their child in a physiological study (without a prospect of direct benefit) related to sudden infant death syndrome. All those who participated reported doing so for altruistic reasons. Just over a quarter of these parents were initially concerned about safety issues but no longer expressed concern after the study. Of the parents who declined to participate, about half cited inconvenience and a quarter cited safety concerns.

In a study that included both parents who agreed (*n* = 221) and parents who did not agree (*n* = 208) to enter their infant in a randomized clinical trial of pertussis vaccine, Canadian researchers concluded that altruistic motivations (a desire to contribute to medical knowledge and to help others) were major factors contributing to parents' willingness to enter their infants into the trial (Langley et al., 1998). The involvement of the family physician was also important to a majority of those who agreed. Concerns about painful procedures and blood drawing were important to parents who did not agree to their child's participation.

Another group of Canadian investigators questioned parents who had agreed (*n* = 103) or declined (*n* = 37) to have their newborn infant included in one of three randomized, controlled clinical trials in a neonatal intensive care unit (Zupancic et al., 1997). (The response rates were between 80 and 85 percent for the two groups.) The researchers reported that parents giving permission for the infant's enrollment were more likely to see the research as probably benefiting their child and less likely to perceive it as risky than were parents not giving permission. Parents who allowed their infants to enter the study were also less likely to view the consent process as too complex, although only a minority in each group gave this response—10 percent of those who gave permission versus 22 percent of those who did not. Nearly all parents who gave permission believed that it was important for children to take part in research because it would help other children. A large majority (84 percent) of the parents who did not give permission also responded positively about the importance of research participation. The two groups did not differ significantly in socioeconomic characteristics.

In a study that included parents permitting and parents not permitting a child's participation in anesthesia research (168 and 78 parents, respectively), Tait and colleagues (1998) reported that parents who did not give permission cited fear for the child's safety and the potential risk to the child as the most important factors in their decision. Very few reported that a lack of understanding of the research was a factor, but 15 percent were concerned about having insufficient time to decide. None reported feeling pressured to agree. Parents who gave permission cited the importance of the research and the low risk to the child as key factors in their decision. The parents who allowed their children to enter the study were more likely to have a child who had participated in a previous study and to have read the consent form completely.

In a statement presented to the committee, a group representing parents of children with asthma noted that parents may simultaneously understand the importance of allowing children to participate in research and be reluctant to allow their own children to serve, in their words, as "guinea pigs"

(AANMA, 2003, p. 2). The statement cited a number of reasons for such reluctance, including concerns about safety, pain, and inconvenience (e.g., disruption of the children's routines and missed work by the parent).

In sum, research suggests that parents have various reasons for permitting their children to participate in research. Some may involve expectations of a direct treatment benefit or perceptions that research participation increases access to care and information. Altruistic motives figure in some parents' agreement to their children's participation in research, usually in studies involving no prospect of benefit. Parents not permitting a child's participation are more likely to cite concerns about safety and pain or discomfort than parents agreeing to participation.

Experience of Illness and Expectation of Benefit

> *There is never enough time . . . in those kinds of situations to make an "informed decision" [about research]. I think that to say . . . that either the parent or the patient is making an "informed decision" is not correct. . . . And, of course, we signed [the form] because that's what you do. . . . It's always at the worst time to be reading this type of material. . . . But parents aren't in control when they're doing this, nor is the child.*
>
> Joseph Lilly, parent, 2003

The circumstances under which parents face making a decision about a child's participation in research may have a profound effect on their ability to evaluate information, ask questions, and make reasoned assessment of the potential harms and potential benefits presented by the proposed research. In particular, the conditions for informed and reasoned choice are threatened when parents are confronting a new diagnosis of a life-threatening medical condition and a crisis situation in which immediate decisions are sought.

Pletsch and Stevens (2001) investigated the factors affecting initial decisions about research participation by mothers of children who had leukemia or diabetes. (The investigation was part of a larger study that also studied children's comprehension and perceptions of research participation, as discussed later in this chapter.) The authors concluded that "the boundaries between research and treatment were unclear or irrelevant" for many of the 24 mothers whose children had cancer (p. 59). The mothers described being in shock and not having time to think. The urgency of the threat to their child dominated their decision making. In contrast, the nine mothers of children with diabetes faced circumstances more supportive of informed decision making. They were more concerned about the risks of research for children whose condition had, for the time being at least, been stabilized. These mothers were able to clearly differentiate between their child's usual care and the research activities. Their families had had time to adjust, to some extent, to the diagnosis and did not confront the need for crisis-driven decision making about the participation of the child in research. They also had had time to develop some expertise in negotiating and working within the health care system.

Kodish and colleagues (1998) reported that pediatric cancer researchers believed that parents' "state of shock" was the major factor interfering with understanding of the participation decision (see also, Simon et al., 2001). These findings are consistent with those of other studies about parents' decision making about clinical care in the face of a child's cancer diagnosis. These studies point to a high state of parental anxiety and the frequent sense of not having a real choice (Ruccione et al., 1991; Hinds et al., 1996; Levi et al., 2000). Levi and colleagues (2000) reported that these stressed parents "did not verbalize distinctions between their understanding of their child's medical treatment, [and] research participation" (p. 3).

Deatrick and colleagues (2002) undertook a retrospective analysis of transcripts of interviews and other information related to an earlier study of decision making by parents (n = 21) of children with advanced cancer about the child's participation in phase 1 trials. All the families were facing situations in which all other treatments with curative intent had failed. More than half the parents (n = 13) reported that they had no choice; as one said, "you have to try everything . . . keep fighting to keep her here with me" (p. 118). As described by the researchers, the parents' expectations included "providing treatment, buying time for another therapy, working a miracle, being altruistic, and delaying death" (p. 117). Some parents were clear that they were hoping for a miracle. At least one parent spoke of the doctor's optimism about the drug as the deciding factor.

Using a combination of interviews and focus groups, Caldwell and colleagues (2003) studied 33 Australian parents whose children's health status ranged from healthy to seriously ill. The investigators reported that parents of ill children, some of whom were or had been involved in clinical trials, saw the greatest potential for direct or personal benefit from the trial. Not surprisingly, these parents were also more knowledgeable about trials. As viewed by one parent whose child had participated in a trial, children not participating were "missing out," whereas participating children were "getting the benefit" (p. 556). Parents of ill children were concerned about "blinded" studies that withheld information about the treatment that their child was receiving. Parents of children with cancer mentioned that they wanted to monitor medications because of past experience with medical errors. (The majority of parents approached by Caldwell and colleagues either declined outright to participate in the interviews or did not participate after indicating that they would.)

Differences between families with different experiences of illness were also reported by Geller and colleagues (2003). They interviewed 37 pairs of parents and children or adolescents about participation in genetic suscepti- bility research. During interviews that asked questions about research that might offer benefit, the parents from families with a history of breast cancer indicated that they would not allow their daughters to refuse participation in potentially beneficial research. In contrast, the parents with a family history of heart disease were more likely to talk about "overriding" the wishes of a child who wanted to participate in a study (p. 266). Parents in both groups strongly agreed that children should not be enrolled against their will in research intended only to gain knowledge.

In the study by Zupancic and colleagues (1997) cited earlier, the inves- tigators reported no differences in perceptions of severity of illness between parents who agreed and those who did not agree to their neonate's partici- pation in clinical trials in the intensive care unit. As described above, par- ents who agreed were more likely than parents who did not agree to believe that the trials would probably benefit their child and were less likely to believe that the trials were risky.

Overall, these studies point to the need for particular care in the design and review of processes for seeking parental permission for research that will involve seriously ill children and high-stress situations. Concerns about the inadequacy of current procedures have led to suggestions that the con- sent process be designed (and tested) as a "continuous" one that involves giving and then repeating information and explanations as research pro- ceeds (see, e.g., Allmark et al., 2003). When a study involves a discrete, one- time intervention and an urgent situation, this approach likely will not be relevant.

Involvement of Children in Discussions and Decisions

The committee found limited information on parent's views about the involvement of their child in discussions and decisions about the child's participation in clinical research. It likewise located little research on the dynamics of family relationships in decisions about research participation or on the consequences for family relationships of different strategies for conducting the permission and assent process.

Based on a questionnaire study of 100 pairs of parents and adolescents at children's hospitals, Sikand and colleagues (1997) reported that 57 per- cent of the adolescent-parent pairs agreed that parents' permission for an adolescent's participation in research was unnecessary for anonymous sur- veys. In other situations, the parents were consistently more likely to favor permission requirements. For example, 78 percent of the parents but only 59 percent of the adolescents favored parents' permission for blood testing for human immunodeficiency virus (HIV) infection, and 62 percent of parents but only 48 percent of teens supported parents' permission for face-to-face interviews. The researchers suggested further research with larger groups to identify factors associated with parent and adolescent views and differences.

In the Australian study by Caldwell and colleagues (2003) cited earlier in this chapter, the investigators reported that parents thought that children's preferences should be considered in decision making about participation in clinical trials. These parents said that they were prepared to let adolescents make decisions about trials involving quality-of-life interventions. They were not, however, prepared to let children or adolescents make the final decision about participating in clinical trials involving life-threatening conditions.

In a small study involving six parent and child pairs interviewed about hypothetical research scenarios, Rossi and colleagues (2003) have reported that parents sometimes but not always considered their child's wishes. No parent wanted the child to be approached for assent before the parent.

The study by Geller and colleagues (2003) cited earlier also found that most parents wanted to make the initial decision about their child's participation in research. When asked about a hypothetical research scenario, parents who were uncomfortable with the research varied in whether they would let the child know about the study. The parents and children differed in their views about how the consent process (i.e., the permission and assent process) should be structured, including whether the parents should be approached first and whether a facilitator should be involved in explaining the study to the family and answering questions. Parents' preferences were influenced by the child's age and the family's style of communication.

In a presentation to the committee, Kodish (2003a) reported that the parents he and his colleagues had interviewed were very clear that the parents and the clinicians should negotiate in advance a child's involvement in discussions and decisions about participation in cancer clinical trials. He also reported that parents were offended by the idea of having their comprehension tested after the consent conference, suggesting that an assessment of parent's comprehension needs to be tactful and discreet.

Independent of parent's attitudes about their children's involvement in discussions and decisions about research participation, it is appropriate to consider how children's involvement might affect the flow of information and the interaction between parents and investigators. Olechnowicz and colleagues (2002) evaluated 85 "informed consent" conferences, comparing those with the child present versus those with the child not present. Of the 34 conferences that concerned children over age 7 years, the child was present during 14. The investigators reported that parents asked fewer questions when the child was included in the conference. In addition, when the child was not present, clinicians were more likely to use quantitative descriptions of the child's prognosis (Kodish, 2003a). To the extent that asking questions is a key element in informative communication, this finding raises some concerns and points to an issue for further investigation.

Based on their findings, Geller and colleagues (2003) concluded that the challenges for researchers are both to assess family communication (especially to identify families that do not communicate well) and to "harness a spirit of connectedness while minimizing undue influences on children by parents or the researchers" (p. 269). The investigators argued for a model of shared decision making that, first, gave parents and children adequate time to ask questions, discuss views, and clarify preferences and, second, gave "children the opportunity to exercise their right to refuse participation without parental influence" (p. 270). The researchers also recommended further research to assess strategies to accommodate differences in parent and child characteristics and respect family relationships while still providing safeguards that give children a voice.

The committee agrees that more research would be helpful to understand parent and child views about children's participation in discussions and decisions about participation in research. It also encourages more research on the effects on communication of including children in initial discussions of research participation and, more generally, the effects of different ways of structuring the permission and assent process. Such research should help guide investigators and IRBs in developing procedures that both support parental roles and family relationships and provide for the developmentally appropriate and respectful involvement of children in discussions and decisions about research participation.

The Role of Physicians

Research findings are limited and somewhat mixed on parents' views of the physician's role in decision making about a child's participation in research. In the study by Zupancic and colleagues (1997) cited above, the investigators reported that one-third of parents (including those who did not agree to participation) agreed with the statement, "I would prefer to have the doctors advise me whether my baby should be in the study, rather than asking me to decide" (p. 3). Investigators in another Canadian study found that parents believed in the necessity of research but often believed that their own knowledge was limited, so they needed to depend on their baby's doctor (Singhal et al., 2002). A subsequent study, which involved a different group of parents from the same Canadian research site, found that when parents were explicitly asked who should make the decision about enrolling the newborn, nearly all parents rejected the option of having the physician decide (Burgess et al., 2003).

In his presentation to the committee, Kodish (2003a) reported that trust was an important theme in interviews with parents about their decisions on their child's participation in research. As expressed by one parent, "if I have to put my faith in a human, it has to be the doc. So, I have to trust her unconditionally." Nonetheless, although parents saw a clinician's presentation of participation in a clinical trial as an implicit recommendation, they wanted an explicit recommendation only upon their own request.

Reporting on a study of 64 Australian parents questioned after completion of a clinical trial, Harth and Thong (1995) found that 15 percent of parents viewed strict informed-consent procedures as unnecessary because they would follow the doctor's advice. A majority thought being in a hospital-based trial involved little or no risk, and few realized that the study was to assess safety as well as efficacy. Only one-third of the parents were aware that they could withdraw their child from the trial. These results suggest deficits in the consent and permission process, even if the parental bias is to rely on the doctor's advice.

In a study of decisions about cancer treatment (not research), Pyke-Grimm and colleagues (1999) studied the preferences of 58 Canadian parents about the role of physicians in decision making. They found that parents most preferred collaborative decision making between families and physicians, with a minority of participants preferring either a passive role (of parents) or active involvement. The investigators also reported that parents placed more emphasis on their needs for "concrete" information than on information about possible emotional or family consequences. Parents' views about their information needs were highly variable, which led the investigators to stress that the provision of information needed to be tailored to the individual families. This is possible in a well-designed consent and permission process.

In another study that examined parents' preferences for clinician involvement in decisions about clinical care (not research) during elective surgical procedures, Tait and colleagues (2001) showed parents generally preferred a process of shared decision making with the anesthetist. A significant fraction, however, wanted a more active role; those parents were less satisfied with their child's care.

Although limited, these findings generally support the movement in recent decades away from medical paternalism toward a collaborative model of decision making about medical care and research participation. They also suggest that investigators should be sensitive to and respectful of differences in parents' decision-making styles and preferences. At the same time, investigators must be mindful of the potential for undue influence based on power and information imbalances between investigators and parents. They also must still fulfill their ethical obligations to offer the information and explanations that parents need to provide informed, voluntary permission. As Kodish observed (2003a), all this can make for a "very delicate pas de deux" between investigator and parent.

Views and Results of the Consent and Permission Process

Several studies have sought parents' views on the importance of different aspects of the consent and permission process. In another article from their study of parents' agreement to children's participation in a clinical anesthesia or surgery study, Tait and colleagues (2002) asked 184 parents and 38 investigators to rank elements of informed consent by importance. Both groups considered information about risk to be the most important element. Parents, however, put more emphasis than investigators on information about potential benefits (to their child or other children) and less emphasis on voluntary agreement.

Tait and colleagues (2003a)—in another study involving permission for clinical anesthesia or surgery research—found that although parents perceived their own understanding of elements of research "consent" as high, independent assessors were less positive. The investigators reported that consenting parents showed more understanding than those who did not consent. Factors related to parents' understanding included education level, the clarity of the disclosure information, whether their child had previously been involved in a research study, and parental attention to disclosure and consent forms.

Kodish and colleagues (1998) reported that parents found discussion with staff more helpful than the consent and form. Although they found the whole process somewhat confusing, most parents believed that the amount of information provided was appropriate. In contrast, about half of the investigators surveyed thought that too much information was presented.

In the study by Hayman and colleagues (2001) cited earlier in this chapter, the investigators reported that 85 percent of the parents who agreed to enroll their child in research believed that the verbal explanation was the most useful source of information about the trial. All the parents said they understood the study's purpose and procedures. Only 6 percent wanted more information about the study.

A small pilot study of parental decision making in cancer clinical trials found that parents were generally satisfied with the "informed-consent" process, despite their distress, the time pressures, and the amount of information presented to them (Kupst et al., 2003). During interviews after the consent discussions, parents recalled information about the diagnosis, intervention, and survival statistics but were less clear about the research procedures, including randomization. The parents expressed a wish for more information about alternatives to the trial intervention and about research aspects of the study.

Kodish and colleagues (2004) recently reported that 50 percent of parents who had participated in a discussion of their child's participation in a cancer clinical trial did not understand randomization. The lack of understanding was higher among minority parents and parents of lower socioeconomic status. Physicians had explained randomization in 83 percent of the discussions. As the researchers observed, "to make informed consent more effective, future research must seek to improve communication" (Kodish et al., 2004, p. 470).

European research also raises concerns about parental understanding. In an analysis of data from nine European countries on 200 parents giving permission for their neonates' participation in clinical trials, Mason and Allmark (2000) reported that three-quarters of the permissions provided by parents were deficient. The deficiencies were most common for emergency situations. The most frequent problem areas involved the information provided and the parents' understanding of the research. These findings were one impetus for the suggestion for a continuous consent process as mentioned above.

In a study designed to learn more about groups at risk of poorly informed decision making, Simon and colleagues (2003) compared discussions of research participation involving non-English-speaking Latino parents (n = 21), English-speaking minority parents (n = 27), and English-speaking majority (white) parents (n = 60). The research involved cancer clinical trials. The investigators reported that the non-English-speaking parents were significantly less likely than the English-speaking majority group to receive explanations of the consent form, to be provided with as much detailed information or explanation about the trial, and to ask questions about the trial. For example, 48 percent of the non-English-speaking group received explanations of the consent document, whereas 92 percent of the English-speaking group did. In addition, independent raters assessed the explanations and found that they were less successfully provided to the former group than to the latter group. Not surprisingly, the investigators reported that problems with understanding were most frequent among the non-English-speaking parents. Only 14 percent of these parents understood randomization, whereas 60 percent of the English-speaking majority group did; 60 percent of the non-English-speaking group understood that research participation was voluntary, whereas 90 percent of the English-speaking majority group did. In their discussion of the findings, the authors encouraged investigation of the "role of interpreter accuracy and communication-fatigue, which commonly affects both interpreters and the original speakers" (Simon et al., 2003, p. 217).

Implications

Studies of adults asked to provide consent for research participation in their own right and studies of parents asked to provide permission for their child's research participation are generally consistent in a number of respects. They suggest that parents' understanding of research purposes is often incomplete and that the process for seeking parental permission should be improved. Particular care needs to be taken when seeking permission from parents who are just beginning to cope with a child's serious illness or injury and its treatment. In these circumstances, investigators and IRBs should consider structuring parental permission as a continuing process that is sensitive to parents' developing knowledge of their child's diagnosis and prognosis, as well as the treatment options. The process should also take into account how parents' emotional states may affect their understanding and consideration of options.

Given parents' usual reliance on and trust in their child's physician, research pointing to parents' willingness to defer to the physician's judgment about research participation is not surprising. It reinforces the need for investigators and IRBs to be particularly attentive to the potential for undue influence or conflict of interest when the child's physician is also the investigator responsible for seeking informed consent.

The needs of non-English-speaking parents warrant further attention. Qualified translators or interpreters should be provided, as discussed later in this chapter. Both the discussion and written materials should be adapted to the expected language spoken by the parents to be approached for particular studies as well as to other capacities of the parents.

For most research situations, the presentation of a consent and permission form is ethically secondary to the discussion about research participation. This discussion should include opportunities for the parents to ask questions and—when appropriate—probing by investigators so that they feel comfortable with the parents' understanding of the proposed research, its requirements, and the rights and protections available to the child and family (e.g., the right to withdraw from the research). The research reviewed by the committee does not explicitly identify situations in which the parents fail to protect their child adequately, but investigators must also be alert to this possibility.

In addition to materials describing an individual research protocol, research institutions, collaborative research groups, and research sponsors should consider developing more general guidance to help parents think about their child's participation in research. Box 5.2 lists some questions that might be included in such guidance. Parents may also be referred to more detailed guidance that has been developed for adults considering participation in clinical trials (see, e.g., ECRI, 2002).

BOX 5.2
Questions Parents May Want to Ask When Considering Their Child's Participation in Clinical Research

- What is the purpose of the research? Who is paying for it?
- Where will the research be done? How long will it last?
- What kinds of procedures and/or tests will be involved? How will they differ from what would happen if my child doesn't participate?
- What are the possible short-term and long-term harms and benefits (if any) of the study? How do they compare with treatments that my child is receiving or might receive without being in the research?
- Will the research procedure(s) hurt? If so, for how long? What can be done to prevent or limit pain? Are there other side effects?
- What will I have to do? What will my child have to do?
- Will I have to pay anything if my child is part of the study? Will my child or I be paid anything for participating?
- Who do I call with questions or in an emergency? What will happen if something goes wrong?
- What will I be told during the study and after it is finished?
- How can I withdraw my child from the study? Will that affect my child's care?
- Who will know that my child is in the study? What information will they get?

SOURCES: Adapted from Children's Hospital of Philadelphia, 2002; Children's Hospital Boston, no date; and ECRI, 2002.

CHILDREN'S AND ADOLESCENTS' COMREHENSION OF RESEARCH PARTICIPATION

At age 14, my parents brought me to the National Institutes of Health for care . . . I was encouraged to participate in clinical research. . . . I welcomed the chance to interact with CF [cystic fibrosis] physicians and researchers on a more professional level. . . . My initiation into clinical research as a teenager was one of deliberation and independence—the first time I became a partner in my health . . . It was a wonderful learning experience.
Suzanne Pattee, Cystic Fibrosis Foundation, 2003

Children and adolescents who participate in clinical research may have vastly different experiences and perceptions of their experiences depending on the nature of the research and their own medical, psychological, and social circumstances. Some may not really understand that they are participating in research or may be reluctant participants. Others—like Suzanne Pattee—may find it to be a positive experience that gives them a greater sense of control over their situation.

Although the literature is not extensive, the committee identified some research that is relevant to assessments of what children and adolescents understand about research participation and when and how their agreement to participate in research should be sought. A more extensive literature on children's general cognitive or decision-making capacities also has implications for these assessments.

Development of Cognitive Capacities in General

Studies continue to expand understanding of the patterns of cognitive development and variation in children and adults. Many psychologists agree, in general, that children's cognitive development follows a fairly regular course, although they disagree about many specifics. In a highly simplified account, as described by followers of Piaget,[6] children first develop sensory and motor skills (from approximately birth to age 2 years) and then begin to use language and images (to approximately ages 6 or 7 years), develop certain concrete reasoning and problem-solving abilities (to approximately age 11 or 12 years), and, lastly, acquire more advanced capacities to think and reason about complex, abstract concepts, relationships, and processes (adolescence). Other psychologists put more emphasis than Piaget and his followers on the role of cultural and social factors in children's development, in particular, children's interactions with parents, other adults, and peers (see, e.g., Vygotsky, 1978; and Doolittle, 1997). Still others take an information-processing approach that focuses on maturation of the sensory capacities, encoding abilities (attentiveness to and retention of information relevant to a task), and information retrieval skills (Siegler, 1991).

Particularly for more abstract concepts and reasoning capacities, research suggests that both adolescents and adults vary considerably in their capacities. It also suggests that culture, context, experience and training affect both the pace and the eventual adult level of cognitive development and performance (see, e.g., Capon and Kuhn, 1982; Chi and Ceci, 1987; Nisbett et al., 1987; Chien et al., 1996; Morris and Sloutsky, 1998; Segall et al., 1999; and Klaczynski and Robinson, 2000; etc.). These findings reinforce the argument for viewing informed consent (as well as permission

---

[6]The basics of Piaget's conceptualization of development are covered in Inhelder and Piaget, 1958; Piaget and Inhelder, 1969; and Grisso and Vierling, 1978. For those citing Piagetian concepts in the context of children's comprehension of and decisions about medical care and similar important matters, see, for example, Weithorn and Campbell, 1982; Garrison, 1991; Ambuel and Rappaport, 1992; Leiken, 1993; Wertz et al., 1994; Britner et al., 1998; and Broome, 1999.

and, as appropriate, assent) as a process that should stress careful explanation; provide opportunities for questions; and take into account the language, cultural, and other characteristics of prospective research participants. Although IRB policies and other sources often require assent starting at age 7 years, investigators should treat children as individuals and consider when it may be reasonable and respectful to provide children under that age with simple information about what will happen.

Table 5.1 depicts Broome's summary of how the general theoretical and research literature on children's development relates to the more specific question of children's developing capacity to understand and make decisions about research participation. It refers to social and emotional as well as cognitive factors.

TABLE 5.1 Developmental Differences Influencing a Child's Participation in Research

Age Group	Understanding of Research	Voluntariness	Autonomy
Preschooler (2-6 yr)	• Processes information in concrete, egocentric ways	• Understanding is specific to self • Seeks to know what others want	• Is dependent on parents • Believes health care providers hold absolute authority
School-aged (7-12 yr)	• Is more likely to see locus of control as external, which influences ability to acquire or seek information • Understanding is based on previous experience	• 7- to 9-yr-olds are less conforming to pressure than 10- to 14-yr-olds • <8-yr-olds are authority oriented; avoid punishment	• Medical authority is respected • Is rule bound; likes to comply • Decides about propriety of decision based on whether it satisfies self or others close to self
Adolescent (13-18 yr)	• Can see value of others' perspectives • Can weigh alternatives • Can entertain alternative treatments and risks simultaneously • Are hypothetical thinkers	• Need for approval decreases • Compares own actions with those similar to self	• Understands that medical authority is dependent on patient's agreement to comply • Judges merits of action on ability to help others

SOURCE: Broome, 1999. Used with permission.

Understanding of Research Participation

[P]ediatric researchers should not underestimate the awareness and maturity that some children possess when addressing issues of concern to them.

Geller et al., 2003, p. 269

I would like to see the age limits completely scrapped and maturity brought in. As you grow up your age has a stereotype. I'm trying to escape from that stereotype.

Robin, age 13, (quoted in Alderson, 1993, p. 9)

Recent years have seen an increasing interest in determining what children and adolescents comprehend about research participation and using that knowledge to guide decisions about when and how to seek children's agreement to participate in research. The findings are not entirely consistent, and each study has limitations in terms of the methods and the populations studied that affect generalizations. For example, most of the studies involved healthy middle-class children, although some included children with different kinds of medical problems. The focus was usually on children's intellectual or cognitive capacities rather than their emotional state or development. One exception involves studies of gravely ill children (Bluebond-Langner, 1978; Bluebond-Langner et al., in press). The possible effects of mental disorders (e.g., depression) on children's involvement in discussions and decisions about research participation have received little attention.

Some studies that the committee reviewed presented children with hypothetical research situations; others took place in the context of actual clinical research or other psychosocial research (i.e., research not involving the study of research understanding as such). Studies varied in the complexity of the hypothetical or real situations facing children and also in the way in which information was presented (e.g., in writing or orally). Few studies have included children as young as age 7 years, the age at which many IRBs and others advise that assent first be sought (see, e.g., AAP, 1995).

Some of the research reviewed below examined children's understanding of or agreement to medical care rather than research participation. Findings from these studies are relevant to the extent that they relate to children's and adolescent's knowledge of their medical condition (if any) and their understanding of medical procedures or other dimensions of clinical care (e.g., the potential harms and benefits of different treatments) that are identical or similar to those used for clinical research.

Very little research has investigated the actual process of obtaining children's assent to research participation. One study, already discussed above in the section on parents, analyzed 85 informed-consent conferences that concerned research participation by children with cancer (Olechnowicz et al., 2002). (Under federal regulations, assent was not a necessary condition for this research to proceed.) Of the 34 conferences that concerned children over age 7 years, the child was present during 14. The mean age of these children was 14 years (range, 10 to 18 years); the 20 children not included were younger (but their average age was not reported). The study authors reported that the investigators conducting the conferences differed in how they approached the discussion; for example, whether they indicated that the decision should be a family decision, the parents' decision, or "up to" the child (p. 808). During the conferences, older children asked more questions than younger children. Most children, however, talked very little and real discussion was uncommon. The majority of the questions from children focused on the disease and the treatment.

Although it did not assess child or adolescent understanding directly and did not observe the process of assent, another study examined 70 informed-consent documents that were used with adolescents being recruited for genetic research (Weir and Horton, 1995). The investigators concluded that the documents were often confusing and unclear. This is consistent with the findings from evaluations of informed-consent documents for adults. The investigators also concluded that the documents did not reflect "developing ethical and legal standards" for research involving adolescents (p. 347).

Comprehension of Research Purposes, Characteristics, and Possible Consequences

> *I would like to see consent forms be presented in [a clearer] manner. Some of the terms are a little bit ambiguous, especially for the patient, and if you're going to be the one getting treatment, it would seem to me that you would like those things to be clarified.*
> Carolyn Brokowski, research participant (at age 16), 2003

As reviewed below, most studies of children's understanding of the purposes and procedures of research suggest that children under age 9 or 10 years have a limited ability to understand the purposes, risks, and potential benefits of research, especially more complex research. These younger children are better able to grasp the more practical aspects of research (e.g., what they are expected to do) than they are to understand the more abstract dimensions (e.g., expectations of confidentiality). Most studies and summaries conclude that by the age of 14 or 15 adolescents differ little from adults on measures of research comprehension, but some suggest caution about other dimensions of adolescents' understanding and judgment.[7]

Children Compared to Adolescents A few studies suggest that children as young as age 6 or 7 years can comprehend some aspects of research. One study that included 6- to 9-year-olds (studied in groups not individually) concluded that although older children comprehended more about a vaccine study, children as young as 6 years could ask what the investigators viewed as reasonable questions about the research (Lewis et al., 1978). They could comprehend certain basic information about what might happen to them in medical treatment or research and what they were expected to do. A study by Susman and colleagues (1992) of hospitalized young people ages 7 to 20 years did not find important differences between children ages 7 to 13 years and young people ages 14 to 20 years. Both groups did better in understanding concrete features of research (e.g., what they were to do) than in comprehending more abstract features (e.g., alternatives and the right to withdraw). The investigators concluded that emotional factors (e.g., anxiety and a sense of control) were more important than age or cognitive development in affecting the participants' understanding of research participation (Dorn et al., 1995).

Most studies, however, have reported differences in comprehension between younger and older children. For example, in assessing the results of a study of 102 children 7 to 18 years of age, Tait and colleagues (2003b) concluded that children under age 11 years had particularly limited understanding of the study protocol (which involved an anesthesia or a surgery study), the potential benefits, and their right to withdraw from the study. Another study (Nannis, 1991) reported that more than 84 percent of the fifth graders (approximately 11 years old) in the study correctly understood what research was, whereas only 35 percent of the third graders (approximately 9 years old) answered the question correctly. In a study that included only second, fourth, and sixth graders, Hurley and Underwood (2002) reported that few of the participants in their psychological study understood its primary goals, even after a debriefing. They speculate that their results may have reflected the complexity of both the study (which investigated how children coped with peer provocation) and the debriefing.

Broome and colleagues (2001) found that children younger than age 10

---

[7]Some studies of decision making in a legal context have similar conclusions. For example, Bartholomew (1996) concluded that research shows similar decision-making capacities for adults and adolescents over the age of 14, but performance is more variable for younger individuals (see also Ambuel and Rappaport, 1992 and Scott et al., 1995).

years could describe overall goals and potential benefits but did less well in describing research risks. (This study, which also involved a parent component, as discussed earlier, included 24 children and young people with leukemia and 10 children and young people with diabetes; participants were 8 to 22 years of age and were involved in various studies related to their condition.) The investigators also reported that both children and adolescents who could discuss the purpose of the research could not always "translate [that understanding] into an acknowledgement that they themselves were involved in a clinical trial" (Broome et al., 2001, p. 41).

In a study of 18 children ages 5 to 18 years who were involved in nutrition research that did not offer the prospect of direct benefit, Ondrusek and colleagues (1998) concluded that compared with older children and adolescents, children under age 9 years showed deficient understanding of the purpose of the study, its potential harms and benefits, and their right to withdraw. (Children under age 13 years were read information about the study; older participants received a written form with the same information. This difference in presentation might have affected the results.) Younger children were, for example, more likely than older children to relate the research to checking their own health rather than to gaining information that would help sick children. The authors concluded that "the current age of 7 years for initiating assent (in addition to parental consent) is possibly not appropriate and should be reconsidered" (Ondrusek et al., 1998, p. 158).

Based on a study of student understanding of research and research rights (which included 4th, 7th, and 10th graders and college students), Bruzzese and Fisher (2003) reported that a majority of students at each level answered the questions correctly. A sizeable minority of the fourth graders, however, appeared to be confused about the purpose of the research (which was to compare the ability of children in different age groups for their abilities to comprehend the meaning of research). Overall, the study reported a steady increase by age in student's comprehension of the purpose and nature of the study as well as the risks and potential benefits of the study.

In sum, most research indicates that children between ages 6 or 7 years and ages 9 or 10 years can understand the more practical features of research but show a lesser appreciation than older children of the more abstract features of research (e.g., understanding of risks). The committee notes the shortfalls in younger children's understanding of research but believes that evidence does, on balance, support their involvement in age-appropriate discussions of participation in research and their ability to dissent (as provided for by federal regulations) from participation in research that does not present the prospect of a direct benefit. Such participation respects children's developing maturity and emerging autonomy. This is consistent with the moral purpose of assent.

Younger and Older Adolescents Consistent with a continuing maturation of cognitive capacities, most research shows differences between younger and older adolescents in their comprehension of providing informed consent to participate in research. Research on differences between adolescents and adults is more mixed.

A 1981 study by Lewis (involving 108 adolescents in the 7th, 8th, 10th, and 12th grades) looked at adolescents' recognition of risks and future consequences in a hypothetical situation involving peer counseling about cosmetic surgery or a trial of acne medication. She found sizeable differences by age, with the older adolescents showing greater awareness of risk and future consequences. Older adolescents were also more likely to suggest the need for independent professional opinion about the situations presented to them. When Halpern-Felsher and Cauffman (2001) replicated the study, however, they did not find important differences by age in the ability to recognize of risks and future consequences. Their findings are consistent with the findings of studies by Kaser-Boyd and colleagues (1985) and Ambuel and Rappaport (1992).

In their study of competency to consent to medical treatment, which involved 98 participants at ages 9, 14, 18, and 21 years, Weithorn and Campbell (1982, p. 1589) reported that the 14-year-olds in their study did not differ from adults on four standards of competency: understanding, choice, reasoned outcome, and rational reasons. A number of summaries of the literature also suggest that by the age of 14 years, most adolescents possess the "psychological elements of 'intelligent' consent" (Grisso and Vierling, 1978, p. 420; see also Weithorn and Campbell, 1982; Leiken, 1993; Weir and Peters, 1997; Thompson, 2000b).

Others are more cautious about the capacity of adolescents to evaluate participation in research. For example, after reviewing the few studies of age-related differences in judgments of risk, Millstein and Halpern-Felsher (2001) state that, depending on one's perspective, these studies could point either to a "heightened sense of vulnerability [among young people] compared to that among adults" or to a picture of adolescents being less accurate in their judgments than adults (p. 30). After noting the limitations of the available research (e.g., a lack of longitudinal studies that differentiate cohort from developmental influences), they conclude that "the finding of age-related increases in risk identification does call into question the degree to which we should consider adolescents, particularly younger adolescents, competent" (p. 24). Based on their review of the literature on the development of judgmental maturity, Steinberg and Cauffman (1996) concluded that evidence points to greater differences between early adolescents and mid- and later adolescents than between the two older groups. The authors suggested that more research is needed on the cognitive and noncognitive factors associated with mature decision making as needed.

In presenting initial results from an Australian study of 234 participants ages 12, 15, 18, and 21 years who were asked about several medical treatment vignettes, Bartholomew (1996) reported that 12-year-olds showed less evidence of decisional capacity than older participants. In contrast, 15-year-olds did not show significant differences from 18-year olds on measures related to comprehension and the amount of information sought. On other measures that related to reasoning capacities, however, 15-year-olds were more like 12-year-olds than they were like older participants.

A study by Bernhardt and colleagues (2003) of children's views of participation in a genetic susceptibility study suggested that the children (ages 10 to 17 years) did not initially appreciate the study's risks and potential benefits. When conversation encouraged them to "personalize" the possible consequences of genetic testing, they developed a fuller appreciation of the possible risks. This supports the emphasis on discussion in the design of the assent process.

Other research suggests that the development of decision-making capacities continues into adulthood, although "not all of these developmental changes point to increased rationality" (Millstein and Halpern-Felsher, 2001, p. 37). For example, certain biases in decision making may increase with age, including the tendency to reject evidence inconsistent with one's views and accept evidence that supports them (Stanovich and West, 2000; Millstein and Halpern-Felsher, 2001; but see also, Klaczynski and Gordon, 1996 and Klaczynski and Narasimham, 1998).

Although a number of studies indicate that adolescents differ little from adults in certain elements of competent decision making, research overall suggests that abilities to comprehend important dimensions of research participation continue to evolve during adolescence. As the research reviewed earlier in this chapter made clear, adults are not always well informed and often show deficits in understanding related to research participation, especially when they are under stress. Overall, the committee concludes that it is usually advisable for parents to be involved in decision making about research participation for adolescents. Adolescents' capacity to make informed decisions should not, however, be dismissed out of hand, especially when requiring parental permission would endanger adolescents or preclude their participation in research with important potential to benefit them or other adolescents in the future.

Comprehension of Rights in Research

Several studies suggest that younger children have less understanding than adolescents of their rights in research, including rights related to confidentiality and their choice to participate in a study (or withdraw from a study once it has started). For example, Bruzzese and Fisher (2003) asked children in the 4th, 7th and 10th grades to identify violations of research rights in several hypothetical vignettes. The youngest children were least able to identify such situations. In a study of 9-, 15-, and 21-year-old males, Belter and Grisso (1984) concluded that the 9-year-olds were less able to recognize violations of patient rights and less able to protect against such violations than the 15- and 21-year-olds.

With respect to confidentiality specifically, Hurley and Underwood (2002) found that sizeable minorities of second graders in their study did not understand the "fine points of confidentiality," despite repeated explanations in different contexts that information from their study would not be shared with family or school personnel (p. 140). Fourth and sixth graders did better. In their study of children ages 5 to 12 years, Abramovitch and colleagues (1991) likewise found younger children to be more uncertain about confidentiality.

In contrast, Bruzzese and Fisher (2003) reported that a large majority of the students at each grade level (4th, 7th, and 10th grades) in their study understood confidentiality. In discussing the difference between their findings and those of Abramovitch and colleagues (1991), Bruzzese and Fisher (2003) suggested that their repeated explanations of rights—before students took the permission form home to parents and again before the testing began—may have contributed to their better results among the younger children. Hurley and Underwood (2002) also provided repeated explanations, without the expected effects, but the youngest children in the study by Bruzzese and Fisher were older than the youngest children in the two other studies.

On the question of what would happen if they wanted to stop participating in the study, the children in the different age groups studied by Hurley and Underwood (2002) had similar, high levels of accurate responses. In contrast, the study by Ondrusek and colleagues (1998) cited earlier found that children under age 10 years had a low level of understanding that they could withdraw from the study. Even the older children believed that their parents would not like them to withdraw. Abramovitch and colleagues (1991) also found that few children ages 5 to 12 years believed that they had the right to withdraw from the study. In the study by Brusseze and Fisher (2003), fourth and seventh graders were less likely than older adolescents to understand that they had the right to withdraw from the study, although the majority in both groups did indicate accurately that they had that right. The investigators noted that they had, on the basis of findings from previous research, made particular efforts to provide explicit explanations of voluntary participation and how to withdraw from participation.

Bruzzese and Fisher (2003) concluded that providing a brief lesson in the rights of research participants improved understanding of these rights for individuals in each of the grade levels studied as well as for college students. (The investigators compared the responses of the students receiving the research rights lesson with students receiving education about an unrelated topic.) Their findings suggest, however, that even young adults may not be aware of their right to ask questions of investigators. They may also be uncomfortable asking questions in some research situations.

Overall, Hurley and Underwood (2002) also concluded that processes for obtaining assent and debriefing children after research participation were "moderately effective" in helping children understand their rights as research participants (p. 139). Younger children understood less than older children. The authors cautioned that debriefing might "do more harm than good" for younger children who do not understand the information provided (p. 139).

Although her opinions were focused on medical care rather than research, the views of a 7-year-old on how hospitals could make children more comfortable suggest that some very young children do have concepts of responsible action by health professionals. As expressed to her mother (a newspaper columnist), the child set forth several rules (McIntyre, 2002; used with permission; excerpts not in original order):

- "Don't surprise me. Tell me what you are going to do before you do it."
- "Ask my permission before you put any part of your body on mine."
- "Get down on my level. If I'm in the bed sit down."
- "Be honest. I get really upset . . . when they say something isn't going to hurt [and it does]."
- "Always think of a less painful way of doing things."
- "Try to keep the doctors and nurses who come into my room the same."
- "Stop saying it's no 'big deal.' It might not be a big deal to you because it's not happening to you."

To summarize, findings about children's and adolescents' understanding of their rights in research are generally consistent with findings about their comprehension of research purposes and characteristics. Older children and adolescents understand more than younger children. Some studies indicate that careful explanations of research rights can help both younger and older children have an improved understanding of their rights as research participants.

Influence of Experience with Illness

Few studies have directly examined the influence of children's or adolescents' experience with illness on their understanding of research participation. The literature cited above in the general discussion of children's cognitive development suggests that culture, context, and experience as well as age can influence children's cognitive skills and understanding of the world.

In their research on children's experience of grave illness (e.g., cancer recurrence), Bluebond-Langner and colleagues (in press) found "evidence for children's ability to hold several, sometimes contradictory views of their illness and what a particular treatment, drug or trial would offer." The children—and their parents—could recognize that their condition was not curable but still express belief or hope in the possibility of a cure. In the context of grave illness, the views of many children about participation in a clinical trial may be captured in one child's statement: "What choice is there? It is this or nothing." The investigators reported that children's experiences with grave illnesses are more predictive of their understanding of their illness and prognosis than is their age. Earlier qualitative studies suggest that children who have serious chronic illnesses may develop an earlier conceptual understanding of death than healthy children (see, e.g., Bluebond-Langner, 1978; and Sourkes, 1995).

In the study by Broome and colleagues (2001) cited earlier, the investigators found that half of the 24 children with cancer indicated awareness that they were in research, whereas all 10 diabetic children knew they were involved in research and could more clearly differentiate between clinical care for their condition and the treatment-related aspects of the clinical trials in which they were participating. The authors link the differences in understanding to differences in experiences. The children with diabetes had lived with their condition for a longer period, were on a stable treatment regimen, and had been involved in multiple studies since the diagnosis of their condition. As an incentive for their participation in research, these children also received a gift certificate or payment at the end of the studies. In contrast, the children with cancer had more recently received the diagnosis, had little or no previous experience with research, were presented with the option to participate in research soon after receiving the diagnosis under highly stressful circumstances, and were never offered financial incentives to participate in the research. These children were often involved in several studies, and the studies were typically simultaneous and related to each other and their clinical care. Some of the children with cancer were in data collection studies that did not involve an experimental intervention, and some of them may not have understood that this data collection was research. In addition, several of the children with cancer "were removed from the discussions" surrounding their enrollment in research because of pain or the severity of their illness (p. 44).

Parental Influence

As children develop, one mark of increasing maturity is an increasing desire for autonomy in decision making. Voluntary choice and independence in thinking are important dimensions of informed consent. The influence of parents appears to be strongest for younger children but parents influence adolescents as well.

In a study with individuals ages 9 to 10, 14 to 15, and 21 to 25 years that used hypothetical vignettes about medical treatment, investigators reported that considerable deference to parents' preferences was evident at all ages (Scherer, 1991). The youngest children, however, were the most deferential, particularly for vignettes involving more severe and complicated situations. The children gave various reasons for their deference, including respect for parental judgment and knowledge, need for parental support, desire to avoid conflict, and a belief that they had no choice. Based on responses of just the 14- and 15-year-olds in this study, Scherer and Reppucci (1988) reported that deference varied depending on the degree of parental pressure depicted. Abramovitch and colleagues (1991), in their study of participation in psychological research by children ages 5 to 12 years, found children across this age spectrum were concerned about withdrawing from research for fear of disappointing their parents *and* health care professionals.

Based on their interviews with children with cancer and children with diabetes, Broome and Richards (2003) reported that nearly all the children had faith that their parents would protect them. Responses were more mixed on whether parents would support children's choices about research participation, although most thought their parents would take their views into account.

In their study cited earlier, Geller and colleagues (2003) suggested that the older and more mature the child the greater the likelihood that decisions would be made jointly rather than by the parents alone. The children and adolescents that they interviewed generally believed that the decision to participate should be the child's, "unless they're like babies" (p. 264). All, however, wanted to know what their parents thought. A minority (all younger girls) said that they would defer to their parents.

Reporting on a study with 37 adolescents and their parents, Brody and colleagues (2003) found that the two groups agreed approximately three-quarters of the time on decisions involving an asthma research vignette. Both, however, claimed that they had "ultimate responsibility for the participation decision" (p. 79).

Bluebond-Langner and colleagues (in press) have stressed that one complication in determining what gravely ill children understand or want with respect to treatment or participation in research is that these children, in particular, may not express their concerns, wishes, or fears to their parents, clinicians, or investigators. This reticence may reflect not only the children's deference to their parents but also the children's desire to protect their parents from the additional distress of knowing their child's fears or facing the mutual acknowledgment of the prospect of death. The investigators refer to a process of "mutual pretense" that constrains free discussion and questions about treatment or research in the context of grave illness.

Children's dissent or unwillingness to agree to research participation is not well studied. Citing the work of Abramovitch and colleagues (1991), Thompson (2000b) notes that children may find meaningful dissent difficult "not only because of limitations in judgment, but also because their invitation to participate typically occurs in a context of prior parental permission, institutional support (whether the institution is a school, childcare center, hospital, or other setting), and adults' interests in furthering the research enterprise" (pp. 164-165).

When a parent believes that the child should participate in research for altruistic or other reasons and the child does not want to participate, the actual decision about research may involve sensitive discussions with the parent and child. As long as the child is not coerced into assenting, it is reasonable for parents to engage in persuasive discussion, for example, about the importance of helping others. Even young children know what it means to "help" someone, although the ability of children to reason abstractly about altruism develops with age. Children also show empathy, sympathy, and other traits associated with the moral motives for adult altruism (Hoffman, 1990; Eisenberg et al., 2002; Bernhardt et al., 2003). Nonetheless, consistent with the regulations, the child's dissent should override parental assent when the research does not promise direct benefit to the child.

Implications

> *I think that it has to be for children a very interactive process in terms of consent. After I was asked this entire list of questions, I began to question my own first response. I think that just giving a kid a piece of paper, no matter how comprehensible the piece of paper is, is not going to be effective. I think the kid needs to be*

prompted with questions because I would never have thought of those issues, even as a 13-year-old. . . . When I was asked by the researcher did you consider this, what about these consequences, I began to change my idea of whether I would really want to participate in that study.

Sarah Lippincott, research participant, 2003

Although research is limited and findings are not entirely consistent, they support a gradual expansion of the involvement of children in discussions and decisions about research participation. For younger children, the emphasis should be on providing basic information about what will happen, responding to their questions and concerns (including those not explicitly expressed), and—particularly when the research does not offer the prospect of direct benefit—recognizing when children do not want to participate. Even when federal guidelines do not require the child's assent, investigators should still inform children (as appropriate given the circumstances) about what will happen and answer any questions that the child may have.

As children mature, they can participate more fully in discussions and decisions about their participation in research, although the involvement of parents is still required and prudent in most situations. Older adolescents may not have the legal capacity to make decisions in their own right, but the research reviewed here generally suggests that their level of comprehension of research approaches that of adults. Many aspects of the assent process can be similar to the consent process for adults *if* that process has been designed to accommodate people of various educational, social, and cultural backgrounds. For children and adolescents as well as adults, physical incapacity or distress related to serious illness may limit the extent to which they are involved.

Fisher (2003) has described a general approach to assent that aims for a "goodness-of-fit" between children's maturing skills and the assent processes. Because children have limited experience exercising their rights in response to requests from adults (especially in educational, medical, or unfamiliar settings), the assent process should be designed to demonstrate that participation is voluntary and dissent will not be penalized. In some cases, tutorials on research procedures and protections may be an appropriate element of the assent process. Opportunities for supported decision making that involves a parent-child discussion can also be created; a facilitator may be helpful in such a discussion. The broad objective is to create assent contexts and processes that minimize stress, encourage children's involvement in decisions about their participation in research, and ensure that their wishes and concerns are adequately communicated and considered.

Based on their analysis of findings related to both parents and children, Broome and colleagues (2003) similarly argue for variations in the permission and assent process to fit the circumstances, particularly in studies involving adolescents. They conclude that the explanations of research should be provided separately to adolescents and their parents and that parents and adolescents should, when feasible, be provided more time (hours to days) to consider participation in clinical trials related to serious illness. For adolescents and their parents, agreement to research participated should be regarded as a "shared endeavor . . . based on implicit, developmentally based negotiations" (Broome et al., 2003, p. S23).

Among the sensitive issues related to research participation is when adolescents should be free to consent to research participation without parental permission. As noted above, although the DHHS regulations make provisions for the waiver of parental consent when appropriate, the FDA regulations do not. The research reviewed here suggests that the DHHS regulations reasonably provide for waivers, as long as safeguards are provided that are appropriate for the individual adolescent being considered for research participation.

IRB AND INVESTIGATOR POLICIES AND PRACTICES

Information about IRB and investigator policies and practices related to parental permission and child assent to research participation is limited. McWilliams and colleagues (2003) analyzed information from 31 (of a total of 42) cystic fibrosis care centers related to IRB review of a genetic epidemiology study that included children. The genetic study involved the collection of data from medical records and the analysis of a blood sample. Twenty-one of the centers reported that investigators were required to obtain assent from children, but 10 centers reported that assent was not required. Of the 21 centers obtaining assent, 10 used a separate assent form with an explanation of the study, whereas the rest provided for initials or a signature on an adult consent form. Some centers used distinct parental permission forms. Local templates often did not include information appropriate for genetic studies (e.g., assurances of confidentiality for family members). Few of the approved forms included all the information that has been recommended for inclusion by guidelines on the banking of genetic information. The researchers noted criticisms of IRB preparation to deal with genetic research, quoting Frances Collins's statement that the "IRB Guidebook is dusty and out of date for genetics research" (McWilliams et al., 2003, p. 364, citing Collins, 2001, online, unpaged).

Mammel and Kaplan (1995) undertook a national survey of IRB chairs to describe policies for obtaining the agreement of adolescents to participate in research; they received usable responses from 30 percent of the 600

IRB chairs contacted. Of those responding, 70 percent said that the IRB required parental permission for all minors involved in studies; that is, they did not allow waivers of parental permission for certain kinds of research involving adolescents. IRBs that reviewed more than 10 protocols involving "adolescents" a year were less likely to have this blanket requirement (p. 323). Approximately one-third of the respondents said that their IRB would waive parental permission for a study that involved anonymous testing of adolescents for HIV infection.

A statement to the committee by the Allergy and Asthma Network included observations on the experiences of one office-based researcher, who reported that sponsors often did not provided assent materials and that protocols were "often approved without an assent document being reviewed by the IRB" (White, 2003, p. 7). In this physician's view, adolescents generally needed a simplified version of the consent document to help them understand the research.

Several studies have documented considerable variability in the practices of IRBs related to informed consent. In a study supported by NIH, researchers surveyed the chairs of nearly 500 IRBs that had conducted at least 10 protocol reviews in 1995 (Bell et al., 1998). More than a third of respondents reported that their IRBs had suspended or terminated a research project; of this group, just over 20 percent of the actions had been based on investigator failure to obtain informed consent. When questioned about their priorities for the initial review of protocols, about 20 percent of IRB chairs indicated that consent forms were a priority and another 11 percent mentioned informed-consent procedures. When questioned about deficiencies in protocols during the initial review, 60 percent of IRB chairs said that excessively technical language in the consent form was often a problem. Less than 10 percent said that they often saw problems with other aspects of consent forms (e.g., understatement of risks or benefits) or with the consent process. More than half, however, said that they sometimes found problems with consent processes that did not "promote comprehension" (p. 62). For multisite studies that originated at another institution, more than half the chairs reported that their IRBs had required modifications in the (model) consent form. Almost 90 percent of the chairs and administrators said that the failure of investigators to provide an acceptable consent form with their initial submission was a problem. "Issues relative to assent procedures" had been encountered by almost 90 percent of the IRB chairs (p. 22).

For the survey just cited, Bell and colleagues (1998) also questioned investigators and administrators associated with 300 IRBs. Among the investigators who reported that they had modified a research protocol in response to IRB concerns, more than three-quarters reported that they had to modify the consent form and one-fifth mentioned that they had to modify the consent process. Responses from investigators questioned about informed-consent practices indicated that the median time spent in discussion related to consent was 20 minutes (mean of 30 minutes). Nearly one-third of the investigators reported that they spent 10 minutes or less on consent. Investigators from institutions with high volumes of research spent more time, on average, in these discussions (means, 34 versus 25 minutes). About half the investigators indicated that they shared responsibility for discussions of consent with other members of the research team, whereas a third took sole responsibility for that activity.

In a study of 16 institutions involved in a single multicenter trial of treatment for patients with acute lung injury, Silverman and colleagues (2001) found that only 3 institutions had prepared forms for the study that included all the information that is specified in the federal regulations. The reading levels for the forms varied from the 8th to the 13th (college freshmen) grade. One of the 16 IRBs waived the requirement for informed consent.

Burman and colleagues (2003) used independent reviewers to evaluate changes made in consent forms for two multicenter tuberculosis studies. The researchers concluded that 85 percent of the changes altered "wording without affecting meaning," that 11 percent of the changes introduced errors, and that two-thirds of the locally approved forms had at least one error related either to the protocol or to federal regulations (Burman et al., 2003). Another study that involved 44 institutions reported that only eight applications for IRB approval were approved without changes and that 91 percent of the changes requested in the other applications involved consent forms (Stair et al., 2001).

In its summary of common findings of noncompliance after investigation of complaints, OHRP listed several topics under the heading of informed consent, including failure to obtain legally effective consent and various deficiencies in consent documents (OHRP, 2002d). None of the listed findings explicitly mentioned children's assent or parent's permission.

Overall, these surveys and studies suggest room for improvement in the processes for obtaining informed consent, permission, and assent. The following discussion focuses on steps to strengthen the processes related to permission and assent.

IMPROVING PROCESSES FOR REQUESTING PERMISSION AND ASSENT

Accomplishing the goal of real understanding as a precondition to a meaningful decision to participate [in research] will require a sea change in [review board] and investigator perception and practice.

Institute of Medicine, 2003a

Informed consent is widely regarded as a cornerstone of ethical research. Because children usually do not have the legal capacity or maturity to provide informed consent, the concepts of parental permission and child assent have been developed as a foundation for ethical research involving children. (Again, in this report, the term *parent* covers guardians as well.)

Taken together, a considerable body of research—albeit imperfect—points to important shortfalls in the current processes for seeking permission and assent. It also points to some directions for improvements, while underscoring the challenges of securing informed agreement, especially under conditions of stress, desperation, and crisis. On the basis of its experience and judgment as well as its review of the research literature, the committee developed the conclusions and recommendations presented below.

Focus on Permission and Assent as Processes

We have to make sure that in our attempts to protect children we aren't making the consent process so onerous and paper heavy that we're actually prohibiting or inhibiting new studies from opening, or conversely scaring families away.

Lise Yasui, parent, 2003

As discussed earlier, informed consent—and, by extension, permission and assent—should be viewed as a process, not a form. Committee experience and the limited evidence about IRB practices suggests reason for continued concern that investigators and IRBs devote disproportionate attention to consent forms, while paying less attention to the overall process for seeking consent and ensuring, insofar as possible, that consent is informed, reasoned, and voluntary.

This committee reiterates the importance of placing more emphasis on the design and implementation of ethical processes for seeking parents' permission and children's assent to a child's participation in research. Discussions about research participation should allow sufficient time for questions and, if necessary, further explanations. Such discussions should always precede the presentation of forms. Before any forms are presented for signature, investigators and others involved in the process of requesting permission and assent should feel comfortable that the parents and, when appropriate, the children have an adequate understanding of the course to which they are agreeing.

Recommendation 5.1: To focus attention on the process of requesting parents' permission and children's assent to research participation, investigators should provide and IRBs should review protocol descriptions of

- who will request permission and assent;
- how and when permission and assent will be requested;
- who should be contacted if parents have questions or concerns about the research; and
- for studies that extend over considerable periods of time, when and how permission and assent may be requested again, for example, as children reach important developmental milestones.

A one-time process for requesting permission and assent may be all that is needed for many studies, for example, those involving a single encounter or a brief hospital stay and routine follow-up. Other studies should provide for periodic revisiting of the parents' and children's agreement to the child's participation in research. This may occur yearly or more frequently, depending on the nature of the research and, possibly, changes in the child's health status. For example, if children come in for testing every 6 months, particularly for research that does not have the prospect of benefiting them directly, it usually will be appropriate to check that they want to continue to participate. (Some children will signal their unwillingness to continue by persuading their parents not to bring them in for the testing.) In addition, if the research changes in ways that could affect the parents' and children's assessment of the risks in relation to the potential benefits, permission and assent should also be sought again.

For children with serious medical conditions, the initiation of permission and assent procedures for clinical research is often inextricably intertwined with decisions about basic clinical care. Discussions of research participation may occur close in time to a family's first being told of the child's diagnosis or learning about a setback in the child's response to treatment. These discussions may also cover acute care that is not part of the research protocol. In these circumstances, permission and assent should be conceptualized as continuing processes that are sensitive to parents' developing knowledge of their child's condition and their shifting emotional reactions to the diagnosis, prognosis, and treatment options. The processes also should be sensitive to changes in the child's cognition, emotions, and physical health that may alter the balance between research risks and burdens in relation to potential benefits. Such changes may also affect whether it is possible or appropriate to involve the child in discussions and decisions about research participation.

Recommendation 5.2: When appropriate for research involving children with acute illnesses or injuries, investigators and institutional review boards should provide for ongoing processes for permission and assent that will accommodate a family's evolving understanding of the child's condition, the child's emotional state and decision-making capacity, and the child's changing medical and psychological status. These processes are not matters of signing or updating forms but, rather, of continuing communication based on appreciation of the difficult and even overwhelming circumstances in which parents may be asked to make grave decisions about their child's future.

Informed Parental Permission

Parents will inevitably vary in their levels of understanding of their child's health status, the difference between clinical care and clinical research, and other matters critical to informed decision making. To some extent, but not entirely, this variation may reflect differences in educational and reading levels and, possibly, proficiency in English. Sociocultural differences may also shape how parents understand and engage in the process of deciding about their child's participation in research. Regardless of the study population, consent and permission forms and processes should avoid language that creates or reinforces confusion about the difference between research and clinical care.

In designing and reviewing procedures and related written materials for seeking parental permission, investigators and IRBs should consider what is known or expected about the educational, language, cultural, and other relevant characteristics of the populations to be involved in particular studies. Studies consistently indicate that informed-consent materials are geared to individuals with reading skills at levels higher than those that many prospective research participants or the parents of prospective child participants possess. Some research also suggests that most information in consent documents can be presented in much simpler language that will still convey information essential for decision making. For groups with low levels of literacy, investigators and IRBs should consider the use of information tools (e.g., simple graphics and oral explanations or special videos) that do not depend on written documents. Again, investigators should view the presentation of consent, permission, or assent forms as the end of the process, not the beginning.

When language barriers exist, investigators should see that the consent forms translated from English to other languages are adequate and that the content is equivalent to that in the original. As necessary for a meaningful process of seeking parental permission, investigators should use interpreters who have the knowledge, language skills, and awareness of cultural factors that are necessary both to translate information about clinical research and to assess the level of understanding of that information by the participant of the participant's parents. In support of effective communication with patients, accreditation standards and various federal and state policies now expect hospitals to have available interpreters of the languages frequently used by their constituent groups of patients (see, e.g., Perkins et al., 1998;

OCR, 2000; and Somers, 2003). Except in a clear emergency when no acceptable alternatives exist, children should not serve as interpreters for their parents. The practice may compromise parent-child relations and increase the risk of misinformation.

Investigators using translators in hospital and other settings should also be sensitive to issues of confidentiality. Particularly in small ethnic communities, those who can appropriately act as interpreters may have business or social relationships with prospective research participants and their families (Fisher et al., 2002).

The committee recognizes the cost implications for clinical studies of provisions for adequate translation and interpretation services and materials otherwise appropriate to the language skills of target research populations. To support investigators in meeting their ethical obligations as part of the permission and assent process, research sponsors should recognize these costs.

> **Recommendation 5.3: Investigators—with assistance and oversight from institutional review boards, research institutions, and research sponsors—should design procedures for seeking parental permission for a child's participation in research that are sensitive to educational, cultural, and other differences among families and include provisions for**
>
> **• educating—not merely presenting information to—parents about issues critical to informed decision making and, as appropriate, assessing the degree to which these critical issues are understood;**
> **• writing consent and permission materials in the simplest language that still conveys essential information about the study; and**
> **• providing competent, trained translators and interpreters, when needed, and otherwise assisting parents with limited English-language proficiency with making informed decisions.**

Particularly when a child has a serious medical condition, parents may be concerned that their child's access to care will be negatively affected if they do not agree to their child's participation in a clinical study. Even though it is not the intent of the investigator, the result may be permission that is less than fully voluntary. Investigators should work with IRBs and research institutions to develop safeguards to ensure that parents understand that their child's normal access to clinical care will not be disrupted if they choose not to permit their child's participation in research or if they choose to withdraw the child after the start of a study.

When no effective standard therapy exists or standard therapies have failed, parents may see participation in a clinical trial as the only option offering any prospect of extending or improving their child's life. In these situations, investigators still have an obligation to discuss the expected or possible burdens that research participation may impose on the child, to offer their best assessment of the prospect of benefit, and to explain what relevant options for palliative care may be available within or outside the research setting.

Waiver of Parental Permission

As described earlier and consistent with the recommendation of the National Commission, DHHS regulations permit IRBs to waive parental or guardian permission for a child's participation in research when such permission (1) is not a reasonable requirement to protect the child and (2) is not inconsistent with federal or state laws. The regulations also require the substitution of an appropriate protective mechanism when a parental waiver is approved. The FDA regulations do not allow such waivers, even when the research involves, for example, abused or neglected children who would thereby be denied the potential benefits of research participation.

For a variety of reasons, it is generally desirable to seek parental involvement in decisions about children's and adolescents' participation in research, especially when the research involves a clinical trial or presents more than minimal risk. In some situations, however, requiring parental permission could put a child or an adolescent at risk of violence, expulsion from the home, or other harm. This could impede some important research. For example, researchers trying to identify risk factors for HIV infection among different groups of adolescents might be successful in encouraging some teens to involve their parents but be unable to recruit those teens who are most fearful of violent parental reactions. Such reactions may be part of a family dynamic that is, itself, a risk factor.

In addition, some adolescents have no parents or guardians and are not wards of the state, and others are runaways or "throw-aways" (adolescents who are evicted from or asked to leave the home by their parents) (Blustein et al., 1999). Research to understand the circumstances of these adolescents—including their health status—is unlikely to be feasible if parental permission is required. Likewise, it may not be possible to enroll these adolescents in clinical studies that have the prospect of direct benefit.

In some cases, an adolescent for whom parental permission is not feasible may be able to receive an investigational product outside a trial if the product (e.g., an antidepressant) is approved for other uses or age groups. (Such use will still require either parental consent or a judgment that such consent is not required under applicable laws.) Although this approach may, on balance, be prudent and may potentially benefit the individual adolescent, it will not advance knowledge to benefit future adolescents.

Committee experience and some research suggest that many IRBs are reluctant to consider waivers of parental permission for adolescent's participation in research even though the proposed waivers are consistent with DHHS regulations and relevant state laws. Restrictive IRB policies and practices can be just as constraining as current FDA policies, thereby limiting research that can benefit adolescents.

Again, parental involvement and permission is usually advisable, especially for research involving more than minimal risk. IRBs should not, however, employ a blanket policy of denying protocols that provide for waivers of parental permission. Rather, they should consider protocols on their merits taking into account their purposes and rationales (e.g., parental neglect, fear of parental violence), the basis for assessing the adolescent's capabilities to make decisions, proposed safeguards, and applicable federal and state policies.

Recommendation 5.4: Institutional review boards should consider granting waivers of parental permission for adolescent participation in research when

- **the research is important to the health and well-being of adolescents and it cannot reasonably or practically be carried out without the waiver (consistent with 45 CFR 46.116(d) and 45 CFR 408(c)) or**
- **the research involves treatments that state laws permit adolescents to receive without parental permission (consistent with the definition of children at 46 CFR 402(a))**

and when

- **the investigator has presented evidence that the adolescents are capable of understanding the research and their rights as research participants and**
- **the research protocol includes appropriate safeguards to protect the interests of the adolescent consistent with the risk presented by the research.**

The committee agrees with the National Human Research Protections Advisory Committee (NHRPAC) (Marshall, 2001) and the Society for Adolescent Medicine (SAM, 1995) that FDA's restrictive policy hampers important research involving adolescents. As discussed earlier in this chapter, the committee believes that FDA's statute provides discretion when parental permission is not feasible or it is contrary to the child's best interests. Furthermore, as NHRPAC has noted, the FDA regulations define children with reference to state laws that apply in the locale where the research takes place, which reasonably means that the age of consent (i.e., when parental permission is not required) depends on the law of that state. States also permit minors to consent to treatment in their own right under a range of circumstances, although these provisions do not explicitly mention research.

202 ETHICAL CONDUCT OF CLINICAL RESEARCH INVOLVING CHILDREN

Recommendation 5.5: The Food and Drug Administration should adopt policies consistent with federal regulations at 45 CFR 46.408(c) that allow institutional review boards with appropriate expertise to waive requirements for parental permission in research, provided that additional, appropriate safeguards are in place to protect the child's or the adolescent's welfare.

OHRP, FDA, and NIH should cooperate to develop guidance for investigators and IRBs on the additional safeguards that should be in place when a waiver of parental permission is sought and obtained. The safeguards should fit the risks associated with specific studies. In making recommendations about health research with adolescents that involves only minimal risk, the Society for Adolescent Medicine advises that IRBs should find that the research meets several conditions (SAM, 1995). Box 5.3 provides an example of questions devised by one IRB based on this advice. Beyond these questions, IRBs and investigators should be familiar with state policies relevant to the medical treatment of minors without parental permission.

In some cases, safeguards might involve a research ombudsman or independent advocate who would review the adolescent's situation, identify relevant state laws, observe or participate in the consent discussion (including, unless inappropriate in the circumstances, discussion of the desirability of parental involvement), perhaps hear the views of a nonparent relative or other adult who is providing support and guidance, and document the

---

BOX 5.3
Questions and Information for Investigators Seeking Waiver of Parental Permission for Adolescent's Participation in Research

- Please specify why the research could not be practically conducted without a waiver and why parental permission is not a reasonable requirement.
- Are the risks associated with this protocol minimal? Please specify why.
- The IRB requires assurance that the waiver of parental permission will not adversely affect the rights and welfare of the subjects.
- How will you ensure the privacy and confidentiality of the study subjects?
- Investigators must encourage each adolescent to seek the support of a parent or another adult prior to participation. How will this be accomplished? The informed consent must also address this issue.
- Investigators must establish procedures to allow adolescents to seek assistance on a confidential basis after completing surveys containing questionnaires that may raise issues for which adolescents may desire further information or assistance. Please specify how this will be accomplished.

SOURCE: Children's Hospital Boston, no date

reason for waiving parental permission. IRBs should consider the guidelines from the Society for Adolescent Medicine. For research involving more than minimal risk, they advise (among other protections) that IRBs determine that someone other than the investigator will assist the adolescent by identifying an adult familiar with his or her situation, committed to his or her well-being, and willing to offer appropriate emotional support. Further, the Society recommends that an appropriately trained professional (e.g., psychologist or masters level social worker), who is not involved in the study should confirm

> the capacity of the adolescent as a mature minor to give informed consent by finding evidence of: (a) cognitive ability to comprehend the objectives and requirements of the research and other important considerations (e.g., the voluntary nature of participation, the potential of risks and benefits) as would be required for a competent adult; (b) reasonable judgment as evidenced by the ability to address problems, to foresee the long-term consequences of action or inaction, and to evaluate the validity of information; and (c) personal responsibility to be able to comply with the requirements of the research protocol, especially those designed to ensure individual safety. (SAM, 1995, p. 266.)

Finally, it is important for regulators and institutions to develop appropriate policies and procedures for waiving parental permission and child assent to permit research involving children who have acute, unanticipated health problems (e.g., extreme prematurity or head trauma) when parents are not immediately available or not medically competent to provide permission and when the child is incapacitated. Consistent with OHRP and FDA policies and regulations on emergency research, IRBs should develop policies and procedures for simultaneously protecting the well-being of the affected children and the rights of the parents while still permitting the acquisition of new knowledge concerning the most frequent causes of child morbidity and mortality in the United States, which are—for children beyond infancy—intentional and unintentional injuries. The committee recognizes that many institutions have been unwilling to consider such research out of concern about adverse outcomes and the concurrent legal liability associated with these outcomes.

Children's Assent or Dissent in the Context of the Family

Rather than viewing the process of requesting a child's agreement to participation in clinical research as an independent event, investigators and IRB members should adopt a family systems perspective. In the committee's experience and as indicated in some of the research reviewed above, parents often want to decide whether their child will be approached about research participation. Children are usually not approached unless parents are willing to consider the child's participation.

In some cases, parents may agree to a child's participation in research with the expectation that the child, once approached, may not want to participate and that the child's wishes will be accepted. In other situations, parents and children may negotiate decisions about research participation, with the views of adolescents tending to have more weight. Sometimes, parents may expect their wishes for the child to participate in research to prevail over a child's wish not to participate in research, especially when the research has the prospect of benefiting an ill child. Federal regulations governing research involving children appropriately do not require the child's assent when research offers the prospect of an important direct benefit that is available only in the context of the research" (45 CFR 46.408(a); 21 CFR 50.55 (c)(2)). Investigators should avoid suggesting to children that they can make the participation decision when their parents can override their wishes.

Nonetheless, even when it can be overridden, a child's dissent should not be regarded as simply inferior to the parents' views and decisions but, rather, should be viewed as reflecting a different and still important point of view. Investigators or others involved in the assent process should work with parents to help them understand children's views and treat them respectfully. It will usually be better for all involved if agreement between parent and child—especially an older child or adolescent—can be achieved. This may involve a developmentally variable process of negotiation. As discussed earlier, it may sometimes be reasonable—as part of a respectful and noncoercive assent process with parental agreement—for investigators to come back to a child who says "no" to see whether he or she may feel differently later.

In rare instances, understanding and respect may lead an investigator or clinician involved with the child's care to advocate—with great sensitivity to the family's wishes and values—on behalf of a dissenting older child or adolescent when the assent process reveals compelling reasons for encouraging parents to consider accepting rather than overriding the dissent. One such situation may arise when a mature adolescent who has a grave medical problem that has been unresponsive to treatment asks not to be subjected to a burdensome investigative procedure that offers at most a remote prospect of meaningful benefit. When parents are desperate to do something or fear feeling guilty in the future if they refuse proposed interventions, they may find it difficult to fully consider the burdens that research participation is likely to impose on their child.

When research does not have the prospect of direct benefit to the child, the committee interprets the regulatory requirements that "adequate provisions are made to solicit the child's assent" to mean that the child's dissent overrides parental permission. Investigators should be alert to nonverbal indications of children's wishes about research participation, particularly when children may be reluctant to distress their parents by voicing disagreement. The federal regulations specify that failure to object to participation should not, by itself, be construed as assent. Again, in the committee's view, a child's dissent does not preclude investigators seeking the child's assent at another time, as long as such practices are respectful and not coercive and parents are involved and supportive.

Some research has the potential to reveal sensitive information about a child or, more often, an adolescent that might provoke negative, even punitive, parental reactions. Investigators should be sensitive to this potential and should determine when adolescents and possibly younger children should be told about the kinds of information that may be shared with their parents if they agree to participate in research. Researchers studying adolescents have been concerned that the federal privacy regulations (see Appendix C) may allow parents to have access to information about adolescents that would otherwise be held confidential. The regulations defer to state laws on parental access to the health records of minors, which means that research-related personal information may be protected in some states and not in others.

Recommendation 5.6: In designing and reviewing procedures for seeking a child's assent to participation in research, investigators and institutional review boards should aim to create assent processes that consider and respect the child and the family as a unit as well as individually. The process for requesting assent should

• be developmentally appropriate given the ages and other characteristics of the children to be approached;
• provide opportunities for children to express and discuss their willingness or unwillingness to participate;
• clarify for parents and children (as appropriate) the degree of control that each will have over the participation decision; and
• when appropriate, describe to children and parents the kinds of information about the child that will or will not be shared with the parents.

Age-Appropriate Assent Processes

The construction of age-appropriate assent materials and procedures should be informed by the literature on cognitive development in general and on child and adolescent capacities for assent in particular. For children and adolescents at all ages, the assent process should be designed to be an empowering and respectful experience.

The research on children's cognitive, intellectual, social, and emotional development and their understanding of research participation provides somewhat mixed directions on the question of a minimum age for seeking affirmative assent. As long as investigators and IRB members recognize that the assent process for young children should be age appropriate and quite simple, it is not unreasonable for investigators to be asked to seek assent for children as young as age 7 years. (Such an age-defined policy may be useful for practical reasons, but investigators should also be encouraged to provide simple explanations for children younger than that age who seem to be capable of understanding basic information.)

For younger children (to age 9 or 10), assent information and procedures can be limited and can focus on a subset of the information required for adults. For example, the discussion and, if appropriate, written material or assent form for younger children should explain in simple language

- what the study is about and whether it might help (e.g., "We want to see whether a new medicine will or won't help children like you who have earaches." or "We want to understand your illness better.");
- what will happen and when (e.g., "You will have to come to the clinic once a week for 8 weeks to have a shot, you will not be allowed to eat for 12 hours, and then the following things will happen: . . .");
- what discomfort there might be and what will be done to minimize it (e.g., "Your head may hurt after the test and you may need to stay in bed for a day." "You will get a cream on your skin that will keep you from feeling the shot." or "You will have someone to whom you can talk about your feelings.");
- who will answer the child's questions during the study; and
- whether an option to say "no" exists (e.g., "You do not have to be in this study and no one will be mad at you." or "If you say "yes" and then change your mind, that is okay.").

With the increasing age of the child, assent information should become correspondingly more substantive and specific and should use language appropriate to the cognitive and emotional maturity of the child or adolescent. The nearer an adolescent is to the age of majority, the more the assent process should resemble a well-designed informed-consent process for adults. Most research suggests that by age 14 or 15 years adolescents are similar to adults in their ability to comprehend the meaning of participation in research, although they may still be maturing in other areas of understanding and decision making. If consent forms for adults are written to be easily read by those with reading skills at less than a high school level, they may be appropriate to use as the assent form for middle to older adolescents. As for adults, in designing assent processes and written information for children and adolescents, investigators should take into account the expected language competencies and preferences of the groups to be included in the research. For emancipated and mature minors who are making decisions in their own right, the process for seeking assent should still be sensitive to the level of maturity of these adolescents (e.g., their attitudes about risk taking) and appropriate safeguards should be provided.

Discretion in Documenting Assent

As described above, federal regulations permit oral presentation of assent information and allow the IRB to use discretion about the way in which assent is documented. Although the guidelines on pediatric drug research adopted by ICH (and issued as FDA guidance) are more specific (requiring signatures on assent forms for participants of "appropriate intellectual maturity" [FDA, 2000b, p. 13]), they, too, allow some discretion and should not be rigidly interpreted.

On the basis of the literature reviewed in this chapter, the committee suggests that requiring a child's signature on an assent form may be developmentally inappropriate for younger children (e.g., those under age 9 or 10 years). A signature requirement may confuse rather than inform a child, and a child may even experience this situation as intimidating or coercive.

> Recommendation 5.7: Guidance and education for investigators and members of institutional review boards should make clear that federal regulations allow discretion—based on children's developmental maturity—about the way in which information is presented to children and the manner in which assent is documented. Investigators and institutional review board members should apply that knowledge in determining what procedures will best serve the goals of assent for particular research protocols and populations.

While allowing for discretion with individual children or adolescents, IRBs and institutions can provide guidance about age-appropriate options for documenting assent. For example, in addition to developing sample age-appropriate information and assent materials for younger children, institutions can suggest that investigators use their judgment in determining when it is appropriate and respectful to ask younger children to sign simple assent forms. If investigators have developed an adult consent or permission form that is suitable for use with adolescents, the form could be used to document adolescent assent. Alternatively, then adolescents could sign a simpler assent form that includes age-appropriate information beyond that included on the form for younger children.

Investigator Knowledge and Skills

Developmentally appropriate and family-sensitive procedures for obtaining children's assent and parents' permission for a child's participation in research require communication skills and knowledge of child psychology and family dynamics. Education in these skills may not be part of the standard training for clinical researchers, including some investigators who conduct studies that include children. Investigators and other team members who are experienced in communicating with children and families will usually be better prepared to undertake these procedures than those who work entirely or mainly with adults. Even experienced pediatric researchers may, however, benefit from formal training in both the regulations related to permission and assent and the means of implementing permission and assent as "a process, not a form."

> Recommendation 5.8: To increase investigator competence in communicating with children and parents about research participation, educational programs for investigators and research staff who expect to do research involving children should include training and evaluation in developmentally appropriate and family-sensitive processes for seeking permission and assent.

Directions for Research

Although the committee was encouraged to find some research on parental permission and child assent, much of that research involves very small numbers of participants and other limitations. The range of pediatric conditions and research experiences covered by studies of permission and assent is also fairly limited.

Better evidence about how parents and children of different ages comprehend various dimensions of research and research participation is needed to help investigators and IRBs devise ethical and effective processes for explaining research and seeking permission and assent. To the same end, more research is needed to describe how permission and assent are actually sought in different contexts, how processes vary, and what processes appear to better serve the goals underlying the requirements for permission and assent, given the variations in research purposes and populations.

> Recommendation 5.9: Federal agencies, private foundations, and advocacy groups should encourage and support research on existing and innovative permission and assent processes and information materials to support improvements in these processes and guide the education of investigators and institutional review board members.

One template or model for permission and assent clearly will not fit all parents and children, and certain research contexts (e.g., acute serious illness) will make reasoned reflection and decision making more difficult. Some topics that should be considered for investigation include:

- current practices for seeking permission and assent for different types of research and for children of different ages and with different conditions (e.g., mild chronic conditions or life-threatening diseases);
- the effect on the flow of information of different processes for seeking permission and assent (e.g., approaching the parent first, involving both the parent and the child in the first meeting, or including a facilitator or research advocate for certain kinds of research);
- the consequences for communication, comprehension, and decision making of parents and children with different characteristics (e.g., education level, language, and cultural background) and different research purposes or contexts; and
- the opportunities that children actually are given to dissent, the way in which they express a reluctance or an unwillingness to participate in research, and the reactions of parents and investigators.

In addition, the committee encourages public and private support for research on innovative ways to improve permission and assent processes generally. One starting point would be research on shared decision making between clinicians and patients and methods for improving patient understanding of and decision making about clinical services (see, e.g., O'Connor et al., 1999; Deyo et al., 2000; and Volk et al., 2003). Depending on the research and the circumstances, strategies might include interactive videos, computer programs, and Internet resources.

As described in Appendix B, policies on research participation by wards of the state are poorly documented. The committee encourages a systematic effort to document state policies, their rationales, and their application as a basis for further discussion of the appropriateness of these policies and practices. Some state policies and practices that were an understandable reaction to historical abuses and controversies may now go beyond the provisions and protection of federal regulations in ways that unduly restrict research participation that could benefit the population of children and adolescents who are wards of the state.

CONCLUSION

Both ethical principles and legal requirements place strong emphasis on having competent adults provide informed consent for their participation in research. Because children are usually not legally or intellectually competent to provide consent, an alternative approach has been devised that relies on parental permission and, when appropriate, children's assent to participation in research.

For adults agreeing to clinical research in their own right and for parents agreeing to a child's participation in clinical research, studies suggest that truly informed consent or permission is unlikely to be completely achieved for all individuals in all research situations. Parents who are asked to provide permission for their child's participation in clinical trials are, in particular, often making decisions under great stress and time pressure. Some prefer to trust the physician's assessment rather than make their own, and investigators must be acutely sensitive to the influence that they wield in discussions with parents of ill or injured children. A significant minority of parents may misunderstand the purpose of research, especially when the research tests an intervention for a medical condition. Nonetheless, the goal of having parents provide informed permission remains an important protection for children, both when participation in research is initially sought and throughout the course of a study.

The capacity to make voluntary, informed decisions clearly evolves from birth through adolescence and into adulthood. It also clearly varies among individuals of the same age. The goal should be to involve children in discussions and decisions about research participation as appropriate, given their cognitive and emotional maturity and psychological state. Involving children in discussions and decision making respects their emerging maturity, helps them prepare for participation in research, and gives them an opportunity to express their concerns and objections—and, possibly, influence what happens to them.

This chapter has discussed some circumstances that may raise concerns about undue or even coercive influences on family decision making, for example, when a child's physician is also the investigator seeking agreement to the child's participation in research. Payments to parents or children related to research participation have also raised questions about the potential for undue influence. The next chapter examines these questions.

6

PAYMENTS RELATED TO
CHILDREN'S PARTICIPATION IN
CLINICAL RESEARCH

Interviewer: What if I offer you money [to participate in a study]?
10Y[ear-old]: Well, I don't know. It wouldn't really make a differ-
ence to me.
Interviewer: It wouldn't? What about a lot of money?
10Y (laughs): Probably, a little difference.
Interviewer: So, so what is a lot of money?
10Y: Ah well, the drug study that we did was a hundred and thirty
dollars, I think.
Interviewer: Was that a lot of money?
10Y: For me it is!
Interviewer: So did you decide (to participate) based on how much
money that was?
10Y: No, not really.
Interviewer: No? Would you have done it if I didn't offer you any
money?
10Y: Sure.

Robert M. Nelson, unpublished interview, 1999

Because enrolling sufficient numbers of children in clinical research is often a significant challenge, investigators and research sponsors have tried various strategies to recruit more children. These strategies include expanding studies to more sites, using new methods such as Internet listings to publicize trials, and offering payments or gifts to children and parents to make participation less burdensome or more attractive. Although they are often appropriate and desirable, payments related to research participation may raise ethical questions. The researcher asking the questions above was probing for how much influence payment might have on a child's decisions about research participation. Despite the child's last response, the answers overall provide somewhat conflicting signals about how strongly money might affect the child's decision making.

In preparing this report, the Institute of Medicine (IOM) was charged with considering "whether payment (financial or otherwise) may be made to a child, parent, guardian, or legally authorized representative for the participation of the child in research." This chapter describes the different kinds of payments offered to parents and children, reviews the ethical concerns about such payments, and describes the regulations or guidance provided by federal agencies and others to investigators, institutional review boards (IRBs), and sponsors of research. It also reviews the very limited literature on the use and effects of payments and other incentives. Although they are not payments for research participation as such, the chapter also considers policies and practices on compensation to participants for research-related injuries and payments to physicians for recruiting children to clinical studies.

TYPES OF PAYMENTS RELATED TO RESEARCH PARTICIPATION

Wendler and colleagues (2002) have distinguished four types of payment related to participation in research:

- reimbursements for expenses (e.g., parking or bus fare);
- compensation for the time and inconvenience involved in research participation (e.g., payment at minimum wage for some or all of the hours required of a research participant);
- appreciation payments at token levels (e.g., $25, toys, gift certificates, or movie coupons); and
- incentive payments that offer amounts for participation in research that are not limited to reimbursement, compensation, or token levels.

The committee found the above categories helpful in distinguishing differences among types of payments and discussing payment practices that may unduly influence decisions about research participation. Often, however, research protocols lump payments into one sum, which can make it difficult to determine whether a payment (and how much of payment) is intended to reimburse expenses, compensate for time, express appreciation, or provide an additional incentive for research participation. An explicit identification of the purpose of a payment may help investigators and IRBs evaluate that purpose and also consider reasonable variations in payment practices or amounts, including those that arise from differences in research sites. For example, parking expenses for a 2-hour research visit at a city hospital could run more than $20, whereas parking at a suburban hospital might be free.

For purposes of this report, "nonfinancial payments" include gifts such as toys, computer games, and books. Gifts are usually—but not always—nominal in value and are typically given as tokens of appreciation. Other forms of nonfinancial payment might include services that investigators offer to parents or children to make research participation more attractive or less burdensome (e.g., additional health information or medical monitoring or tours of a research laboratory). One rationale for using movie coupons, gift certificates, or other noncash tokens of appreciation in certain studies, for example, studies involving adolescents at risk for illegal drug use, is to prevent them from using the cash for purposes that might be harmful to their health (e.g., to buy drugs).

In general, the committee believed that it is appropriate and fair to permit investigators to provide payments to parents and children for expenses related to a child's participation in research that they would not otherwise incur. Parents and children, especially if they are economically disadvantaged, should not be asked to bear costs that result solely from research participation.

As discussed below, payments may be determined in different ways, but no payment should be so large or be timed in such a way as to unduly influence parents' or children's decisions about research participation. For example, providing a small payment at the end of the study may encourage completion, but making the entire payment contingent on completing a study could distort a parent's or a child's decision about continued participation in a study. Payments should not influence parents' or children's decisions to participate in research when such participation is not in a child's best interest.

ETHICAL PRINCIPLES AND REGULATORY POLICIES

Ethical Concerns About Payments to Children and Parents

As discussed in Chapter 5, ethical standards for participation in research require that the agreement to participate be freely given, that is, be neither coerced nor unduly influenced by psychological, financial, or other pressure. The major concern about financial incentives—as defined above—is that they may distort decisions about research participation, especially for economically disadvantaged individuals or families. Because parents have the authority to permit a child's participation in research, safeguards against coercion or undue influence on parents are important to ensure that the child's best interests are protected. This chapter focuses on payments, but undue influence on decisions about research participation can come in other forms, including psychological pressure from personal physicians who are also investigators with a stake in the research.

In the words of the *Belmont Report*, undue influence occurs "through an offer of an excessive, unwarranted, inappropriate or improper reward or other overture in order to obtain compliance" (National Commission,

1978a, p. 14). Guidance from the U.S. Department of Health and Human Services (DHHS) stated that "[a]n offer one could not refuse is essentially coercive (or 'undue')" (OPRR, 1993, online, unpaged). Faden and Beauchamp (1986) argue, however, that if coercion is defined as the use of a threat of punishment or harm to influence choice, then payment is not coercion as such. The committee agrees with this distinction.

Unfortunately, no bright line distinguishes proper and reasonable payments to parents and children from payments that are inappropriate. A mix of group or individual circumstances may determine when a particular type or level of payment crosses the line. What is excessive in one situation may not be in another, and reasonable people may sometimes differ in their judgments.

Although payments to research participants may have different purposes, for example, fairness, payments may also be intended to influence enrollment decisions. Thus, expense reimbursement for transportation and parking costs may both be fair and also encourage some people to participate in research (especially research with no prospect of benefiting them) when they might otherwise be reluctant to do so. Reimbursement for expenses is not thought to pose the risk of unduly influencing parents' or children's decision making. (To minimize paperwork and discretionary judgments about appropriate expense levels, flat payments, e.g., $20 per research visit, may be made to cover reasonable local transportation costs and other minor outlays.)

With respect to compensation payments, Wendler and colleagues (2002) note that determining the appropriate compensation for time and inconvenience poses several problems. To cite just one problem, an amount that neutralizes the burden of research participation for one family may exceed it for another and, thereby, act as an inducement. To avoid the unintentional creation of incentives for low-income individuals, some have argued for setting compensation at the level for essential unskilled jobs or at minimum wage (see, e.g., Dickert and Grady, 1999; and Dickert et al., 2002). If, however, parents are not employed or are employed less than full-time (as is more likely in low-income areas), then paying them at minimum wage to bring their child in for a study might be judged to be little different from paying the parent for the child's participation. If such payments are proposed for studies that focus on low-income populations, IRBs should assess the potential for undue influence. An alternative strategy might be to provide night and weekend hours to accommodate research participation by working families who cannot afford to take time off from work.

Is it ethical to pay parents purely for the use of their child in research (i.e., to offer an incentive payment as defined above)? Most sources that the committee consulted either explicitly opposed such payments to parents or omitted such payments from the categories of payments that they endorsed (see, e.g., Grodin and Glantz, 1994 and the discussion of organizational statements later in this chapter). The committee agrees that such incentive payments are not appropriate in pediatric studies.

Some have argued that any token payment to children for participating in research should not be discussed with them until after research is completed for fear of unduly influencing their decisions (AAP, 1995). Wendler and colleagues (2002) disagree, arguing that this practice requires investigators to conceal "pertinent" information as part of the process of seeking permission and assent and, thereby, risk deceiving parents or children who inquire about payment (Wendler et al., 2002, p. 168). On balance, the committee agrees that it is best to mention token or other payments during the permission and assent processes.

Federal Regulations and Other Policies on Payment Related to Research Participation

Federal regulations on the protection of human participants in research do not explicitly mention payments related to participation. They do state that informed consent must be sought "only under circumstances . . . that minimize the possibility of coercion or undue influence" (45 CFR 46.116; 21 CFR 50.20). This provision is generally interpreted by federal officials and IRBs to require an assessment of whether any payments related to research participation are substantial enough that they might distort decision making.

Participants must also be provided "a statement that participation is voluntary, that refusal to participate will involve no penalty or loss of benefits to which the subject is otherwise entitled, and that the subject may discontinue participation at any time without penalty or loss of benefits" (45 CFR 46.116(a)(8); 21 CFR 50.25(a)(8)). However, federal regulations also require investigators to describe "the consequences of a subject's decision to withdraw from the research and procedures for orderly termination of participation by the subject" (45 CFR 46.116(b)(4); 21 CFR 50.25(b)(4)). This implies that researchers must explain to parents (and, sometimes, children or adolescents) how withdrawing from the study would affect any payments that they were to have received; for example, a bonus payment for completing the study.

Office for Human Research Protections

The Office for Human Research Protections (OHRP) supplements federal regulations with guidance on a variety of topics. Its primary guidance on payment to research participants appears to be provided by *Protecting Human Research Subjects: Institutional Review Board Guidebook*, which was last revised more than a decade ago (OPRR, 1993). The guidebook outlines the major issues that IRBs should consider in reviewing payment provisions in a research protocol. It also refers readers to a Food and Drug Administration (FDA) information sheet on payment to research subjects (discussed below). In the section on analysis of study risks and benefits, the document emphasizes that payments to research participants should not be considered in assessing whether a protocol's risks are reasonable in relation to its potential benefits (OPRR, 1993, Ch. 3, online, unpaged).

The guidebook does not offer specific guidance about payments related to children's participation in research. Much of the guidance is relevant to pediatric research, but some does not apply. For example, the additional protections provided to child research participants would likely preclude approval of the kinds of higher-risk studies that might, for healthy adult volunteers, provide larger-than-usual incentive payments for the acceptance of greater research risk. (Some IRBs do not permit such risk-related incentive payments for adults participants in research.)

The IRB guidebook stresses that IRBs are responsible for ensuring that consent is not coerced or unduly influenced but is truly voluntary. "Offers that are too attractive may blind prospective subjects to the risks or impair their ability to exercise proper judgment" and "may prompt subjects to lie or conceal information that, if known, would disqualify them from enrolling—or continuing—as participants in a research project" (OPRR, 1993, Ch. 3, online, unpaged). In the discussion of IRB evaluation of incentives for enrollment in studies that involve risk or discomfort, the guidebook notes that there are disagreements among the IRB members about what practices are appropriate.

As IRBs assess proposed payments to research participants, the guidebook advises them to consider not only a participant's health status, employment status, and education level but also his or her financial, emotional, and community resources. This advice also applies to the consideration of payments to parents of prospective child research participants.

On its website, OHRP summarizes "common findings" about noncompliance with federal regulations based on the compliance determination letters that it has sent to institutions (http://ohrp.osophs.dhhs.gov/references/findings.pdf). The list of common findings under the heading "informed consent" includes "enrollment procedures that did not minimize the possibility of undue influence or coercion" (OHRP, 2002c, online, unpaged). One letter of determination included, among many issues, a concern that the IRB had not recognized that free care could result in undue influence on subjects or families (McNeilly, 2001).

Food and Drug Administration

The FDA's primary guidance document for investigators provides some specific advice about the timing of payments and the information to be provided by investigators to IRBs and research participants (FDA, 1998d). The advice does not mention payments to parents or children. In general, payment should accrue during the course of a study (e.g., per visit) and should not be contingent upon completion of the study (although a small bonus for completion is acceptable). Protocols should provide IRBs with details about the type, level, and timing of payments to participants at the time of initial review and the details should also be included in the informed consent form. The guidance does not include specific details or examples to illustrate unacceptable practices.

The FDA has also issued as guidance the report *E11 Clinical Investigation of Medicinal Products in the Pediatric Population*, which was developed by the International Conference on Harmonisation (FDA, 2000b; ICH, 2000b). The guidelines recommend that "[r]ecruitment of study participants should occur in a manner free from inappropriate inducements either to the parent(s) or legal guardian or the study participant" (FDA, 2000b, p. 12). The guidelines state that expense reimbursement and subsistence costs may be included in protocol design, but these payments should be reviewed by the ethics review board. The guidelines of the Council for International Organizations of Medical Sciences state that a "guardian asked to give permission on behalf of an incompetent person should be offered no recompense other than a refund of travel and related expenses" (CIOMS, 2002, Guideline 7).

USE OF PAYMENTS IN RESEARCH INVOLVING CHILDREN

Little systematic information is available about the use of various kinds of payments or other incentives for participation in either adult or pediatric studies. A commentary on the ethics of paying for children's participation in research cited a review of data from a clinical trials listing service that suggested that a quarter of pediatric trials provided for payments (Wendler et al., 2002). The largest amount mentioned was $1,500 to cover time and travel costs for families participating in a study of a psoriasis drug, but details about how this amount was determined were not provided.

Trial listings and recruitment notices often describe payments very generally without making clear whether they are restricted to reimbursement for expenses or compensation for time. This lack of specificity may be intended—and, indeed, required by IRBs or research institutions—to discourage initial expressions of participant interest in research participation based primarily on the promise of payments beyond expenses. Some IRBs or research institutions prohibit mention of the actual amount of a payment in a recruitment notice, allowing only a general statement about the type of payment that will be provided (e.g., "reimbursement for expenses").

In a study comparing research involving children with cancer and research involving children with diabetes, Broome and colleagues (2001) found that participants in cancer studies were never offered financial incentives (in the words of the investigators). In contrast, participants in diabetes research listed financial incentives as a key reason for participating.

For research protocols that offer a potential of direct benefit, particularly in an acute-care situation, the view seems to be that investigators do not need to include any incentives because parents' desire to have access to the investigational drug or procedure is the driving force in decision making. In addition many of the costs normally associated with research participation (e.g., parking and transportation) would be incurred anyway in connection with clinical care for an acute problem.

The policies of one research consortium provide an example of reasonable payment for the time spent by participants in research. The Therapeutic Development Network (TDN) of the Cystic Fibrosis Foundation approves payment for time and expenses. It cautions that such payment "should not be excessive and should not be perceived as an inducement to participate" (TDN, 2003, p. F-2.).

For time spent in research, TDN suggests that study participants be reimbursed as follows:

- Inpatient study: $150 per full day
- Outpatient study:

<2 hours	$ 25.00
2 to <4 hours	$ 50.00
4 to <8 hours	$ 75.00
8 to 12 hours	$100.00

These TDN payment guidelines are monitored regularly and are changed on the basis of cost-of-living increases, IRB feedback, and parent and patient input. The guidelines do not sanction varying payment based on the risk presented by a study. TDN has received favorable comments from several IRBs regarding the helpfulness of its standardized approach that is consistent across studies and sensitive to ethical issues regarding payment. Flexibility in applying the guidelines is provided as a safeguard. The guidelines clearly state that the local IRB has the final decision regarding the actual payments at each site.

A recent review of 127 studies (not limited to health research) involving adolescents reported that 55 percent of all studies and 40 percent of health studies provided for payments (Borzekowski et al., 2003). Fifty percent were paid in cash and 38 percent with vouchers. The mean payment value per research session was $26 (range, $1 to $100), and the average total amount for research involving multiple sessions was $82 (range, $1 to $600).

One recent study looked specifically but somewhat indirectly at practices in pediatric research through a survey of IRB chairs who reported that their institutions conducted some pediatric research (Weise et al., 2002). Of the 128 IRB chairs included in the analysis (response rate, 36 percent), two-thirds reported that their institutions had approved at least one protocol that offered payment to the parents of children who were research participants. Ten percent reported that they had not approved any studies that offered payment, and just over 20 percent reported that no protocols involving payment had been submitted. The IRB chairs reported that payments for studies at their institutions ranged between $1 and $1,000 for cash payments and between $10 and $500 for bonds. (The median minimum amount of cash payment was $10, and the median maximum amount of cash payment was $100.) The great majority reported that payment was discussed before the child's enrollment in the research protocol. IRBs that reviewed a larger percentage of pediatric protocols were more likely than other IRBs to require investigators to make changes in their plans for paying research participants or their parents. The article did not clearly distinguish among reimbursement, compensation, appreciation, and incentive payments and did not provide study details; for example, how payment amounts were determined.

In another study, researchers in the Clinical Bioethics unit at the National Institutes of Health surveyed individuals at 32 organizations who were involved in developing, conducting, or reviewing clinical research (Dickert et al., 2002). The organizations included academic research centers, drug companies, contract research organizations, and independent IRBs. Although the study did not focus specifically on pediatric research, the results raise concerns about the adequacy of institutional information and policies on payment. According to the investigators, only one respondent reported that no studies involved payments to research participants, and another respondent had no information. As discussed further below, only 38 percent of the organizations reported having policies on payments related to research participation. Less than one in five of the organizations had any systematic way of tracking studies involving payments, and thus, most could not provide a "confident estimate" of the proportion of studies in which subjects were paid. The results did not distinguish among types of payment. However, in a discussion of institutional guidance about payment practices, the authors report that "most organizations said that subjects were paid for the time (87 percent), inconvenience (84 percent), or travel (68 percent) associated with research participation" and "[t]hirty-two percent reported that subjects were paid for incurring risk" (Dickert et al., 2002, p. 370).

IRB POLICIES AND PRACTICES

In the study by Weise and colleagues (2002) cited earlier, only 6 of 128 of the IRB chairs whose responses were included in the analysis reported that their IRBs had written policies about payments to research participants. Of the five written policies reviewed by the authors, all permitted payment related to expenses or burdens associated with participation. Two of the written policies reviewed prohibited payments as "inducements" but provided neither further explanations nor examples of the types of payments that would constitute inducements.

Of the organizations in the study by Dickert and colleagues (2002) cited earlier, 38 percent of the organizations that were included in the analysis reported that they had written policies on payment to research participants. Of the 17 IRBs included in the study, 9 had written policies on payment. Some organizations (31 percent) approved payments only for the parents; a smaller group (19 percent) approved payments only for the child; 42 percent approved payments for both. Almost half the organizations had some restrictions on how payments could be described (e.g., prohibiting mention of specific payment amounts). None reported that they forbade any mention of payment in recruiting advertisements. One, however, prohibited reference to payment in pediatric studies.

Consistent with the survey findings, the institutional payment policies varied among the unrepresentative examples reviewed by the committee. Most policies were consistent with the guidance provided by DHHS (e.g., full payment should not be contingent on completion of a study), but they were sometimes less detailed. Some mentioned the ethical concerns underlying the policies. At the University of California at Los Angeles, for example, the policy notes that children "are in a dependent relationship to adults and easily manipulated in an academic or clinical setting" and that "incentives or rewards for participation may be used but should not be so valuable, within the value system of the child, as to sway their legitimate reluctance to participate" (UCLA, 1997, sec. 6-6).

At the Children's Hospital Boston, the policy on payment explicitly states that "[i]t is sometimes desirable to provide subjects and their parents compensation for their participation in research projects" (e.g., taxi fare, babysitting fees, lunch, cash remuneration in lieu of expense payments, parenting books, and infant formula but not lotteries or prize drawings). Children themselves should be given a small toy or gift certificate when possible. The policy emphasizes that "[i]n all instances, compensation should not be so large as to act as an inducement for subjects to participate regardless of how minimal the risk may be" (Children's Hospital Boston, 2003, unpaged).

STATEMENTS OF PROFESSIONAL ORGANIZATIONS

In its 1995 statement on the ethical conduct of drug studies with pediatric populations, the Committee on Drugs of the American Academy of Pediatrics (AAP) stated that remuneration, compensation, and indemnification are ethical payment practices based on current societal standards. It also observed that "serious ethical questions arise when payment is offered to adults acting on behalf of minors in return for allowing minors to participate as research subjects" (AAP, 1995, p. 293). As noted and questioned earlier in this chapter, the statement recommended that investigators refrain from discussing gifts or appreciation payments with children until after the research is completed.

In its 2003 statement to the Institute of Medicine (IOM) committee, AAP emphasized that "parents should not profit from placing their child in research," even when the research does not present "significant risk" (AAP, 2003, p. 12). In contrast, for research that involves no burden to the child beyond inconvenience (i.e., no discomfort, unpleasantness, or tangible risk), "remuneration may be a major incentive for participation and completion of the study and it is appropriate in this context to compensate children for their efforts in a manner comparable to compensating adult research subjects," as long as the payment is not used to coerce (unduly influence) children or their parents into agreeing to participation (p. 12). Research projects may also waive treatment costs if the IRB and investigators judge that such payment-in-kind will not "be coercive of participation."

Other organizations presented statements to the IOM committee in which they indicated that it is appropriate to reimburse expenses or compensate for time or inconvenience. These organizations include the Association of Medical School Pediatric Department Chairs, the Cystic Fibrosis Foundation, the Society for Pediatric Research (which mentioned only "expenses"), the Allergy & Asthma Network/Mothers of Asthmatics, Public Citizen's Health Research Group, and the Genetic Alliance. None of these groups explicitly endorsed incentive payments to parents or children.

OTHER CONCERNS ABOUT PAYMENT RELATED TO CHILDREN'S RESEARCH PARTICIPATION

Compensation for Research-Related Injuries

If an adult or child suffers a research-related injury that is not the result of malfeasance or negligence, that person has no legal avenue to recover

treatment costs or lost earnings. However, provisions to compensate research participants for research-related injuries may be a factor for parents
who are deciding whether to enroll their child in research.

For research involving more than minimal risk, federal regulations require that informed-consent forms include information about whether compensation or medical treatment may be available in the event of a research-
related injury, how to get further information, and whom to contact in the
event of such an injury (45 CFR 46.116 (a)(6 and 7);21 CFR 50.25(a)(6
and 7)). No federal regulations require compensation for research-related
injuries.

The Council for International Organizations of Medical Sciences has
endorsed the provision of compensation for physical injuries related to
research. Specifically, their guidelines state that "[i]nvestigators should ensure that research subjects who suffer injury as a result of their participation are entitled to free medical treatment for such injury and to such
financial or other assistance as would compensate them equitably for any
resultant impairment, disability or handicap. In the case of death as a result
of their participation, their dependants are entitled to compensation"
(CIOMS, 2002, Guideline 19, online, unpaged). In addition, investigators
are not to ask research participants to waive these rights. Several foreign
countries have policies providing for some compensation for research-related injuries (IOM, 2003a).

The IOM report *Responsible Research* identified some government
agencies (e.g., the Veterans Administration and the National Institutes of
Health (NIH) Clinical Center) that provide or cover short-term medical
expenses for research-related injuries (IOM, 2003a). It located only one
private organization, the University of Washington that paid long-term
medical costs related to such injuries. The report recommended that organizations conducting research cover at least medical and rehabilitation costs
for research participants who are injured as a direct result of participating
in research, without regard to fault. It also recommended that DHHS collect data on the incidence of research-related injuries and analyze their
costs. In addition, organizations that accredit IRBs include such compensation as a requirement of accreditation.

Payments to Physicians for Recruiting Child Research Participants

Although the committee was not asked to examine the issue of payment
to clinicians for enrolling child patients in research, this is an increasingly
important issue in pediatric research. In the research context, a finder's fee
is a payment (or sometimes a nonfinancial reward) that is made to a clinician in exchange for referring or recruiting a research participant and that is

not directly linked to the reasonable costs of identifying potential research subjects (e.g., searching medical records). The finder's fee may be contingent on the actual participation of the referred individual in the research, and the provision of such a fee may or may not be disclosed to the referred patient. The ethical concern is that physicians who accept finder's fees have a conflict of interest that may lead them to make recommendations that are not in their patients' best interests and may undermine the trust between patient and physician, whether or not the payment is disclosed to the patient (see, e.g., Flegel, 1997 and Goldner, 2000).

The American Medical Association has explicitly condemned the practice of paying finders' fees and similar incentives to physicians who recruit their patients for clinical trials (AMA, 1994, 1999). A 2000 report from the Office of the Inspector General of DHHS questioned the practice and noted that many IRBs do not review these kinds of recruitment practices (OIG, 2000b). It recommended that federal agencies clarify that IRBs have the authority to review such practices. It also recommended that FDA and OHRP cooperate to provide guidance to IRBs about these and other recruiting practices. Current IRB policies are not catalogued anywhere, but an informal review of institutional web sites indicates that policies vary. Some IRBs or research institutions ban the offering or accepting of finder's fees, whereas, others discourage but do not forbid them. Finder's fees are illegal in some states.

The recruitment by physician-investigators of their own patients as research participants also raises concerns. It is an attractive and convenient research strategy, especially given the challenges of recruiting sufficient numbers of children for pediatric studies. Nonetheless, it raises ethical questions. As described by the National Bioethics Advisory Commission, this is one of the situations that IRBs should "recognize and avoid," as it creates susceptibility to harm or coercion (NBAC, 2001b, p. iv). The committee agrees. In addition, the practice may blur the distinction for a patient between research and treatment and contribute to the therapeutic misconception as discussed in Chapter 5.

IMPROVING PRACTICES AND POLICIES ON PAYMENT RELATED TO CHILDREN'S PARTICIPATION IN RESEARCH

Payments to parents and children can be ethical elements of research involving children if these payments are established, reviewed, and implemented in a thoughtful and consistent manner and adhere to the principles of ethical research. Investigators, sponsors, and IRBs should be vigilant in scrutinizing financial payments for the possibility of undue influence on parents' or children's decision making. They should also be alert to nonfinancial practices that may distort decision making, for example, inappropriate advertising or solicitations for research participation by primary care physicians that take advantage of the trust that families place in them.

At the same time, IRBs should be receptive to investigators' creative but ethically responsible efforts to reduce financial barriers that may discourage parents, especially economically disadvantaged parents, from agreeing to their child's participation in research. These efforts should be considered in the broader context of strategies to respect and accommodate the legitimate needs of families, especially families already stressed by a child's serious illness.

Because little information exists on how parents and children perceive and respond to different payment practices, investigators and IRBs lack useful information to guide them in making decisions about what practices threaten parent or child judgment. Given current efforts to increase the number of children involved in research, federal policymakers should solicit ideas for studies that could illuminate the ethical and practical implications of different kinds of payments related to children's participation in research. A variety of methods may be appropriate for such studies, including focus groups; surveys; and interviews of investigators, parents, and older children or adolescents. Evaluations of the use of study or consent monitors might also provide insights into investigator behaviors (e.g., whether and how payment is discussed) and parent and child responses.

Written Institutional Policies on Payment

Even in the absence of data about the impact of payment practices on parent and child judgments, IRBs and research institutions should develop written policies on payments related to research participation. By developing such policies, IRBs can consider how different practices may serve or compromise ethical principles for the conduct of human research outside of the context of an individual protocol. Such a deliberation will not eliminate uncertainty or subjectivity in decision making about payment practices, but it should help achieve a fairer and more consistent approach to decision making about individual protocols.

Although written policies can not cover every contingency presented by actual research protocols, they should be detailed enough to provide investigators with useful guidance as to what is and what is not acceptable for pediatric studies. In addition, examples of wording about payments that the IRB has approved for consent and permission forms can be helpful to investigators.

In addition to requiring that protocols include descriptive details about proposed payments (e.g., use of a bonus for completion of a study), IRBs should require that researchers present, as part of a protocol, the rationale for why any payments that they propose to make to parents or children are appropriate. Researchers should also explain how payment amounts are determined (e.g., taking the age of the child participants into account in selecting gifts of appreciation).

> Recommendation 6.1: Institutional review boards, research institutions, and sponsors of research that includes children and adolescents should adopt explicit written policies on acceptable and unacceptable types and amounts of payments related to research participation. These policies should specify that investigators
>
> • disclose the amount, the recipient, the timing, and the purpose (e.g., an expense reimbursement or a token of appreciation to a child) of any payments as part of the process of seeking parents' permission and, as appropriate, children's assent to research participation;
> • avoid emphasis on payments or descriptions of payments as benefits of participating in research during the permission or assent process; and
> • obtain institutional review board approval for the disclosure of information about payments in advertisements and in permission and assent forms and procedures.

In general, any type of payment related to a child's participation in research should be discussed during the process of seeking parental permission. Information about payment should also be included in the consent and permission form. When appropriate, payments to children or adolescents should likewise be discussed during the process of seeking their agreement to research participation. That discussion should be appropriate to the child's maturity, psychological condition, and other characteristics. Although descriptions of payment arrangements in permission and assent forms should be scrutinized by IRBs, failure to provide information on approved arrangements could discourage low-income parents from permitting their child's participation in research and could also deter adolescents from agreeing to participate in research. In addition, parents may expect certain kinds of payments on the basis of their knowledge or perceptions of other studies and may feel misled if they discover at the end of the study that they are being paid differently.

Categories of Acceptable Payments

Certain types of payments to parents or adolescents are usually if not always acceptable, for example, reimbursement for reasonable expenses that are necessary for research participation. The specifics may vary, but examples of reasonable expenses are costs of transportation to the research site, parking, lodging, meals, and babysitting. Other payments are never appropriate in pediatric research, for example, paying parents for the use of their child in research.

Compensation to parents for lost wages or time may be appropriate under carefully scrutinized circumstances. One objective of IRB and institutional policies on payments related to children's participation in research should be to encourage equal access to study participation regardless of a family's economic status. At the same time, policies should prevent practices that risk exerting an undue influence over the parents' decisions. If a low-income parent cannot afford to lose time from work to take a child to a research site, then some form of compensation (e.g., at the minimum wage) may be reasonable and fair.

For some parents, the barrier may not be lost wages for hours missed but fear of losing their job if they take time off. To respond to the diverse barriers to children's research participation, nonfinancial strategies to equalize participation opportunities should also be considered, for example, adjusting the times or places for research visits. In certain instances, for example, when IRBs allow flexibility in devising arrangements with individual families, it may be appropriate for them to specify that a family or child advocate independently assess the appropriateness of the arrangements and the decision of a family to enroll a child.

> **Recommendation 6.2: In addition to offering small gifts or payments to parents and children as gestures of appreciation, investigators may also—if they minimize the potential for undue influence—act ethically to reduce certain barriers to research participation when they**
>
> • **reimburse reasonable expenses directly related to a child's participation in research;**
> • **provide reasonable, age-appropriate compensation for children based on the time involved in research that does not offer the prospect of direct benefit; and**
> • **offer evening or weekend hours, on-site child care, and other reasonable accommodations for parental work and family commitments.**

Although controversial, it may be appropriate under certain circumstances to pay adult volunteers larger amounts for agreeing to participate in higher-risk research that will not directly benefit them. Likewise, it may be appropriate to pay adults more for engaging in higher-risk work, subject to socially sanctioned health and safety regulations. What is acceptable for competent adults is, however, often not acceptable for children. Child labor laws present a case in point. In general, the issue of risk-related payment should not arise in research involving children because federal regulations (if they are interpreted as recommended in Chapter 4) substantially limit the amount of risk to which children can be exposed in research without the prospect of direct benefit. The potential for harm must be minimal or only slightly more than minimal. Given this appropriate conservatism, the committee believed that it would be inappropriate—even within these narrow boundaries—to allow financial encouragement for children's participation in research based on the level of risk involved. The recommendation above allows, however, for reasonable, age-appropriate compensation for those whose research participation is associated with more time or inconvenience (e.g., for adolescents who must take time away from a job).

Payment for Research-Related Injuries

Consistent with the recommendations of an earlier IOM committee and other groups, this committee also recommends compensation for child participants who are injured in the course of research. Depending on their medical condition, children who are permanently injured as a result of research participation may live with the consequences of an injury for a far longer period than an adult so injured. The committee also agrees that DHHS should collect data on the incidence of research-related injuries and should analyze their costs.

Recommendation 6.3: Research organizations and sponsors should pay the medical and rehabilitation costs for children injured as a direct result of research participation, without regard to fault. Consent and permission documents should disclose to parents (and adolescents, if appropriate) the child's right to compensation and the mechanisms for seeking such compensation.

Payments to Investigators or Others

As described in Chapter 2, FDA and NIH have adopted policies to encourage investigators and research sponsors to include children in research. Chapter 2 also described the challenges that pediatric investigators face, including recruiting sufficient numbers of children for many kinds of studies. Given the combination of government policies and existing recruitment problems in some areas of research, policymakers, research institutions, and IRBs should be attentive to the recruitment practices proposed in pediatric protocols and should strongly discourage or forbid bonuses or similar financial incentives to physicians for enrolling their pediatric patients in research.

Recommendation 6.4: Investigators and their staffs may appropriately be reimbursed for the costs associated with conducting research. Payments in the form of finder's fees or bonuses for enrolling a specific number of children or adolescents are unethical and should not be permitted.

CONCLUSION

Payments related to research participation have a role to play in reducing barriers and equalizing access to research participation. The primary concern is that certain types or levels of payment may unduly influence a parent's or child's judgment about research participation and encourage decisions that are not in the child's best interest. Payments to physicians for enrolling children in research also raise questions about undue influence and conflict of interest. Such payments should be limited to reimbursement for costs related to the conduct of research.

Although the specifics of an individual protocol may affect judgments about what payment practices are appropriate, IRBs should develop written policies to provide basic guidance for investigators and IRB members in developing or reviewing protocols and reduce inconsistent, ad hoc judgments. The process of developing written policies should encourage more systematic reflection on the fit between different payment practices and the ethical standards for clinical research involving children.

7

REGULATORY COMPLIANCE, ACCREDITATION, AND QUALITY IMPROVEMENT

[T]o preserve public trust in research, the scientific community must go beyond a culture of compliance—it must strive for a culture of conscience—one in which we do the right thing not because we are required to, but because it is the right thing to do, a refrain now echoed frequently throughout the research community.

Greg Koski, 2002, p. 1

The late 1990s saw considerable public concern about the extent to which investigators and IRBs were following federal regulations to protect human participants in research. Chapter 1 summarized some of the consequences, which included the reorganizing and refocusing of federal government units responsible for regulatory oversight and the well-publicized, temporary suspensions of federally supported human research in a number of prominent universities for deficiencies in their programs for protecting research participants. By the time that Greg Koski (outgoing director of the Office for Human Research Protections) offered the challenge quoted above, the emphasis on compliance per se had expanded to recognize that a strong, broadly shared commitment to acting on the values underlying the regulations would be a far more powerful and consistent motivator of ethical performance than simply a commitment to compliance.

This chapter examines one element in the statement of task for this study: the compliance with and enforcement of the federal regulations. It also examines accreditation programs and quality improvement initiatives that promote voluntary efforts to exceed and not just to meet regulatory requirements.

Technically, the federal regulations on protections for human participants in research apply only to federally conducted, supported, or regulated research. Many research institutions have gone further to establish the regulations as the standard for all human research. One of the recommendations in the final chapter of this report is that all clinical research involving children should occur under the umbrella of a formal human research protection program regardless of source of funding or regulation under the Federal Food, Drug, and Cosmetic Act. (Consistent with earlier chapters, this report refers to the regulations found in 45 CFR 46 as the DHHS regulations and the regulations found in 21 CFR 50 and 56 as the FDA regulations.)

Some of the failure to comply with the federal regulations is not due to obvious shortcomings on the part of investigators, members of institutional review boards (IRBs), or others. Rather, it reflects, in part, the ambiguity and lack of clarity in the regulations themselves. The federal government must bear some responsibility for the wide range of interpretations of important elements of the regulations. This report, particularly Chapter 4, attempts to clarify some key terms and concepts in the regulations. It also recommends that the government provide more interpretive guidance and provide examples of procedures and studies that illustrate permissible research involving infants, children, and adolescents. Such guidance should help investigators and IRBs better understand their responsibilities and the boundaries between acceptable and unacceptable practices, although differences in judgment will undoubtedly remain.

Unfortunately, the committee found a particular dearth of information about compliance with the regulations as they relate to children. As a result, the group could not reach firm conclusions about compliance. One of the recommendations in this chapter is for government agencies and IRBs to collect and analyze information specific to children that will begin to allow assessment of the performance of investigators, IRBs, research institutions, research sponsors, and federal regulators. Having used its authority to establish regulations, the federal government has an obligation to collect information and take other actions to assess the extent to which they are being appropriately monitored and implemented.

CONTINUED CONCERN ABOUT OVERSIGHT OF RESEARCH INVOLVING HUMANS

As described in Chapter 1, policies and programs to protect human participants in research have evolved over several decades, often in response to public outcries over publicized instances of unethical or questionable research practices. The first stages of that evolution involved recognizing problems, placing them within an ethical framework, and developing standards and public policies for the ethical conduct of human research. Over time, policies became more formal as the government adopted regulations and expanded their scope, for example, by adding special protections for vulnerable populations, such as children and prisoners.

In the last decade and a half, concern has increasingly focused on the implementation of the regulations at all levels—the investigator, IRB, research institution, and government levels—and on the adequacy of resources devoted to this task. A series of reports have noted progress in human research protections but have also described deficiencies in their implementation and have made recommendations for improvement.

No report has, however, focused explicitly on problems in implementing the federal regulations protecting child participants in research. In the committee's experience, however, the problems identified for human research protection programs generally extend to implementation of research protections for children. Indeed, the problems may be amplified in pediatric research for the reasons identified throughout this report. These reasons include the particular challenges of designing and conducting pediatric research, the limited amount of such research in many institutions, and the difficult or ambiguous concepts included in the regulations governing child participants in research.

Government Reports on Human Research Protection Regulations and Programs

A 1996 report by the General Accounting Office (GAO; an arm of the U.S. Congress) concluded that the regulatory oversight of biomedical and behavioral research had reduced the likelihood of abuses of human research participants. Nonetheless, it warned that no system of research protections can be foolproof and that limited resources and other constraints threatened the effectiveness of both local review boards and federal oversight (GAO, 1996). The report stressed the need for continued vigilance in protecting human participants in research and warned against overreliance on investigators' voluntary compliance with regulatory requirements. A 2001 statement from the GAO noted several areas of progress since its earlier report but expressed continuing concern that the "pace of some actions is too slow" and "gaps remain" (Heinrich, 2001, p. 12). In addition to reiterating concerns about inadequate oversight resources at both the federal and local levels, it cited problems with insufficient guidance on informed consent and unclear requirements for adverse event reporting. That same year, another GAO report urged more forceful direction from the U.S. Department of Health and Human Services (DHHS) regarding the prevention and management of financial conflicts of interest that threatened the integrity of biomedical research (GAO, 2001).

The DHHS Office of the Inspector General (OIG) has issued several critical reports on national and local oversight of human research. Taken together, three reports issued in 1998 characterized IRBs as being inundated with proposals, hurried in their reviews, beset by pressures on their independent judgment, and short of resources, including not only paid staff but also community (nonscientific) representation and clinical expertise from volunteers prepared to take time away from revenue-generating activities (OIG, 1998a, b, c). The OIG argued that the regulatory and oversight system often focused on less important issues while it ignored major ethical issues and concerns. The 1998 reports made a number of recommendations for federal action. Two years later, the OIG concluded that DHHS had increased its enforcement efforts and taken other promising steps but had not acted on most of the earlier recommendations (OIG, 2000a). The OIG acknowledged that some of the improvements that it had recommended would take legislative action.

In a comprehensive report in 2001, the National Bioethics Advisory Commission (NBAC) argued (among other criticisms) that growth in the scope and scale of human research had outpaced the system for protecting participants in that research (NBAC, 2001b). For the entire system, "scarce [financial and human] resources limit the functioning of the oversight system at every level (NBAC, 2001b, p. 8). Noting that "any system of sanctions can only be as good as the monitoring and investigating processes that are used to determine their need," the report observed that some agencies, such as DHHS, "conduct only 'for cause' investigations, generally because limited budgets do not permit more proactive monitoring" (NBAC, 2001b, pp. 12-13). (As discussed later in this chapter, the Office for Human Research Protections [OHRP] now undertakes occasional "not-for-cause" evaluations.)

The 2001 NBAC report noted the failure of all federal agencies that conduct or fund research involving children to adopt the special protections application to children found in Subpart D of the DHHS regulations. As described in Chapter 3, only the Department of Education, the Central Intelligence Agency, and the Social Security Administration have adopted Subpart D. The NBAC report also pointed to the inconsistent interpretation of research protection regulations across federal agencies.

As discussed in Chapters 1 and 3, an increasing amount of pediatric research funded by American companies is being conducted in other countries. In another report issued in 2001, NBAC examined ethical issues in international research. The report noted that DHHS has never "determined formally that guidelines or rules from any other countries afford protections equal to those provided by U.S. human regulations" (NBAC, 2001a, p. 14). It also detailed criticisms from foreign investigators and others about the excessive burdens imposed by the United States' research protection regulations. NBAC commended OHRP for recent efforts to make certain rules applying to foreign research less burdensome (e.g., permitting foreign institutions to abide by other ethical standards or guidelines identified in this report). It also recommended that an independent body evaluate the new policies after a suitable period. Such an evaluation should examine research involving children.

In the same year as the Commission's report, the DHHS OIG issued a critical report stating that the Food and Drug Administration (FDA) "receives minimal information on the performance of foreign institutional review boards . . . [and] has an inadequate database on the people and entities involved in foreign research" (OIG, 2001, p. ii). It argued that it is not sufficient to depend on foreign investigators' statements that will they comply with protections for human research participants.

Other Reports and Attention

Several reports from the Institute of Medicine (IOM) have offered recommendations for improving the ethical conduct and oversight of research involving human participants. One of the strongest statements about the difficulties of assessing system performance came in the report *Responsible Research* (IOM, 2003a). It noted that a lack of information on current protection activities and results had "repeatedly confounded" analysis but went on to say that "the evidence is abundant regarding the significant strains and weaknesses of the current system" and that "major reforms are in order" (IOM, 2003a, p. 4).

Congress has twice included provisions in legislation calling for reports that would, among other topics, discuss the appropriateness of the regulations on protecting child participants in research and the monitoring and enforcement of compliance with them. This report responds to the most recent legislation (the Best Pharmaceuticals for Children Act of 2002). In a report called for in earlier legislation, the Children's Health Act of 2000 (P.L. 106-310), DHHS concluded that the federal regulations are "sound, effective, and well-crafted, and when implemented properly by IRBs and investigators, provide adequate and appropriate protections for children of all ages and maturity levels" (DHHS, 2001, p. iii). The DHHS report did not include explicit findings on IRB or investigator implementation of or compliance with the regulations but observed that "problems and concerns related to research involving children generally have resulted from a failure to implement the existing regulations appropriately and consistently, not from fundamental deficiencies of the regulations" (DHHS, 2001, p. iii).

(The body of the report, which had to be finished on a short, 6-month timetable, was 22 pages in length, excluding the summary.)

In addition to sometimes critical reports on the system for protecting human participants in research, the system has also come under public scrutiny and criticism after the deaths of several research participants. For example, a story in the New York Times about the death of Ellen Roche, a healthy volunteer at Johns Hopkins University, reported that information about the research "sketch[ed] a picture of an experiment that went amiss" (Altman, 2001, p. A16). The story also described the difficulties in obtaining information about the circumstances surrounding the death. The September 1999 death of Jesse Gelsinger in a gene therapy trial likewise prompted many critical stories (see, e.g., Halim, 2000 and Stolberg, 1999).

As noted above, federal officials have temporarily suspended or restricted federally funded or regulated research at several major academic institutions (see Exhibit 3.1 of NBAC, 2001b, pp. 54–56). Although some criticized these actions as being too extreme, they dramatically underscored a new commitment by officials to identify and correct deficiencies in the protection of human participants in research and recognized this protection as "an absolutely critical foundation" of research involving humans (Koski, 2001, p. 1). Federal officials have also undertaken a number of more positive actions to improve the protection of human participants in research, as discussed below.

GOVERNMENT OVERSIGHT OF REGULATIONS PROTECTING CHILD PARTICIPANTS IN RESEARCH

The committee that prepared the IOM report *Responsible Research* (IOM, 2003a) found that government data on compliance with policies on protection of human research participants were very limited. The present committee found that data specific to clinical research involving children were even more limited. Most of what follows describes the government's compliance monitoring and enforcement activities in general. OHRP was able to provide some data on compliance problems related to clinical research involving children, but FDA could not.

As described in Chapter 1, both DHHS and FDA have reorganized their human research protection programs following the above-cited criticisms of the oversight of human research protections and the widely publicized instances of questionable or deficient research conduct. In June 2000, the Office for Protection from Research Risks became the more explicitly named Office for Human Research Protections (OHRP), and DHHS moved the unit from the National Institutes of Health (NIH) to the Office of the Secretary of DHHS (DHHS, 2000). In March 2001, the FDA established the Good Clinical Practices Program within the Office of Science and Health

Coordination in the Office of the Commissioner. The program essentially has the lead for policy issues related to human subject protection, although individual centers (e.g., the Center for Drug Evaluation Research) still maintain their own medical policy and bioresearch monitoring units relevant to their jurisdictions (David Lepay, M.D., Ph.D., Food and Drug Administration, personal communication, October 4, 2003). As described below, OHRP and FDA use different strategies to monitor compliance with regulations for the protection of human participants in research.

Oversight by the Office for Human Research Protections

Even when regulators necessarily rely on voluntary compliance with regulations and adopt a quality improvement perspective that encourages excellence and not merely compliance, regulators must still have methods suitable for monitoring and enforcing adherence to the regulations for which they are responsible. The OHRP strategy for compliance oversight relies primarily on the investigation of allegations of institutional noncompliance or other problems (Koski, 2000).

Since 1990, the agency has conducted more than 750 investigations of such allegations (Carome, 2003). In 1998 and 1999, the office's actions against institutions holding an OHRP-approved assurance increased significantly, particularly for academic medical centers which saw one action in 1997 and 14 in 1999 (Burman et al., 2001). (An assurance states an institution's formal commitment to protect human research participants.) In 2002, OHRP announced the expansion of "not-for-cause" evaluations, in part to obtain a more representative picture of institutional performance. Since 2001, the agency has undertaken eight such evaluations (Carome, 2003).

If OHRP staff determine that the office has jurisdiction to act on an allegation or an indication of a compliance problem at an institution, the usual first step in evaluating the problem involves sending a letter to the institution that explains the office's concerns and its investigation process. The letter asks the institution to investigate the situation and submit its findings along with relevant documentation such as IRB policies and meeting minutes. OHRP staff may subsequently request additional information and documents. They may also interview institutional officers, IRB members, investigators, or others. Sometimes they conduct an on-site evaluation.

Once its assessment is complete, OHRP issues a "determination letter" that describes the agency's conclusions, which may include findings of noncompliance and a list of corrective steps to be taken. If the institution investigated responds that it has already taken action on the basis of its own evaluation, the letter will note whether the actions are satisfactory. If an institution is in compliance, the agency may still suggest improvements in policies and practices.

If OHRP finds an institution to be in serious noncompliance, the institution's authorization to conduct federally funded research may be restricted or even suspended. For very serious misconduct, investigators or institutions may be debarred from participating in federally funded research. To date, OHRP has not recommended this sanction (Carome, 2003). OHRP can also recommend that NIH or other peer review groups be notified of an institution's or an investigator's noncompliance before the review of new federal funding awards or requests for applications for awards from that institution or investigator.

Each determination letter is posted on the OHRP website. The office has also compiled information on common findings of noncompliance in several areas, including (1) initial, continuing, and expedited reviews; (2) informed consent; (3) IRB membership, expertise, workload, and resources; and (4) documentation of IRB activities and findings.

In a presentation to the committee, OHRP staff reported an analysis of noncompliance findings from 269 determination letters sent to 155 institutions (including some units of NIH) between October 1, 1998, and June 30, 2002 (Carome, 2003). The letters contained 1,120 citations of noncompliance or deficiencies. More than 90 percent of the institutions investigated were found to have at least one finding of noncompliance or deficiency. The median number was 4, with a range of 0 to 53.

Of the 155 institutions receiving letters of determination, more than 80 percent conducted research involving children. One-fifth of the institutions were cited for an IRB's failure to make the required findings for research involving children (e.g., whether the research involved minimal risk or a prospect of direct benefit) (Carome, 2003). Of the total of 1,120 citations, 3.5 percent involved a failure to document findings related to proposed pediatric studies. More than three-quarters of the 18 institutions that OHRP visited on-site had such deficiencies.

Oversight by the Food and Drug Administration

FDA monitors compliance with a substantial array of regulations to ensure the safety and effectiveness of a wide range of medical products, including drugs, medical devices, and biologic products (e.g., vaccines, products derived from blood or human cells, and tissues for transplantation). As noted in Chapter 3, the FDA regulations on human research protections are nearly identical to the DHHS regulations. In addition to regulations, FDA issues guidance documents, *E6 Good Clinical Practice: Consolidated Practice* (FDA, 1996a) and *E11 Clinical Investigation of Medicinal Products in the Pediatric Population* (FDA, 2000b), both of which were developed by the International Conference on Harmonisation (ICH) (ICH, 1996, 2000b). Compliance with the guidance documents is not required if a regulated firm or institution can show that it follows satisfactory alternative practices.

Overall, about 70 percent of FDA-regulated research is commercially funded, and more than half of the regulated research is conducted outside academic institutions. These sites include nonacademic hospitals, clinics, and physicians' offices that may not have their own IRB. Many protocols are reviewed by independent, commercial IRBs that are not affiliated with academic or other institutions and that are distant from the research sites. FDA has prepared specific guidance for such IRB reviews (FDA, 1998c). It has also provided guidance for IRB reviews of "cooperative" research studies that involve multiple sites and delegation of IRB review to a single lead site (FDA, 1998b).

FDA has a more intensive and direct process for monitoring regulatory compliance than does OHRP. It reviews information submitted to it and conducts on-site inspections. This review and monitoring program covers much more than compliance with protections for human research participants. Notably, it covers compliance with scientific and quality standards to ensure that drugs and other products are safe and effective.

Depending on the specific product and its characteristics, FDA reviews may occur at several stages, for example, when a company seeks permission to study a drug in clinical trials with humans, while it is conducting the study, when the company seeks permission to market the drug, when the agency requires further studies once a drug is approved for marketing, and following reports of adverse events. Given the complexity of FDA reviews, review teams typically include physicians, pharmacologists, statisticians, and others. They review new research protocols, revisions in protocols, safety reports, and other data (e.g., from animal or laboratory studies). FDA reviewers can recommend that study protocols be revised or suspended or that additional laboratory or other data be collected.

FDA also conducts approximately 1,100 on-site inspections yearly (Lepay, 2003). About two-thirds of these inspections involve clinical investigators, and approximately one-quarter involve IRBs. Most of the inspections involve routine surveillance, but some are prompted by complaints or problems identified during the review of written information. Depending on what prompted the inspection, FDA staff may review written procedures and data, conduct interviews, and undertake forensic studies. As with OHRP, most problems identified are resolved through voluntary actions, without penalties or sanctions.

FDA could not readily provide information on inspection findings or problems found during the review of written materials that involved pediatric studies, its rules on pediatric trials, or ICH guidelines on pediatric studies. However, FDA is currently establishing a mechanism whereby the

Division of Scientific Investigations in FDA's Center for Drug Evaluation and Research will be notified of all studies done under the pediatric exclusivity provision (David Lepay, M.D., Ph.D., Food and Drug Administration, personal communication, December 15, 2003). Given the government's application of incentives to increase the numbers of pediatric clinical trials, the committee believes that special attention by FDA's new Office of Pediatric Therapeutics to inspection and other findings related to pediatric studies is warranted.

Institutional and Sponsor Oversight of Compliance

Research institutions have the responsibility for ensuring institutional compliance with a wide range of federal regulations involving not only the protection of human research participants but also a number of other research concerns, including conflicts of interest; research misconduct; and research involving animals, biohazards, or radioactive materials. These responsibilities are important and complex enough that institutions have usually created compliance offices to monitor such research-related regulations. Except in institutions that focus exclusively or nearly exclusively on pediatric research, compliance with regulations for pediatric studies does not appear to be a particular focus.

Research sponsors, particularly commercial companies that have a large economic stake in ensuring that their clinical trials meet all FDA standards, typically have active programs for monitoring trials for both safety and compliance with FDA regulations and guidance documents. Sponsors have increasingly relied on contract research organizations to undertake some or most activities related to clinical trials, including ensuring compliance with federal regulations. In response to the competition for clinical trials business from such organizations, academic children's medical centers have been developing more extensive infrastructures for supporting commercially sponsored clinical trials, again, including the monitoring of compliance with FDA regulations and guidelines.

Improving Data on Federal Oversight of Pediatric Research, Regulatory Protections, and Safety in Clinical Trials

The dearth of information about human research and human research protections in general and about pediatric research and research protections for children in particular makes it impossible to describe adequately the application of these regulations, much less evaluate compliance. As one of its recommendations for strengthening the system for protecting human participants in research, the IOM report *Responsible Research* proposed that the DHHS commission studies "to gather baseline data on the current system . . . and to assess whether the system is improving over time" (IOM, 2003a, p. 164). The report noted that such information could not be compiled immediately and that some data could be collected through special studies and sample surveys rather than ongoing data collection mechanisms. This committee agrees that this kind of information is needed and emphasizes that it should cover studies involving children and compliance with the regulations governing such studies.

> Recommendation 7.1: To help identify what further guidance, education, or other steps may be needed to protect child participants in research, the U.S. Department of Health and Human Services—with direction from the U.S. Congress, if necessary—should develop and implement a plan for gathering and reporting data on
>
> • research involving children, including the categorization of studies by the relevant section of federal regulations (45 CFR 46.404 to 407 and 21 CFR 50.51 to 54), and
> • implementation of the regulations that govern research involving children, including data from the Office for Human Research Protections and the Food and Drug Administration on their inquiries, investigations, and sanctions related to such research.

The categories of possible information suggested for a federal database are listed in Box 7.1 (which also includes annotations related to pediatric research). These categories include data on the types of research with humans being conducted as well as information on FDA and OHRP activities.

The committee understands that such data collection responsibilities will require a considerable investment of resources by OHRP and, particularly, FDA, given the latter's more extensive oversight activities. It also may require legislation to give DHHS the authority to collect this information without approval from the Office of Management and Budget. Nonetheless, in calling for this study, Congress has already recognized the particular concerns presented by research involving children and the regulations applicable to this research. If necessary, it should be prepared to direct the collection of baseline data on research that includes children and the implementation of research protections for children.

COMPLIANCE IN THE CONTEXT OF VOLUNTARY ACTION, QUALITY IMPROVEMENT, AND ACCREDITATION

"Remember . . . when things go bad, you'll wish you did a better job. And so will we!"

Elizabeth Hohmann, IRB chair

BOX 7.1
Potential Data for a Federal Database on the System for Protecting Adult and Child Participants in Research

- A taxonomy of research institutions: the number of institutions conducting human research, including research involving infants, children, and adolescents, and the number and different types of studies (e.g., studies that include children) reviewed and approved or disapproved by IRBs.
- A taxonomy of review boards: the number of existing IRBs and the fraction of them that are primarily devoted to studies of particular types (e.g., studies involving children).
- A taxonomy of studies with adults and children: the numbers and distributions of investigations by type of study, for example, clinical trials of various stages, health services research, epidemiological and statistical investigations, cross-sectional and longitudinal surveys, and behavioral and social science experiments.
- The numbers of infant, child, and adolescent participants involved in research and, among them, how many are involved in research by category of research identified in Sections 404, 405, 406, or 407 of 45 CFR 46 and how many are enrolled in studies not under IRB review or any other form of review.
- The fraction of studies that involve children and present more than minimal risk for which formal safety monitoring boards have been established.
- The types and numbers of inquiries, investigations, and sanctions by the FDA and OHRP for studies that include children.
- A taxonomy of research harms and injuries applicable to infants, children, and adolescents, including physical, psychological, and social domains.
- The types and numbers of serious and unanticipated adverse events attributable to studies involving children and the types and numbers of research injuries attributable to such studies or to failures of participant protection by age of the child.

SOURCE: Adapted from IOM (2003a, Box 6.1)

A truism of public policy is that "policies don't implement themselves." Passing legislation or issuing regulations is only one step along the path from policy objectives to desired results. Formal enforcement mechanisms are, likewise, only one dimension of implementation.

For most public policies, including those concerned with the protection of child participants in research, the path to desired results depends in large measure on voluntary actions by private individuals and organizations. These actions may have a mix of motivations, including ethical beliefs, commitment to scientific integrity, professionalism, self-interest, peer pressure, and a socialized willingness to follow the law. Various strategies exist to promote voluntary action on behalf of ethical and policy goals. The discussion here focuses on two: quality improvement initiatives and accreditation.

Quality Improvement

To encourage voluntary action and to promote not just compliance but excellence, health care policymakers and institutional leaders have increasingly recognized the precepts of quality improvement pioneered in industry (see, e.g., Berwick, 1989; IOM, 1990, 2001; and Nelson et al., 1998). Rather than focusing primarily on penalizing errors or regulatory noncompliance, policymakers and managers have paid greater attention, first, to identifying and correcting the system-level factors that contribute to problems and, second, to creating environments that make the desired actions easier or more rewarding to perform or both.

As noted in Chapter 1, OHRP created a quality improvement initiative in 2002, in part, in response to criticisms from DHHS and congressional investigators (OHRP, 2002b). Although the office has reorganized the administrative placement of responsibilities for the activity, the initiative is to continue (OHRP, 2003).[1]

The office has developed, as a first step, a voluntary self-assessment instrument for research institutions and independent IRBs (OHRP, 2002d). The instrument, which has not yet been approved by the Office of Management and Budget, includes three questions (of 97) that ask about research involving children.

Question 51: Does your IRB include awareness of, through consultation or representation on the IRB as appropriate, the additional concerns or issues of research involving vulnerable populations (such as, children, prisoners, women who are pregnant, persons with mental disabilities, or persons who are economically or educationally disadvantaged)?

Question 55: When some or all of the subjects are likely to be vulnerable to coercion or undue influence (such as, children, prisoners, women who are pregnant, persons with mental disabilities, or persons who are economically or educationally disadvantaged), does your IRB consider and require that additional safeguards be included in the study to protect the rights and welfare of the subjects?

---

[1]The Division of Assurances and Quality Improvement has been abolished and the responsibilities for quality improvement have been added to the Division of Education and Development.

Question 74: For research involving children, do the minutes document IRB findings in accordance with Subpart D of 45 CFR 46? (OHRP, 2002d).

Later stages of the quality improvement project are to include OHRP consultation with IRBs on improvements in institutional performance (with performance data held confidential) and the sharing of "best practices" among IRBs (OHRP, 2002d). Internally, OHRP has taken steps to ease bureaucratic hassles (e.g., by simplifying the process for obtaining the "assurances" described in Chapter 3), improve its information base (e.g., by developing a registration mechanism for IRBs), and increase investigator and IRB awareness of research participant protection policies through educational programs. OHRP has also promoted voluntary quality improvement in IRB performance by encouraging accreditation (see the next section).

Local and national quality improvement efforts should, if successful, strengthen the overall system of human research protections within which the policies for children are embedded. The committee commends OHRP's quality improvement initiative and encourages DHHS to provide the resources and leadership to follow through in the directions identified. As part of this process, explicit provisions for improving the design, conduct, and review of research involving children should be included.

Quality improvement efforts are hindered by a lack of data, just as are regulatory compliance and oversight activities. The report *Responsible Research* (IOM, 2003a) recommended that research sponsors initiate and fund research to develop criteria for evaluating and improving the performance of human research protection programs. It noted that there is little experience in quality improvement initiatives that directly relates to such programs and that most efforts to date have focused on process criteria rather than outcome measures. The report identified several categories of data that might be included in a database to support quality assurance and improvement in human research protections programs. These are listed in Box 7.2 with annotations relevant to pediatric studies.

When organizations that sponsor or conduct pediatric studies develop quality improvement plans for programs to protect human research participants, they should identify priorities related to research involving infants, children, and adolescents. Organizations that are not involved with significant amounts of pediatric research should still include such research in their quality improvement plans even if such research would not be otherwise identified by priority-setting exercises aimed at high-volume or high-risk studies.

BOX 7.2
Examples of What Might Be Included in a Quality Assurance Database Related to Studies Involving Infants, Children, and Adolescents

- Resources allocated to the human research protection program (e.g., budget, full-time equivalent employees, and space) and resources dedicated to pediatric issues specifically
- Number and percentage of ongoing protocols that include children
- Target sample size for each protocol that includes children and the number of participants of different ages actually enrolled
- Types of studies being conducted (e.g., a clinical trial, observational study, or survey)
- Numbers and types of adverse events involving children and any related protocol modifications
- Sentinel events (not only deaths but also injuries and serious procedural errors) that raise safety concerns
- Duration of studies
- Dates of protocol submission, approval, and continuing review for each study
- Expertise in child health represented on the IRB(s) or sought through consultation by the IRB(s) for studies involving children
- Dates of data safety monitoring board or data monitoring committee actions, as relevant
- Principal investigators and collaborators
- Research staff profiles and delegated responsibilities
- Documentation of training in research ethics and regulations related to research involving children

SOURCE: Adapted from IOM (2003a, Box 6.3)

Compliance and Voluntary Accreditation

In 2001, the IOM report *Preserving Public Trust* recommended the implementation of pilot projects to test programs of nongovernmental accreditation for programs to protect human participants in research (IOM, 2001). The rationale was to promote voluntary quality assurance and improvement efforts; direct greater attention to outcome measures; and encourage an evolving and cooperative process of identifying deficiencies, providing feedback on performance, and recognizing excellent performance. Since publication of that report, efforts to develop and implement accreditation programs have moved well along, and some organizations have won accreditation.

During public meetings, this IOM committee heard from two organizations working to develop and implement such accreditation programs. One is the Association for the Accreditation of Human Research Protection Programs (AAHRPP).[2] The other organization is the Partnership for Human Research Protection, Inc. (PHRP), which is a collaboration between the Joint Commission on Accreditation of Healthcare Organizations and the National Committee for Quality Assurance. Most of the standards adopted by these organizations focus on human research generally, but both have some statements that concern research involving children.

In its statement to the committee, AAHRPP said that 52 of its 100 standards and elements are relevant to research involving children and are specifically evaluated when an institution conducts research involving children (AAHRPP, 2003). For example, the standards and elements require a meaningful consent process based on the type of research, the age of the children, the circumstances or risks under which the research will be conducted, and explicit IRB policies and procedures for obtaining parental permission (or waiving it) and for obtaining children's assent (or waiving it). AAHRPP also requires investigators, the research staff conducting research involving children, and the reviewers of such research to have the expertise appropriate for these roles.

Two policies of PHRP focus on pediatric research specifically (PHRP, 2003). They require evaluation of compliance with regulations on the involvement of children in research, including the review of both organizational policies and actual protocols. Policies on the review of research involving vulnerable populations specify that children be treated as members of vulnerable populations in the IRB's review of research. In addition, the commentary on policies that relate to special IRB expertise notes that IRBs that do not routinely review pediatric studies may need a consultant if they receive a pediatric protocol for review. (The organization does not directly assess the expertise required to review research involving children.)

Consistent with the 2001 IOM report, this committee supports the further development and systematic evaluation of accreditation for human research participant protection programs. The utility of these new programs, which add to the workloads of research institutions and which consume scarce resources, should be assessed and not assumed.

In discussing roles and responsibilities for protecting child participants

---

[2]AAHRPP consists of seven nonprofit founding member organizations: Association of American Medical Colleges, Consortium of Social Science Associations, Federation of American Societies of Experimental Biology, National Association of State Universities and Land Grant Colleges, National Health Council, Public Responsibility in Medicine and Research, and Association of American Universities.

in research, Chapter 8 includes a recommendation about appropriate pediatric expertise for IRBs that review research involving children. For accrediting organizations to assess human research protection programs that encompass pediatric research, accrediting organizations themselves need pediatric expertise.

Recommendation 7.2: Organizations that accredit human research protection programs should

- provide for expertise in child health in their own activities;
- develop explicit provisions for evaluating whether institutional review boards are appropriately constituted and are prepared to review research involving children; and
- involve parents, children, and adolescents who have experience with pediatric clinical research in discussions to identify their concerns with the conduct of research.

In addition, if they are not already doing so, accreditation organizations should examine samples of approved pediatric protocols and protocols that include both adults and children as part of their process of assessing organizations that review pediatric studies.

CONCLUSION

Given available data, little that is definitive can be said about investigator and IRB compliance with the federal regulations on research involving children. Nonetheless, survey information cited in this and other chapters, findings from government investigations and site visits, and discussions involving investigators and IRB members suggest reason for concern that some elements of the regulations may be overlooked and others may be so variably interpreted as to go beyond acceptable differences in judgment.

Recent efforts to educate investigators and IRB members about regulatory requirements should help improve compliance. Better guidance about the interpretation of key concepts in the regulations—as recommended throughout this report—should likewise be useful. If federal quality improvement initiatives progress as initially proposed, they may not only help investigators and IRBs better understand their responsibilities but reduce certain procedural burdens that contribute little to meeting the goals of the regulations. Voluntary accreditation has the potential to provide further guidance and feedback to IRBs, improve knowledge of IRB practices and results, and encourage excellence. In addition, federal officials need better baseline data on clinical research involving children and implementation of research protections for children to help identify what further guidance, monitoring, or other steps may be needed to meet policy objectives.

8

RESPONSIBLE RESEARCH INVOLVING CHILDREN

*[T]hose who participate as subjects of research studies should
share in the accolades usually accorded great scientists. . . . [They]
deserve to be fully informed, treated with respect, listened to, and
protected from foreseeable harm.*

Institute of Medicine, 2003a, p. 29

A robust system for protecting human participants in research in
general is a necessary but not sufficient foundation for protecting
child research participants in particular. Meeting the special ethical
and legal standards for protecting infants, children and adolescents who
participate in research demands additional resources and attention beyond
that required for protecting adults. Such additional commitments are particularly important given recent requirements or incentives to increase the
amount of research involving children. Between 1997 and 2001, the number of industry-sponsored pediatric clinical trials and the number of child
participants in such trials increased by an estimated three-fold (Dembner,
2001; Milne, 2002).

In some cases, the special ethical and regulatory protections for children may preclude potentially important clinical studies that would be
approved for adult participation. This prospect can put pressure on those
involved in developing or reviewing studies that include infants, children,
or adolescents. A strong system of protections for adult and child partici-

pants in research will provide support and guidance for all involved to help them fulfill their legal and ethical responsibilities in such situations.

This chapter considers the final element in the committee's statement of task, which relates to the unique roles and responsibilities of institutional review boards (IRBs) in reviewing research involving infants, children, and adolescents. Consistent with the report's system perspective, the chapter also looks at the roles and responsibilities of other key parties, including investigators, research institutions, federal agencies, and public and private research sponsors. For a more comprehensive resource on ways to improve the structure and functioning of the national system for protecting human participants in research, readers may consult the analyses and recommendations in the 2003 Institute of Medicine (IOM) report *Responsible Research* (IOM, 2003a).

Although this chapter focuses on those who conduct, review, fund, and regulate research, the committee recognizes the important role of parents. They have a most intimate and profound duty and desire to protect and promote their child's safety and well-being in research, as in all realms of life. Chapter 5, in particular, has discussed how investigators, IRBs, and others can effectively and compassionately support parents in fulfilling their responsibilities and, thereby, help them to feel that they have done the right thing for their child, whatever their choices about the child's participation in research. Once parents have agreed to their child's participation in research, they—and older children and adolescents—may sometimes have crucial responsibilities for following the research protocol (e.g., administering medicines or bringing the child in for research appointments). Investigators need to make sure that parents and older children and adolescents understand any such responsibilities before they agree to research participation and that they have appropriate support in adhering to the protocol during the course of the research.

As a general statement of concern about the responsible conduct of clinical research involving children, the committee notes that the regulations offering special protections to child participants in research do not cover all research. They apply only to clinical research that is conducted, supported, and regulated by the U.S. Department of Health and Human Services (DHHS) or that is covered by the policies of research institutions that extend these regulations to other studies conducted under their auspices. If other agencies undertake or support clinical research that includes children, they too should formally adopt these regulations, and private organizations not otherwise covered by the rules should likewise abide by them. Furthermore, institutions involved in significant innovation in clinical care for children should ensure that patients are protected by safeguards equivalent to those that federal regulations provide to research participants.

The committee believes that all research that includes infants, children, and adolescents should occur under the oversight of a formal program for the protection of human research participants. In this, it follows the 2003 IOM report cited above and the 2001 report of the National Bioethics Advisory Commission (NBAC, 2001b).

> **Recommendation 8.1: Federal law should require that all clinical research involving infants, children, and adolescents be conducted under the oversight of a formal program for protecting human participants in research.**

The committee recognizes that legitimate questions exist about the federal government's authority to require such oversight. Thus, it also encourages state governments to exercise their authority to regulate research—but to do so in ways that are consistent with federal policies and compatible with multicenter studies.

ROLES AND RESPONSIBILITIES

Because the relationship between the investigator and the research participant is so critical to participant protection, this section begins with a summary discussion of the roles and responsibilities of investigators who conduct research involving infants, children, or adolescents. The discussion then turns to the roles and responsibilities of IRBs and research institutions. Later sections consider the roles and responsibilities of federal agencies and research sponsors.

Investigators and the Research Team

> *[In addition to participants' knowledge that they are participating in research], there is the more reliable safeguard provided by the presence of an intelligent, informed, conscientious, compassionate, responsible investigator.*
>
> Henry Beecher, 1966, p. 1360

As observed by Edmund Pellegrino (1992), this statement by Henry Beecher serves as a definition of "the character traits of the morally responsible investigator" (p. 1). In clinical research, the investigator has the ultimate responsibility for ensuring the safety, rights, and welfare of individuals participating in research and for seeing that all members of the research team meet the requirements for valid, ethical research. This is the case whether the investigator has a major role in designing the research or uses a design developed by a research sponsor or others. Likewise, he or she is responsible for the safety and welfare of child participants in research, whether the study includes only children or also includes adults.

Box 8.1 summarizes some of the major responsibilities of clinical investigators who conduct research that includes infants, children, or adolescents. To varying degrees, research institutions, sponsors of research, and regulators understand—or should understand—that investigators' success in fulfilling their responsibilities depends significantly on supportive administrative, financial, educational, and other systems, both local and national. The infrastructure provided by these systems should extend from the initial education of investigators through the eventual dissemination of research findings and likewise should encompass all relevant settings and types of practice.

BOX 8.1
Key Responsibilities of Investigators for the
Ethical Conduct of Clinical Research Involving
Infants, Children, and Adolescents

- Achieve and maintain appropriate training, credentials, and skills to perform or supervise all clinical and research procedures required for a study that includes children.
- Achieve and maintain appropriate training and knowledge to meet the ethical and regulatory requirements for conducting research that includes children.
- Ensure that research protocols involving children conform to ethical and scientific standards for such research.
- Submit proposals and proposal amendments for scientific and ethical review and approval before beginning or modifying research and, as required, during the course of research.
- Conduct the study in accord with the approved protocol.
- Disclose potential conflicts of interest to appropriate parties.
- Ensure that the processes for securing parents' permission and children's assent to research participation meet ethical and regulatory standards and are effective and active through the duration of the study. Provide rationale and propose appropriate protections consistent with federal and state laws if a waiver of parent permission is sought.
- Communicate with children participating in research in developmentally appropriate ways and with guidance from their parents about what will happen to them throughout the course of the research.
- Support appropriate safety monitoring and reporting of adverse events.
- Report protocol violations, errors, and problems as required to research sponsors, regulators, or IRBs.
- Disclose research results to the scientific community and the public.
- Communicate research results, as appropriate, to research participants or participant communities.

SOURCE: Adapted from IOM, Responsible Research: A Systems Approach to Protecting Research Participants. Washington, D.C.: National Academy Press, (2003a, Box 4.1).

The committee commends recent efforts by research institutions, sponsors, and federal agencies to strengthen education in research ethics for investigators. Unless an educational program is narrowly tailored to investigators who will not study children, it should specifically cover ethical principles and standards for the conduct of research involving children.

Pellegrino and others have argued that ethical values, behavior, and character can be taught to clinicians and researchers, although this can be challenging when the surrounding environment is, in some respects, not friendly to these values and virtues (see, e.g., Pellegrino, 1992; Ludmerer, 1999; and Siegler, 2002). Again, this challenge underscores the importance of having a supportive system to stand with and behind the ethical investigator. For example, given the special ethical responsibilities of pediatric investigators and the critical need for studies that contribute to generalizeable knowledge to improve children's health, these investigators may face a serious ethical dilemma if research sponsors seek to prevent or limit publication of their findings. Consistent with the IOM report *Responsible Research* (2003a), research institutions should help investigators avoid such dilemmas by approving contracts with research sponsors *only* if they provide for public disclosure of the findings from properly conducted research. The next section of this report suggests other ways in which IRBs and research institutions, in particular, can make it easier for researchers who study children to know and to do what is ethically and scientifically responsible.

As discussed in Chapter 2, it is also important to have sufficient numbers of pediatric investigators who have the necessary preparation to design and conduct valid and ethical research involving infants, children, and adolescents. The National Institutes of Health (NIH) and pediatric professional societies have taken steps to strengthen the education of pediatric investigators, and these efforts should be sustained.

Recommendation 8.2: To strengthen the base of qualified pediatric clinical investigators, federal and state policymakers and research institutions should support
   • **education in the fundamentals of pediatric clinical research, including research ethics, in all educational programs for pediatric subspecialists and**
   • **additional advanced education in pediatric clinical research, including research ethics, for those who seek careers in this field of research.**

Although professional societies are not normally considered to be part of the system for protecting human participants in research, they too have a role to play in developing ethical standards for human research and helping clinical investigators understand and uphold these standards in practice.

Thus, it is important for organizations such as the American Academy of Pediatrics, the Society for Pediatric Research, and the Society for Adolescent Medicine to remain attentive not only to the need for research but to the need for continued vigilance in protecting infant, child, and adolescent participants in research.

Institutional Review Boards and Research Institutions

IRBs are the cornerstone of a system in which other entities, such as research sponsors, also have obligations to protect research participants.

Institute of Medicine, 2003a, p. 70

Much of the administrative infrastructure and activity that contribute to competent and ethical IRB and research institution performance will support equally the protection of adult and child participants in research. Beyond this foundation, however, both the research institutions that conduct research involving children and the local, central, or independent IRBs that review such research have further ethical and legal responsibilities that demand special attention. Box 8.2 summarizes these responsibilities, which begin with educating IRB members, investigators, and others about their ethical and legal responsibilities for protecting child participants in research.

The effective performance of IRB responsibilities can be threatened by the accretion of additional responsibilities for activities such as managing institutional risk related to research activities, assessing potential investigator or institutional conflicts of interest, and overseeing institutional compliance with a range of other research-related policies. Given the magnitude of the tasks involved in effectively overseeing the ethical aspects of human research, research institutions will best promote the objectives of this oversight by assigning other tasks to units other than the IRB as recommended in *Responsible Research* (IOM, 2003a). That report also argued for keeping IRBs (what it termed research ethics review boards) focused on the ethical dimensions of human research through the development of "distinct mechanisms" to provide separate, prior reviews of protocols for scientific merit and financial conflicts of interest. The results of these two separate reviews would then inform the final determinations made by the IRB.

Expertise in Child Health and Research

A critical obligation of IRBs is to bring appropriate expertise to the review of research involving infants, children, and adolescents. The federal regulations on children do not, however, explicitly require that IRBs in-

> **BOX 8.2**
> **Key Ethical and Legal Responsibilities of IRBs and Research Institutions Involved with Clinical Research That Includes Infants, Children, and Adolescents**
>
> • Educate IRB members and, as needed, IRB pediatric consultants about the ethical, legal, and scientific standards for approving research involving children and their appropriate interpretation.
> • Educate investigators who conduct research that includes infants, children, or adolescents about their special ethical, legal, and scientific responsibilities.
> • Apply ethical and regulatory standards for the initial and continuing review and approval of research protocols involving children, including careful evaluation and categorization of research risks.
> • Provide for adequate expertise in child health and research in the review of protocols that include children, including assessment of whether those conducting the studies have adequate pediatric expertise.
> • Make available reference materials and resources on research involving children, including information on research ethics, as part of IRB or research administration websites and educational programs.
> • Conduct ongoing assessments to guide improvements in IRB performance in reviewing and monitoring research involving children.
> • Develop explicit policies or guidelines on important topics for which additional guidance to IRB members or investigators is needed (see Box 8.3).

clude a member with such expertise. IRBs with publicly accessible web sites that list members of biomedical IRBs generally show at least one pediatrician member or, less often, a pediatric nurse or other child health expert. The sites usually provide little indication of any formal provisions for securing additional expertise. In the committee's experience, these provisions are highly variable.

As more children participate in clinical trials and other research, the need is growing for both investigator and IRB expertise in the biological, medical, behavioral, and emotional dimensions of research involving infants, children, and adolescents. Given concerns cited earlier about the adequate supply of trained and experienced pediatric investigators, this can pose an additional challenge for IRBs and research institutions. In some cases, research institutions may have to reach beyond their own boundaries to fulfill their responsibilities, for example, by using outside consultants or referring protocols to IRBs that have the requisite expertise.

IRBs that review research involving children are not the only entities that need expertise in child health and research. As noted in Chapter 3, when a data safety and monitoring board or a data monitoring committee is established to monitor research that involves infants, children, or adolescents, it should include pediatric expertise appropriate for the condition and population included. For certain long-term genetic studies, monitoring bodies may include individuals familiar with the impact of genetic information on the long-term psychological status of children and family members involved in such studies. In addition, as proposed in Chapter 7, agencies that accredit IRBs will require expertise in child health and research to establish standards for IRB review of research that includes children.

The following recommendation focuses specifically on IRBs. It applies to independent, central, and other IRBs as well as local IRBs affiliated with biomedical research institutions.

Recommendation 8.3: Institutional review boards (IRBs) that review protocols for clinical research involving infants, children, and adolescents should have adequate expertise in child health care and research. They should have at least three individuals with such expertise present as members or alternates during meetings in which a research protocol involving children is reviewed. Among them, these individuals—who may be generalists or specialists—should have expertise in pediatric clinical care and research, the psychosocial dimensions of child and adolescent health care and research, and the ethics of research involving children. As appropriate for specific studies, IRBs should consult with other child health experts and with parents, children, adolescents, and community members who can provide relevant family or community perspectives.

Although IRBs that review research protocols involving children can and should rely on consultants to provide additional expertise relevant to particular studies, their own membership should include core expertise in general pediatrics; child development (cognitive, emotional, and social); and the ethical, regulatory, methodologic, and psychosocial dimensions of research involving infants, children, and adolescents. The committee expects that an IRB will require at least three members or alternates with broad pediatric expertise to cover these core areas. Some IRBs may find this difficult and may choose to refer proposals for research involving to children to IRBs that do have the appropriate expertise. A referring IRB should still review proposals for issues related to local conditions and concerns.

An earlier IOM committee recommended allocating one-quarter of the membership of review boards to individuals who are not scientists, not affiliated with the research institution, and able to represent the perspectives of research participants or the community (IOM, 2003a). This committee agrees and further advises that standing pediatric advisory committees and pediatric IRBs include at least one nonscientist, unaffiliated member who can represent *explicitly* the perspectives of parents and children. (The presence of IRB members who also happen to be parents as well as scientists, ethicists, or clinicians does not suffice.)

Depending on the focus of individual protocols, IRBs may also consult with parents and children affected by the condition proposed for study to obtain additional insights and guidance. These community and family perspectives are important for such tasks as comprehensively assessing a study's potential harms and benefits (including effects on the relevant ethnic and other communities); considering the adequacy of personnel and sites for working with children; and evaluating the provisions for informing families before, during, and after the completion of research (Dresser, 2001). All members of IRBs and advisory committees should be prepared to consider relevant community interests in research that includes children, especially research involving sensitive issues such as genetic predisposition to a disease.

Given the great range of clinical studies involving infants, children, and adolescents, even IRBs that specialize in the review of such studies will need to use consultants because some protocols will present issues outside the expertise of the group's members. Depending on a study's focus and setting, consultants may include various kinds of pediatric medical subspecialists, child and adolescent psychologists, child life specialists, pediatric nurses and nurse researchers, and others experienced in the care and study of infants, children, and adolescents with the condition covered by the protocol. Except for certain studies involving older adolescents (e.g., some anti-human immunodeficiency virus [HIV] drug trials), adult subspecialists usually cannot provide appropriate pediatric expertise.

The rosters of pediatric consultants will need to be large enough to provide timely reviews of protocols, consistent with the IRB and institutional workload. The consultants may support multiple IRBs that review all types of biomedical research for institutions operating on that model.

Although many children's hospitals are part of academic medical centers and have IRBs that focus almost entirely on pediatric studies, some IRBs are associated with general children's hospitals or medical groups that are not part of academic medical centers and whose personnel have limited direct experience with the design and conduct of pediatric clinical trials or other complex studies involving children. For these IRBs, expertise in trial design and methods may need to be obtained through consultants or the referral of protocols to appropriately constituted IRBs. That is, expertise is required in pediatric research as well as in pediatric medical conditions and clinical care.

Noting the scarcity of expertise in pediatric research in their statement to the committee, the Society for Pediatric Research and American Pediatric Society recommended creating ways to pool pediatric research resources, for example, through regional pediatric advisory committees or review bodies that could assist local IRBs (SPR and APS, 2003). This could be particularly helpful for rural and other institutions that are not part of academic medical centers. Such arrangements could also help institutions cooperate to increase the efficiency of reviews for multicenter studies. Moves in this direction would be assisted by the development of model affiliation or contractual arrangements that deal with liability concerns, costs, and similar practical matters.

IRB Attention to Special Protections for Children

Again, no systematic documentation exists on the extent to which IRB members understand and fulfill their responsibilities in reviewing studies that include children. In considering IRBs' unique roles and responsibilities, the committee—beyond reference to ethical and regulatory standards—had to rely largely on its members' judgment and experience, including their participation in such activities as regional and national meetings on human research protection, on-site or telephone consultations with IRB members and administrators, accreditation activities, and discussions of IRB reviews of multisite research projects.

The committee also checked research institution websites to see what they included about research involving children. (Some IRBs restrict access to their web sites to investigators, IRB members, and others affiliated with the institution. No comprehensive listing of relevant, publicly accessible sites is available to allow a systematic sampling.) In an informal review of publicly accessible websites of institutions that conduct research involving children, the committee found that several sites displayed little information or guidance about special requirements related to such research. In some cases, useful institutional information or guidance on research involving children was available but was not easily located or clearly identifiable, for example, in website indexes that provide links to IRB policies, guidance, and other resources. As noted in Chapter 1, the 1978 *Belmont Report* of the National Commission for the Protection of Human Subjects of Biomedical and Behavioral Research is widely available on websites, but the committee could not find any site with the Commission's 1977 report *Research Involving Children*. It, too, should be accessible through local IRB websites as well as through the websites of the Office for Human Research Protections (OHRP) and the Food and Drug Administration (FDA).

Website design is a topic beyond the scope of this study, but the committee encourages IRBs and research institutions to design these sites and other resources so that investigators and IRB members will find it easy to locate policies and guidance related to research involving children. For example, the table of contents of the manual of IRB policies and procedures should identify a section on children. That section either should include all relevant policies and information related to child research or should provide clear cross-references to other sections that contain relevant informa-

BOX 8.3
Suggested Elements of IRB and Research Institution
Guidance on Clinical Research Involving Infants,
Children, and Adolescents

- Easily identified references and Internet links to DHHS and FDA regulations and guidance specific to children
- Easily identified descriptions of state policies (including known but not written policies of administrative agencies) relevant to the conduct of research involving children and to minors' ability to participate in research without parental permission
  - Age of majority statutes
  - Emancipated or mature minor policies and judicial decisions
  - Policies involving wards of the state and foster children
  - Other
- Clearly labeled checklist of information and requirements for research involving children, including identification of the applicable category of research under 45 CFR 46 Subpart D and 21 CFR 50 and 56
- Institutional policies or guidance on the qualifications of investigators or other members of the research team
  - Experience with child health care and/or research
  - Role of child health experts in the different components of research
- Guidance for the scientific rationale sections of protocols involving children
  - Necessity for the research to include infants, children, or adolescents
  - Data from relevant laboratory, animal, and adult studies
  - Data from studies with adolescents or older children prior to studies with infants or younger children

tion. State policies on emancipated and mature minors should be cited in the sections of IRB manuals that discuss parental permission and children's assent. To underscore the special ethical character of parents' permission and children's assent, policy manuals and other resources should use those terms rather than the term informed consent.

Box 8.3 lists information specific to the responsible conduct of research involving children that should be easily identifiable among the resources for investigators and IRB members provide by research institution and IRBs. More generally, institutions and IRBs may also wish to check the recently updated guidelines from the Council for International Organizations of Medical Sciences (CIOMS, 2002) discussed in Chapters 1 and 3. The guidelines include a particularly detailed appendix that lists information and explanations that should be included in a human research protocol (or associated documents). Such lists and other tools should help increase the

- Rationale for placebo-controlled trial
- Other criteria related to federal regulations
- Policies and guidance (national and local) for parental permission and child assent processes
  - Provisions of regulations for permission and assent
  - Role, when appropriate, of independent permission or assent monitors, taping of permission or assent discussions, avoidance of children as translators, and other steps to improve processes for seeking permission and assent
  - Criteria for the waiver of parental permission and provisions for appropriate safeguards
  - Other institutional policies or guidance related to the permission process
  - Minimum suggested age for seeking child assent
  - Provisions for adolescent consent rather than assent
  - Policies on age-appropriate methods of documenting assent
  - Sample age-appropriate assent forms or scripts
  - Other policies or guidance related to the assent process
- Policies and guidance (national and local) on
  - Payments to children or parents related to research participation
  - Advertising of studies that include children
  - Payments to physicians for enrolling children in studies
- Appropriate expertise on data and safety monitoring boards or data monitoring committees for studies involving children and policies on establishment of such boards or committees, even when not required, for studies involving more than minimal risk
  - Guidance on data access and publication provisions in contracts with commercial research sponsors of research that includes children

efficiency of the review process by helping investigators submit protocols that do not have be returned because they lack essential information and explanations (e.g., why a protocol providing a waiver of parental permission is justified).

Perhaps more troubling than difficulties in locating information, some institutions (including some children's hospitals) have protocol checklists or application forms that include no items specific to protections for child research participants (and no obvious alternative document with the relevant items). Other institutions have forms that omit certain elements in the federal regulations (e.g., that research involving a minor increase over minimal risk and no direct benefit must be likely to generate vital knowledge about the child's disorder or condition). Failure to include such elements may increase the likelihood that not only investigators but also IRB reviewers will overlook some required protections for children.

As described in Chapter 7, federal agencies have found deficiencies in IRB practices related to research involving children, particularly in the description of the basis for IRB decisions in the meeting minutes. In addition to improving guidance for investigators, IRBs can—as recommended in Chapter 4—strengthen their own evaluations by preparing more complete written explanations of the bases for their judgments about protocols, particularly protocols that raise complex scientific and ethical questions.

Although deficiencies in IRB minutes may reflect poor documentation rather than inadequate analysis, it may also signal inattention by the IRB and research institution both to their responsibilities for assessing research involving children and to the specific regulatory requirements for the approval of such research.[1] Protocol checklists or approval application forms that include items or attachments specific to research involving children help highlight—for reviewers as well as investigators—the ethical and regulatory standards for approving and conducting such research.

> **Recommendation 8.4: For their policy manuals, websites, and other resources, institutional review boards (IRBs) and research institutions should provide easily understood and easily located information that directs investigator and IRB member attention to the ethical principles and special regulatory requirements that apply to the conduct and review of research that includes infants, children, and adolescents.**

Box 8.4 provides an example of the items related specifically to children that might be included in a protocol checklist or application form or provided as an easily identified attachment. Depending on the other information and support readily available to investigators, an IRB and research institution might opt for a shorter form that emphasizes the risk categories.

Development of Supplementary Institutional Policies and Guidance

IRBs, research institutions, and research sponsors must pay meticulous attention to federal regulatory requirements relating to research involving children, provide information and education about these requirements, and establish administrative systems that support adherence to the requirements. Beyond these fundamentals, however, IRBs, research institutions, and re-

---

[1]One study that investigated IRB requirements for consent forms concluded that the inclusion by an IRB of recommended provisions for the use of biological samples was associated with higher volume of protocols reviewed by the IRB and with reliance by the IRB on the 1999 National Bioethics Advisory Commission report on biological samples and the 1993 DHHS manual for IRBs (White and Gamm, 2002).

BOX 8.4
Example of Protocol Checklist for Investigators That
Highlights Requirements for IRB Approval of Research
Involving Children

Purpose: To direct the attention of investigators and IRB members to the ethical and regulatory standards for research involving children, this checklist asks investigators to answer the following questions about their research. The items in this checklist supplement those included in the general protocol checklist. The text of protocols should include appropriate explanations.

Level of Risk: Please check the level of risk presented by the research and note the associated conditions and the requirements for additional information and for parental permission and child assent. See additional requirements and guidance on *permission and assent* in Section x. See also requirements and guidance related to *minimization of risk and other investigator responsibilities* at Section y.

___Minimal Risk research that does not involve risk (potential for physical, emotional, social, or similar harm) greater than that encountered by average, normal, healthy children during daily life or during the performance of routine physical or psychological examinations or tests.

Only one parent or the legal guardian needs to give permission.
Child's affirmative assent is required for children capable of providing it.
Please describe:
What are the processes for obtaining parental permission and children's assent?

___Greater than Minimal Risk research that holds out the prospect of direct benefit to the child.

Only one parent or the legal guardian needs to give permission.
The child's assent is not a requirement if the prospect of direct benefit is important to the child's health or well-being and is available only in the context of the research.
Please explain:
What is the evidence or other basis for proposing that this research has the prospect of direct benefit?
How is the risk presented by the research justified by the anticipated benefit to the children?
How is the relation of the anticipated benefit to the risk at least as favorable to the subjects as that presented by available alternative approaches?
What earlier studies (e.g., involving adults) support the initiation of research with children?
What are the processes for obtaining parental permission and children's assent?
What is the process if the child dissents?

Continued

BOX 8.4 Continued

___Minor Increase over Minimal Risk research that does not hold out a reasonable prospect of direct benefit to the child but is likely to yield generalizeable knowledge about the child's disorder or condition.

Both parents or legal guardians (if there is more than one guardian) must give permission unless one parent or guardian is deceased, unknown, incompetent, or not reasonably available or does not have legal responsibility for the custody of the minor.
The child's affirmative assent is required for children capable of providing it.
Please explain:
In what ways does the research involve a minor increase over minimal risk but not more than that?
In what ways do the procedures involved in the research involve experiences commensurate or similar to experiences inherent in the child's actual or expected medical, dental, psychological, social, or educational situations?
In what ways is the research likely to yield generalizeable knowledge about the children's disorder or condition that is of vital importance for understanding or ameliorating the disorder or condition?
What are the processes for obtaining parental permission and children's assent?

___Other research that does not fit the categories above and is therefore not otherwise approvable but that presents a reasonable opportunity to understand, prevent, or alleviate serious problems affecting the health or welfare of children.

Both parents and legal guardians (if there is more than one guardian) must provide permission.
The Secretary of the U.S. Department of Health and Health Services or the Commissioner of the Food and Drug Administration must approve the research.
Please explain:
Why does this research not fit the categories listed above? In what ways is this research likely to generate knowledge that is vitally important to understanding, preventing, or alleviating a serious problem affecting children's health or welfare? (Note: This IRB considers protocols in this category using the same standard for potential contribution to knowledge as it applies to research involving a minor increase over minimal risk.)

Other special considerations or requirements in research involving children.
Please check as appropriate. The research involves
___Foster children or wards of the state
___Waiver of parental [one or both] permission for some or all of the participants
___Research sites suitable for age groups included in the study
___Research team with pediatric experts appropriate for the age groups included in the study

---

SOURCE: Adapted from forms used by Children's Hospital Boston, and Vanderbilt University.

search sponsors can support responsible research by developing supplementary policies and guidance that further define or clarify ethical research practices. Box 8.3 above suggested several topics for such policy development, including policies on payment related to research participation and processes for seeking permission and assent.

Although it should be brought up to date in some areas, the 1993 IRB manual developed by the Office for Protection from Research Risk, the predecessor of OHRP, provides useful starting points for consideration by IRBs and research institutions (OPRR, 1993). Earlier chapters of this report have also suggested or recommended topics for supplementary IRB policies or guidance.

Review of Multicenter Protocols

As discussed in Chapter 2, multicenter clinical trials have a particularly important role in pediatric studies given the low prevalence of many serious medical conditions in children. Investigators and research sponsors involved in such studies have expressed considerable frustration with the time required to secure approval from IRBs at each study site, especially in view of the considerable variation among IRBs in the time from submission of a protocol to the time of approval of that protocol. For example, in a statement to the committee, the Children's Oncology Group noted that the time to IRB approval for trials under their auspices varies from 4 weeks to more than a year (COG, 2003). Another source of frustration is the variability among IRBs in their decisions or directions about such matters as study design, assent and permission forms and procedures, and assessment of research risks.

Particularly for clinical trials, frustration may be multiplied because research protocols often have already been reviewed by an NIH study section and one or more scientific committees of a cooperative trials group or other research network.[2] A protocol may also be reviewed following IRB approval by committees at institutional General Clinical Research Centers. All may consider ethical and legal issues in their reviews, although that is not the central purpose of these reviews. The IRB is the entity distinctively accountable for reviewing a proposed study's compatibility with ethical standards and federal regulations on the protection of child participants in research.

---

[2]NIH no longer requires IRB approval before peer review, although a grant cannot be awarded without such approval (NIH, 2000b). Individual NIH institutes may decide that certain categories of research require IRB approval before submission of an application. Peer reviewers are to consider protections for human research participants in their reviews.

Several studies have reported considerable variability in IRB decisions about research protocols (see, e.g., Burman et al., 2001, 2003; Silverman et al., 2001; Stair et al., 2001; Hirshon et al., 2002; and McWilliams et al., 2003). As additional examples of variability, Tables 8.1 and 8.2 report selected results of IRB reviews of two protocols for multicenter clinical trials conducted through the Cystic Fibrosis Therapeutics Development Network (Ramsey, 2003). Both trials included adults as well as children. For one protocol involving an early-phase study of the safety and tolerability of an oral pancreatic enzyme product, the time to IRB approval for nine IRBs ranged from 3 to 18 weeks with a median of 5 weeks. Six IRBs gave full approval for the enrollment of children as planned; three IRBs approved the study for adult participants only, although one gave approval to include children following appeal. For a second protocol for a randomized, double-blind, placebo-controlled study to investigate the safety, tolerability, and pharmacokinetics of an anti-inflammatory agent in adult and child patients, four of seven IRBs gave full approval whereas three approved the research for adult participants only. Of the IRBs giving full approval, three categorized the research as involving a minor increase over minimal risk and no direct benefit, but one categorized it as involving more than minimal risk with the prospect of direct benefit.

To cite another example, the REACH (Reaching for Excellence in Adolescent Care and Health) project of the Adolescent Medicine HIV/AIDS Research Network published its experience with IRB determination of risk among 11 investigational sites as reported by site investigators (Rogers et al., 1999). The study involved adolescent subjects between 12 and 18 years of age who were either HIV positive through either sexual activity or drug use or who were HIV negative but engaged in high-risk activity. The objective was to examine the progression of HIV while controlling for the comorbidity of other sexually transmitted diseases. The study procedures included face-to-face interviews, a computerized interview (site blinded), laboratory analysis of clinical samples (blood, urine, blinded drug screen), physical examinations (including gynecological and urogenital examinations), and a wrist radiograph to determine bone age. All REACH sites had a certificate of confidentiality (see Appendix C) from the federal government. The blood volume to be drawn was 100 milliliters (ml) at baseline and annually, 60 ml at 3 and 6 months, and 80 ml at 6 months for HIV-positive subjects and approximately 60 ml at baseline and annually and 50 ml at 6 months for HIV-negative subjects. Four IRBs considered the protocol to present no greater than minimal risk, while one considered it greater than minimal risk. One judged it to present greater than minimal risk for HIV-negative subjects only, and two additional IRBs required changes in order to consider the protocol to be minimal risk. One imposed a screen for anemia prior to blood draws, and the other required that the wrist x-rays

TABLE 8.1 Example 1—Variability in IRB Approval of a Multicenter Research Protocol That Includes Children

Site	IRB Approval Time (wks)	Full Approval	Modified Approval	Comments or Issues
A	7	X		
B	3	X		Approval under Section 406
C	3	X		
D	9		18 yrs only [a]	The IRB was unable to determine if this research fit into any of the required categories because information about the study drug was not sufficient to determine the risk to the subjects. The research was not approved for children.
E	4	X		
F	16	X		Approval under Section 406.
G	3	X		
H	10		18 yrs only	1. Lack of available data from studies with healthy volunteers; approved only for individuals 18 years of age. 2. Individuals 13 to 18 years will be approved in the future, pending a safety review. 3. Clarify how financial reimbursement is distributed between child and parents.
I	18		18 yrs only	The proposed research activity involves patients between the ages of 13 and 45 years. The IRB cannot approve the research for patients younger than age 18 years because of the level of risk for this group.

[a]The application to the IRB was withdrawn because the pediatric cohort was filled.
SOURCE: Ramsey (2003).

TABLE 8.2 Example 2—Variability in IRB Approval of a Multicenter Research Protocol That Includes Children

Site	Full Approval	Modified Approval	Comments/Issues
A		18 yrs only	Greater than minimal risk without direct benefit; not approvable for children
B		18 yrs only	Pediatric approval under 45 CFR 46.406 only after review of safety data from studies with adults
C	X		Approved under 45 CFR 46.406, but blood draws must be <5% of total blood volume
D	X		Minor increase over minimal risk; both parents must sign (under 45 CFR 46.406)
E	X		Minor increase over minimal risk; information gained would contribute to generalizable knowledge
G		18 yrs only [a]	Board deferred approval of the participation of pediatric patients (ages 6 to 17 years) until more information about the effects of the study drug on children becomes available.
I	X		Greater than minimal risk but direct benefit (under 45 CFR 46.405); both parents must provide permission

[a]The IRB application was withdrawn because the pediatric cohort was filled.
SOURCE: Ramsey (2003).

for bone age be deleted for HIV-negative controls (as a condition for waiver of parental permission).

In addition to being frustrating and sometimes costly, inconsistency in IRB judgments may raise ethical concerns. For example, when different IRBs reach different conclusions about research risks or potential benefits and place different conditions on studies, might some children be exposed to higher than acceptable levels of risk? Alternatively, might some children be denied participation in potentially beneficial research?

To some extent, the variability in IRB judgments reflects the uncertainties inherent in (and the reason for) much clinical research. It may also reflect, as discussed in Chapter 2 and 4, the limited data on the less-than-mortal but possibly more-than-minimal harms and discomforts that children may experience from common procedures used in research.

In addition, reasonable people may disagree about how much risk a protocol presents. Chapter 4 made clear that many of the key concepts applied in reviews of research have a substantial subjective component that will lead to variations in decisions, although clearer definitions and education may reduce some of these variations. Furthermore, some variability can be traced to the lack of precision in the regulations themselves (as reviewed in Chapter 4) and the lack of reviewer education about special standards for research involving children. Differences in local culture and institutional policies sometimes play a role. Variability may also be a function of reviewers' lack of expertise in child health care and research. Efforts to improve efficiency should not neglect the need for reviewer education and appropriate pediatric expertise (as recommended above), whether reviews are local, regional, or central.

In some cases, quick IRB approval with no questions asked may be the outcome of an efficient, expert review process. Alternatively, quick approval may sometimes result from a cursory review that does not adequately consider the criteria for approving research involving children, including the risks posed to children. Such an approval may be a relief to investigators and research sponsors but represents a departure from ethical and regulatory standards.

Several groups have proposed steps to change the review of multicenter studies. For example, another IOM committee recently recommended that "[o]ne primary scientific review committee and one primary Research Ethics Review Board should assume the lead review functions [for multicenter studies], with their determinations subject to acceptance by the local committees and boards at participating sites" (IOM, 2003a, p. 102). As described by the earlier committee, acceptance could be refused for serious safety concerns or unique local circumstances.

The National Cancer Institute (NCI) and OHRP are testing a central review model for oncology clinical trials. The central IRB (CIRB) reviews all protocols and then posts the results of each review on its web site along with other relevant information. As described by NCI, "local IRBs have the option to accept the CIRB approval 'as is,' accept it with *de minimus* modifications[3] . . . or they may decide not to accept the CIRB review and require that the investigator submit the protocol for full Board review at their site" (NCI, 2003).

---

[3]As part of a "facilitated review," the local IRB may not delete or contradict elements in a protocol approved by the CIRB, although safety related "stipulations" may be added. Also, certain kinds of local "boilerplate" changes may be considered for inclusion in consent documents to accommodate state or local laws and in certain other cases.

Regardless of the model, central or regional review could be counterproductive for research involving infants, children, or adolescents unless the review organization possesses expertise sufficient to its responsibilities in assessing such research. A critical goal of any streamlined review process should be not only to reduce inefficiency and unproductive redundancy but also to reduce the inexpert review of research involving children and, thereby, improve the quality of reviews.

A different strategy for improving consistency and efficiency in IRB review was taken in an NIH grant-funded project to establish a voluntary national IRB database and information system by use of a secure Internet site (IRBnet, 2003). The primary goals were to (1) support communication among IRBs and investigators and (2) provide standardized guidance for investigators in developing protocols, including protocols involving children. The project will allow the centralized distribution and review of protocols and consent, assent, and permission forms from multiple centers. It will also support the sharing and updating of information about IRB decisions and other developments.

Recommendation 8.5: The federal government, research institutions, research sponsors, and groups of institutional review boards should continue to test and evaluate means to improve the efficiency as well as the quality and consistency of reviews of multicenter studies, including those involving infants, children, and adolescents.

Again, any streamlining strategy that extends to research involving children should be attentive to the special ethical and regulatory requirements for such research. It should provide for expertise in child health and research that is consistent with Recommendation 8.3 and the accompanying discussion. It should also be attentive to the qualifications and characteristics of local investigators and research sites as discussed in Chapter 4. One argument for retaining a meaningful role in protocol review for local IRBs is that a local process seems more likely to engage and educate investigators in the ethical conduct of clinical research, for example, through service as an IRB member or presentation of protocols at an IRB meeting.

Furthermore, the process for reviewing multicenter protocols should become more efficient if, as suggested earlier in this chapter, research institutions and IRBs provide investigators with more specific and easily located guidance on the standards for research involving children. As an anonymous reviewer of this report wrote, "[i]f the local [investigator] is not provided with the tools to make a good and thoughtful IRB application, he will only do so if he's extremely process-savvy. It's not the least bit surprising that IRB responses are all over the proverbial map [for multicenter studies], if the quality of applications [for IRB review] is all over the map."

Sharing Information About IRB Decisions

Although reports are mainly anecdotal, research sponsors are said on some occasions to engage in IRB "shopping." This practice may involve choosing research sites on the basis of expectations about the rigor of IRB review. It may also mean submission of a protocol disapproved by one IRB to another IRB without disclosure of the previous decision. A 1998 study by the DHHS Office of the Inspector General raised concerns about this practice based on interviews involving six university-based IRBs (OIG, 1998b). Citing similar concerns, the FDA issued an advance notice of proposed rulemaking in 2002 to obtain information on IRB practices for the purposes of determining whether investigators and research sponsors should be responsible for disclosing to an IRB the results of any IRB decisions made previously (FDA, 2002b). It also asked for information to help it assess how extensive the problem of IRB shopping was. As of the end of 2003, no final rule had been issued.

This committee believes that the sharing of information about IRB decisions—especially the specific rationales for decisions—would be helpful to IRBs involved in the review of multisite protocols. The NIH project to create a national IRB database (cited earlier) has information sharing as one feature. A narrower approach would involve the posting of information on a sponsor's website listing IRBs that had reviewed or would be reviewing a protocol, the results of the review, the decision outcome, the date, and a contact person at each IRB (Nelson, 2002). IRBs reviewing the same protocol could then query other IRBs to learn, for example, their rationales for negative decisions or modifications. The committee encourages a test of this strategy with a set of NIH-supported or FDA-regulated studies that include children. In addition, the committee encourages the FDA to share the results of its audits of investigators and research sites with the relevant IRBs.

Federal Agencies

For approximately a half century, the federal agencies responsible for conducting and sponsoring biomedical research and for regulating medical products have—sometimes directed by the U.S. Congress—played a major role in developing policies to protect human participants in research. In recent years, they have paid increasing attention to the application of those policies by investigators, IRBs, and research institutions and to the education of these parties about their responsibilities. Federal agencies have also taken some steps to collect better information to guide the evaluation and improvement of system performance.

Box 8.5 summarizes some of the key responsibilities of federal agencies. Although this report has focused primarily on the activities of OHRP and

---

BOX 8.5
Key Responsibilities of Federal Agencies for the
Ethical Conduct of Clinical Research Involving
Infants, Children, and Adolescents

• Provide and promote educational programs for investigators, IRBs, research institutions, and research sponsors on regulations related to research involving children
• Develop additional policy guidance for investigators, IRBs, research institutions, and research sponsors about the application of regulations related to research involving children
• Monitor and enforce compliance with regulations
• Define and collect the data needed to oversee, evaluate, and improve performance nationally and locally and to develop or revise policies
• Report on system goals and performance to policymakers and the public
• Support innovative projects to improve efficiency, reduce inappropriate variability in practices and decisions, and evaluate the effectiveness of policies to protect child participants in research
• Promote cooperation among the government agencies responsible for conducting, funding, and overseeing human research to provide consistent incentives for ethical research conduct and reduce duplicate or conflicting requirements or policies related to research involving children

---

FDA, other agencies, notably NIH, also have roles to play in promoting the protection of human research participant. NIH, for example, has funded research on decision making about children's participation in research. Furthermore, NIH and other agencies also have important responsibilities for other aspects of ethical research conduct related to research participant safety, privacy, and conflict of interest.

Education and Guidance for IRBs and Investigators

Beyond the regulations themselves, the resources made available by OHRP and FDA strongly shape if not dominate local IRB policy manuals and resource links. Although the 1993 IRB Manual and other resources provide some information and guidance about research involving children, the OHRP website does not make it easy to locate resources related to research involving children. For example, under the heading "Policy Guidance," the list of topics does not specifically mention children. The OHRP home page recently added a link to the regulations governing children's participation in research (http://ohrp.osophs.dhhs.gov). OHRP's list of guidance materials includes neither the 1977 report of the National Commission for the Protection of Human Subjects of Biomedical and Behavioral

Research on research involving children nor any other identifiable document on this topic. The agency's website should include links to both that report and the reports of the National Human Research Protection Advisory Committee. It should make all resources related to research involving children easy to identify and locate.

In contrast to the dearth of easily located OHRP resources related to research involving children, the FDA provides considerable information and guidance through the website for its Division of Pediatric Drug Development (http://www.fda.gov/cder/pediatric).[4] The site lists and has links to the FDA's interim regulations on safeguards for children in clinical investigations. It likewise lists and has links to the agency's official guidance on pediatric drug research (i.e., the ethical and scientific guidelines for pediatric research developed by the International Conference on Harmonisation [FDA, 2000b; ICH, 2000b]).[5]

In addition to OHRP and FDA, other agencies that fund or oversee research that includes children should examine their guidance for the ease with which special considerations in the design, conduct, and oversight of such research can be identified. These other agencies include, for example, the Recombinant DNA Advisory Committee (RAC) at the National Institutes of Health. For requirements and topics that they have in common, agencies should also cooperate to provide guidance that is consistent in content.

Recommendation 8.6: The Office for Human Research Protections, the Food and Drug Administration, the National Institutes of Health, and other agencies with relevant responsibilities that include research involving children should each provide—in an easily identifiable document or set of linked documents—comprehensive, consistent, periodically updated guidance to investigators, institutional review boards, and others on the interpretation and application of federal regulations for the protection of child participants in research.

The recent efforts by the federal government to strengthen education in research ethics are an important positive step. These efforts include some workshops and programs devoted specifically to research involving children. OHRP, the FDA, and other agencies should cooperate in the contin-

---

[4]The division is part of the Office of Counter-terrorism and Pediatric Drug Development within the Center for Drug Evaluation and Research. The FDA also has an Office of Pediatric Therapeutics within the Office of the Commissioner.

[5]Guidance from other FDA centers is not so easy to locate. For example, the draft guidance on premarket approval of pediatric medical devices from the Center for Devices and Radiologic Health can be found using the "A to Z Index" for the Center's website, but the agency's home page and links do not mention children.

ued development of such educational programs at the national level for use at all levels by government agencies, research institutions, pediatric academic societies, and other groups. For example, in its statement to the committee, the Society for Pediatric Research noted its eagerness to play a role in disseminating such educational programs (SPR and APS, 2003).

In addition to formal educational programs for investigators and IRBs and the development of up-to-date and easily located guidance for investigators, the committee encourages OHRP to continue to invest in its quality improvement initiative, with attention to the special requirements and challenges of research involving children. For IRBs and research institutions seeking to improve their programs for protecting child research participants, the availability of consultation and other support from OHRP can be valuable both to the local institution and to agency staff in enlarging their appreciation of the various environments in which these programs operate.

Protocols Referred to the Secretary of DHHS

As described in Chapters 3 and 4, under Section 407 of 45 CFR 46, IRBs can refer research proposals to the Secretary of DHHS for review and approval when they find that the proposals are ineligible for approval under other sections of the regulations (Sections 404, 405, and 406) and also appear to offer a "reasonable opportunity to further the understanding, prevention, or alleviation of a serious problem affecting the health or welfare of children." Section 54 of 21 CFR 50 similarly provides for the referral of protocols for review by the Commissioner of the FDA.

In Chapter 4, the committee recommended that those reviewing protocols referred to the Secretary or the Commissioner for review should apply the criterion of "vital importance" in judging the potential contribution to knowledge that could result from the proposed research. It argued that the standard for approving these otherwise-not-approvable protocols should not be weaker than the standard applied to protocols that present more than a minor increase over minimal risk, offer no prospect of direct benefit, and involve children with a disorder or condition.

Box 8.6 lists examples of protocols that have been referred for Section 407 reviews (and, in one case involving a smallpox vaccine, for joint DHHS and FDA review under 21 CFR 50.54). OHRP has returned some protocols on the basis of staff determinations that they clearly do not fit the criteria for referral under Section 407. Issues related to at least two protocols referred to the FDA were resolved before the protocols proceeded to a review panel (David Lepay, M.D., Ph.D., Food and Drug Administration, personal communication, December 15, 2003).

Recently, DHHS has moved to improve significantly the process for reviewing research proposals that IRBs have referred to the Secretary under

---

BOX 8.6
Examples of Protocols Referred for Review by the Secretary of DHHS Under 45 CFR 46.407, by Year of Referral and Institution

1991
The New England Medical Center Hospital: Study of myoblast transfer in Duchenne muscular dystrophy. Not approved but few details are publicly available. (56 FR 49189)

1993
Children's Hospital of Pittsburgh: Proposed study of cognitive function and hypoglycemia (generated through the use of an insulin clamp) in children with insulin-dependent diabetes mellitus. Approved.
(58 FR 40819)

2001
University of Washington: Study of precursors to diabetes in Japanese-American youth. Public comment on departmental recommendation for approval initially requested August 7, 2002 (67 FR 51283-51284). Reopened for public comment in December, 2002 (67 FR 77495). No final decision from the Secretary of DHHS. (http://ohrp.osophs.dhhs.gov/pdjay/pdjayindex.htm)

2002
Harbor-UCLA Medical Center: Test of dilute smallpox vaccine in children ages 2 to 5. Disapproved by the Secretary of DHHS and the Commissioner of FDA for reasons related to expected lack of availability of the vaccine and not to Subpart D requirements.
(67 FR 66403; http://ohrp.osophs.dhhs.gov/dpanel/dpindex.htm)

2003
University of California, Los Angles: Longitudinal study of prolonged HIV infection, antiretroviral therapy, and thymus performance involving comparisons between infected and noninfected children. No final decision from the Secretary of DHHS.
(68 FR 42061; http://ohrp.osophs.dhhs.gov/panels/407-04pnl/pindex.htm)

University of North Carolina: Longitudinal study of newborn infants with cystic fibrosis involving flexible fiber-optic bronchoscopy and procedural sedation. No final decision from the Secretary of DHHS.
(68 FR 35414; http://ohrp.osophs.dhhs.gov/panels/407-02pnl/pindex.htm)

Albert Einstein College of Medicine: Study of the role of metabolism in sleep mechanisms in adolescents. No final decision from the Secretary of DHHS.
(68 FR 35415; http://ohrp.osophs.dhhs.gov/panels/407-03pnl/pindex.htm)

Rhode Island Hospital: Study of the effects of small to moderate amounts of alcohol on sleep, waking performance, and circadian phase. No final decision from the Secretary of DHHS.
(68 FR 17950; http://ohrp.osophs.dhhs.gov/panels/407-01pnl/pindex.htm)

SOURCE: Kopelman and Murphy, (in press) and Office for Human Research Protections (through January 2004).

the Section 407 process. By using its website (as well as publication in the *Federal Register*) to post information and solicit comments about protocols that are under review, the agency has made the process more open to the public and to interested investigators, IRBs, and others. The names and comments of expert reviewers can be read as can other key documents, which may include the initial application for IRB review of the protocol, excerpts from the minutes of the reviewing IRB(s), and relevant correspondence. Previously, it was very difficult to get information even with a Freedom of Information Act request.

The committee commends OHRP for the steps that it has taken to improve the efficiency, effectiveness, and openness of the Section 407 process. It also encourages further reforms. The current process solicits comments from experts but does not provide for the experts to discuss and refine their views, consider and perhaps resolve disagreements, or present their views coherently as a group. A better alternative would be to create a standing Section 407 panel that would meet as needed to consider referred proposals (using topic-specific consultants as appropriate). Although ad hoc panels can provide expert reviews, they do not accumulate experience and insight in the way that a continuing panel would be able to do.

The committee was encouraged that the new Secretary's Advisory Committee on Human Research Protections has identified as one of its priorities the development of recommendations for improving the Section 407 process. The group will consider whether it should constitute a subgroup of the full committee to serve as a standing Section 407 advisory panel.

Recommendation 8.7: The Office for Human Research Protections and the Food and Drug Administration should

- **continue their activities to establish an open and publicly accessible review process for considering research protocols referred by institutional review boards for review under 45 CFR 46.407 and 21 CFR 50.54;**
- **create a standing panel that would meet as needed to consider such proposals; and**
- **provide detailed guidance on the interpretation of the federal regulations governing research involving children to reduce unnecessary referrals of protocols.**

A further concern about the current process is that it is unclear to what extent and for what reasons the agency is declining to consider referred protocols and sending them back to the originating IRB. Committee members are aware of instances of this practice, but the lack of public information deprives IRBs of important insights into agency views and deprives the larger community of interest of the opportunity to evaluate agency decisions. The committee urges OHRP to provide more information about returned proposals and its criteria or reasons for returning them.

An open process for reviews under Section 407 combined with more guidance about the interpretation of the regulations, as recommended in Chapter 4, should help reduce referrals by IRBs of protocols that do not fit the criteria for such review. It should also encourage IRBs to refer protocols when truly appropriately rather than avoid referrals by using overly broad interpretations of the terms such as direct benefit, condition, minimal risk, or minor increase over minimal risk.

Policy Development, Guidance, Data Collection, and Research

The most comprehensive policy recommendation in this report calls for all research involving children to be conducted under the oversight of a formal human research participant protection program. A uniform federal policy is preferable but in the absence of federal action, corresponding state action is encouraged. As encouraged earlier in this chapter, all federal agencies that support or conduct research involving children should adopt the provisions in Subpart D of 45 CFR 46.

Most committee recommendations do not call for new or revised regulations. One that does is the recommendation that FDA make its regulations on the waiver of parental permission for a child's participation in research consistent with those of DHHS.

In general, the recommendations for federal agencies focus on the development of additional guidance for investigators, IRBs, research sponsors, and agency personnel and the collection of additional information to guide the further improvement of policies and programs. In addition to the recommendations in this chapter, the report includes recommendations or suggestions that OHRP, FDA, and NIH—as appropriate given their respective roles and responsibilities—

- develop procedures for identifying, collecting, and reporting basic data on research involving children to provide one foundation for designing further guidance or education for investigators and IRBs;
- create a centralized national registry of research trials involving children (including healthy children);
- provide official guidance for investigators and IRBs based on this committee's interpretation of minimal risk and other key concepts in the regulations on research involving children;
- continue work through the Secretary's Advisory Committee on Human Research Protections to develop consensus assessments of the risk presented by procedures or interventions commonly used in clinical research involving children;

- cooperate to provide more explicit guidance on both the factors that should be considered in decisions about waiver of parent permission and the safeguards that are appropriate for different situations when parental permission is waived;
- join with private foundations and advocacy groups to support research on permission and assent processes and information materials;
- solicit ideas for research that could illuminate the ethical and practical implications of different kinds of payments related to children's participation in research;
- harmonize guidance on safety monitoring for research organizations, including the standardization of requirements and practices for reporting adverse events;
- require that safety monitoring reports be shared with the relevant IRBs to alert them to potential problems with a study under their jurisdictions;
- prepare additional guidance about the elements that should be included in data and safety monitoring plans and provide that all clinical trials—including those supported by NIH—be monitored with the same degree of rigor and scrutiny; and
- require that protocols that include children and that involve more than minimal risk have a plan (not necessarily a board or committee) for monitoring the safety of child research participants and also provide that reports based on this plan be made available to relevant IRBs on a timely basis.

Research Sponsors

Research sponsors—both public and private—have crucial ethical and legal responsibilities for the protection of adult and child participants in research. The conditions that they impose or attempt to impose on the recipients of research funding can either support or undermine the ethical conduct of research and the safety of research participants.

Large commercial sponsors of clinical research typically have well-developed policies and programs for designing, implementing, and monitoring human research consistent with federal regulations and, often, international standards. In fact, in the committee's experience, their monitoring typically exceeds that required or undertaken by government sponsors of research and can serve, in some respects, as a guide to extending oversight by public funders of high-risk clinical studies.

Earlier in this chapter, the committee advised research institutions to approve contracts with research sponsors only if they provide for public disclosure of findings. Research sponsors should likewise refrain from entering into contracts that limit such disclosure. In addition, the committee suggested ways in which the sharing of information about IRB decisions and concerns could be improved, for example, by the posting of information about IRB reviews on sponsors' websites. The results of the FDA investigation of "IRB shopping" by research sponsors may suggest the need for new steps to safeguard the integrity of the system for protecting human research participants.

An important, continuing question about the system for protecting human participants in research involves the costs associated with developing, reviewing, implementing, and monitoring protocols to meet ethical and regulatory standards. As described in another IOM report, "no satisfactory agreement has been reached regarding how the increasing costs of protecting participants should be distributed" (IOM, 2003a, p. 57). That report also notes that recent tragedies and administrative penalties for noncompliance with regulations have prompted significant increases in the resources that research institutions devote to their programs for protecting human research participants. The report commended NIH for providing one-time grants to fund information system and infrastructure improvements. It argued, however, that government agencies should—like private research sponsors—pay directly for initial and continuing IRB review. This committee agrees.

One concern mentioned in Chapter 3 involved monitoring for long-term problems (e.g., the late effects of cancer chemotherapy or irradiation) that arise after research studies are completed. The discussion mentioned the limitations of FDA's postmarket surveillance strategies, which, in any case, apply only to products approved for marketing by the agency. Research sponsors as well as investigators, IRBs, and relevant government agencies should consider potential late adverse effects of investigational therapies and assess what monitoring, end points, and evaluation plans might be advisable for studies with the potential for such harm.

Reflecting a different concern about research-related harms, the committee recommended in Chapter 6 that research organizations and sponsors should pay medical and rehabilitation costs for children injured as a direct result of research participation, without regard to fault. On another point, the committee recommended that research sponsors not cover finder's fees to physicians based on the referral of a child for enrollment in a study.

CONCLUSION

Policies and procedures for protecting adult and child participants in research have evolved over several decades, often prompted by public reports of unethical or questionable research practices. That evolution continues as policymakers, IRBs, research institutions, and investigators find shortfalls in their performance and devise strategies to improve the effectiveness and efficiency of the system for protecting human research participants.

Investigators play a central role in the system for protecting child participants in research. Ensuring that they understand their obligations is a high priority as is further work to build an administrative, financial, and information infrastructure that makes it easier for investigators to know and fulfill their responsibilities. IRBs and research institutions can clearly improve their guidance and tools to help investigators design and implement ethically and scientifically sound clinical studies. Similar improvements by government agencies will, in turn, assist IRBs and research institutions as well as investigators.

Government policymakers can also fund research and demonstration projects to expand the knowledge base for strengthening the performance of the system for protecting child participants in research, for example, by testing strategies to improve the quality and consistency of reviews for multisite research projects and reduce unnecessary burdens and frustrations for their investigators and sponsors. Such improvements will not eliminate tensions between the goal of protecting today's children from research harms and the goal of advancing research that improves the health and well-being of tomorrow's children. They can, however, help all parties feel more confident that the system for protecting child research participants is trying to identify and remove needless burdens on those who undertake these critical investigations.

REFERENCES

AAHRPP (Association for the Accreditation of Human Research Protection Programs, Inc.). 2003. Statement to the Committee on Clinical Research Involving Children. Washington, DC: Institute of Medicine. [Online]. Available: http://www.iom.edu/includes/DBFile. asp?id=14404 [accessed March 11, 2004].

AANMA (Allergy & Asthma Network/Mothers of Asthmatics). 2003. Statement to the Committee on Clinical Research Involving Children. Washington, DC: Institute of Medicine. [Online]. Available: http://www.iom.edu/includes/DBFile.asp?id=13796 [accessed March 11, 2004].

AAP (American Academy of Pediatrics). 1977. Guidelines for the ethical conduct of studies to evaluate drugs in pediatric populations. *Pediatrics* 60(1):91–101.

AAP. 1988. Policy statement: Age limits of pediatrics (RE8116). *Pediatrics* 81(5):736. [Online]. Available: http://www.aap.org/policy/02031.html [accessed March 11, 2004].

AAP. 1995. Guidelines for the ethical conduct of studies to evaluate drugs in pediatric populations. *Pediatrics* 95(2):286–294.

AAP. 2001. Corporal punishment in schools. In: *2001 State Legislation Report*. Elk Grove Village, IL: AAP. Pp. 49–52. [Online]. Available: http://www.aap.org/advocacy/01state legrpt.pdf [accessed March 11, 2004].

AAP. 2003 (July 9). *Participation and Protection of Children in Clinical Research*. Statement to the Committee on Clinical Research Involving Children. Washington, DC: Institute of Medicine.

AAPS (Association of American Physicians & Surgeons, Inc.) v. FDA. 2002. 226 F. Supp. 2d 204, 19689, (D.D.C.). [Online]. Available: http://www.dcd.uscourts.gov/00-02898.pdf [accessed March 11, 2004].

Abramovitch R, Freedman JL, Thoden K, Nikolich C. 1991. Children's capacity to consent to participation in psychological research: Empirical findings. *Child Development* 62(5): 1100–1109.

Aby JS, Pheley AM, Steinberg P. 1996. Motivation for participation in clinical trials of drugs for the treatment of asthma, seasonal allergic rhinitis, and perennial nonallergic rhinitis. *Annals of Allergy, Asthma & Immunology* 76:348–354.

277

ACHRE (Advisory Committee on Human Radiation Experiments). 1995. *Final Report of the Advisory Committee on Human Radiation Experiments*. Washington, DC: U.S. Government Printing Office. Reprint: 1996. New York, NY: Oxford University Press. [Online]. Available: http://tis.eh.doe.gov/ohre/roadmap/achre/report.html [accessed March 11, 2004].

ACS (American Cancer Society). 2003. *Cancer Facts and Figures, 2003*. Atlanta, GA: ACS. [Online]. Available: http://www.cancer.org/downloads/STT/CAFF2003PWSecured.pdf [accessed March 11, 2004].

Ahmadieh H, Javadi MA. 2001. Intra-ocular lens implantation in children. *Current Opinion in Ophthalmology* 12(1):30–34.

Albert T. 2002 (November 18). Federal court overturns FDA pediatric drug testing rule: Bill before the House and Senate would require drug testing in children, but passage is uncertain. *AMedNews*. [Online]. Available: http://www.ama-assn.org/amednews/2002/11/18/gvsc1118.htm [accessed March 11, 2004].

Alderson P. 1993. *Children's Consent to Surgery*. Buckingham, England: Open University Press.

Allmark P, Mason S, Gill AB, Megone C. 2003. Obtaining consent for neonatal research. *Archives of Disease in Childhood. Fetal and Neonatal Edition* 88(3):F166–F167.

Altman LK. 2001 (June 15). Volunteer in asthma study dies after inhaling drug. *New York Times*. P. A16.

AMA (American Medical Association). 1994. *Finder's Fees: Payment for the Referral of Patients to Clinical Research Studies*. Chicago, IL: AMA.

AMA. 1999. Fees splitting: Referrals to health care facilities. *Current Opinions of the Council on Ethical and Judicial Affairs* E-6.03(A-99).

Ambuel B, Rappaport J. 1992. Developmental trends in adolescents' psychological and legal competence to consent to abortion. *Law & Human Behavior* 16(2):129–154.

Amdur RJ, Bankert L. 2003. Adverse Event Reports. In: Amdur RJ. *Institutional Review Board Member Handbook*. Sudbury, MA: Jones & Bartlett Publishers, Inc.

American Heritage. 1992. *American Heritage Dictionary of the English Language*. 3rd ed. Boston, MA: Houghton Mifflin Company.

Angold A, Costello EJ, Erkanli A, Worthman CM. 1999. Pubertal changes in hormone levels and depression in girls. *Psychological Medicine* 29(5):1043–1053.

Annas GJ, Grodin MA, eds. 1992. *The Nazi Doctors and the Nuremburg Code: Human Rights in Human Experimentation*. New York, NY: Oxford University Press.

Annas GJ, Glantz LH, Katz BF. 1977. *Informed Consent to Human Experimentation: The Subject's Dilemma*. New York, NY: HarperInformation. [Online]. Available: http://www.bumc.bu.edu/www/sph/lw/pvl/book/book_content.html [accessed March 11, 2004].

Appelbaum PS, Roth LH, Lidz C. 1982. The therapeutic misconception: Informed consent in psychiatric research. *International Journal of Law and Psychiatry* 5(3–4):319–329.

Arias E, Smith BL. 2003. Deaths: Preliminary data for 2001. In: *National Vital Statistics Reports*. Vol. 51. No. 5. Hyattsville, MD: National Center for Health Statistics. [Online]. Available: http://www.cdc.gov/nchs/data/nvsr/nvsr51/nvsr51_05.pdf [accessed March 11, 2004].

Arrillaga P. 2001 (April 15). Stuck between two worlds: Tribal youth ravaged by violence, drug abuse, depression. *The Los Angeles Times*. P. B1.

ASCP (American Society of Consultant Pharmacists). 1991. *Statement on Drug and Related Research in the Elderly*. Alexandria, VA: ASCP. [Online]. Available: http://www.ascp.com/public/pr/policy/drug.shtml [accessed March 11, 2004].

Baker E, Atwood E, Duffy T. 1988. Cognitive approaches to assessing the readability of text. In: Davison A, Green G, eds. *Linguistic Complexity and Text Comprehension*. Hillsdale, NJ: Lawrence Erlbaum. Pp. 55–83.

Ballentine C. 1981. Taste of raspberries, taste of death: The 1937 elixir sulfanilamide incident. *FDA Consumer Magazine*. [Online]. Available: http://www.fda.gov/oc/history/elixir. html [accessed March 11, 2004].

Bartholomew T. 1996. *Challenging Assumptions About Young People's Competence—Clearing the Pathway to Policy?* Paper presented at the Australian Institute of Family Studies' Fifth Australian Family Research Conference, Brisbane, Australia. Australian Institute of Family Studies. [Online]. Available: http://www.aifs.org.au/institute/afrcpapers/barthol. html [accessed March 11, 2004].

Batalden PB, Nelson EC, Roberts JS. 1994. Linking outcomes measurement to continual improvement: the serial "V" way of thinking about improving clinical care. *Joint Commission Journal on Quality Improvement* 20(4):167–180.

Bayley N. 1993. *Bayley Scales of Infant Development: Birth to Two Years*. 2nd ed. New York, NY: The Psychological Corporation.

Beauchamp TL, Childress JF. 1994. *Principles of Biomedical Ethics*. 4th ed. New York, NY: Oxford University Press.

Beecher HK. 1966. Ethics and clinical research. *New England Journal of Medicine* 274(24):1354–1360. [Online]. Available: http://www.who.int/bulletin/pdf/2001/issue4/vol79.no.4.365-372.pdf [accessed March 11, 2004].

Beecher HK. 1970. *Research and the Individual: Human Studies*. Boston, MA: Little, Brown and Co.

Behrman RE, Kliegman RM, Jenson HB, eds. 2004. *Nelson Textbook of Pediatrics*. 17th ed. Philadelphia, PA: WB Sanders.

Bell J, Whiton J, Connelly S. 1998. *Final Report: Evaluation of NIH Implementation of Section 491 of the Public Health Service Act, Mandating a Program of Protection for Research Subjects*. Arlington, VA: James Bell Associates. [Online]. Available: http://www.washingtonfax.com/samples/docs/bioethics/patients/hsp_final_rpt.pdf [accessed March 11, 2004].

Bellin E, Dubler NN. 2001. The quality improvement—research divide and the need for external oversight. *American Journal of Public Health* 91(9):1512–1517.

Belter RW, Grisso T. 1984. Children's recognition of rights violations in counseling. *Professional Psychology: Research and Practice* 15(6):899–910.

Bernhardt BA, Tambor ES, Fraser G, Wissow LS, Geller G. 2003. Parents' and children's attitudes toward the enrollment of minors in genetic susceptibility research: Implications for informed consent. *American Journal of Medical Genetics* 116A:315–323.

Berwick DM. 1989. Continuous quality improvement as an ideal in health care. *New England Journal of Medicine* 320(1):53–56.

Berwick DM, Godfrey AB, Roessner J. 1990. *Curing Health Care: New Strategies for Quality Improvement*. San Francisco, CA: Jossey-Bass.

Bevan EG, Chee LC, McGhee SM, McInnes GT. 1993. Parents' attitudes to participation in clinical trials. *British Journal of Clinical Pharmacology* 35(2):204–207.

Bleyer WA, Tejeda HA, Murphy SB, Brawley OW, Smith MA, Ungerleider RS. 1997. Equal participation of minority patients in U.S. national pediatric cancer clinical trials. *Journal of Pediatric Hematology and Oncology* 19(5):423–427.

Bluebond-Langner M. 1978. *The Private Worlds of Dying Children*. Princeton, NJ: Princeton University Press.

Bluebond-Langner M, DeCicco A, Belasco J. In press. Involving children in decisions about research and treatment for life shortening illnesses: A proposal for shuttle diplomacy and negotiation. In: Kodish E, ed. *Ethics and Research with Children: A Case-Based Approach.* New York, NY: Oxford University Press.

Blustein J, Levine C, Dubler NN, eds. 1999. *The Adolescent Alone: Decision Making in Health Care in the United States.* Cambridge, United Kingdom: Cambridge University Press.

Bonner GJ, Miles TP. 1997. Participation of African Americans in clinical research. *Neuroepidemiology* 16(6):281–284.

Borzekowski DLG, Rickert VI, Ipp L, Fortenberry JD. 2003. At what price? The current state of subject payment in adolescent research. *Journal of Adolescent Health* 33(5):378–384.

Boseley S. 2003 (June 11). Mood drug Seroxat banned for under-18s. *The Guardian.* [Online]. Available: http://www.guardian.co.uk/uk_news/story/0,3604,974901,00.html [accessed March 11, 2004].

Botkin JR. 2001. Informed consent for the collection of biological samples in household surveys. In: National Research Council. *Cells and Surveys: Should Biological Measures Be Included in Social Science Research?* Washington, DC: National Academy Press. Pp. 276–302.

Bradlyn AS, Varni JW, Hinds PS. 2003. Assessing health-related quality of life in end-of-life care for children and adolescents. In: Institute of Medicine. *When Children Die: Improving Palliative and End-of-Life Care for Children and Their Families.* Washington, DC: The National Academies Press. [Online]. Available: http://books.nap.edu/html/children_die/AppC.pdf [accessed March 11, 2004].

Brainard J. 2003 (October 21). Federal agency says oral history is not subject to rules on human research volunteers. *The Chronicle of Higher Education.* P. A25.

Brazelton TB, Nugent JK, Lester BM. 1987. *Neonatal Behavioral Assessment Scale.* 2nd ed. New York, NY: Wiley.

Brett A, Grodin M. 1991. Ethical aspects of human experimentation in health services research. *Journal of the American Medical Association* 265(14):1854–1857.

Britner PA, LaFleur SJ, Whitehead AJ. 1998. Evaluating juveniles' competence to make abortion decisions: How social science can inform the law. *University of Chicago Law School Roundtable* 5(1):35–62.

Brock DW. 1994. Ethical issues in exposing children to risks in research. In: Grodin MA, Glantz LH, eds. *Children as Research Subjects: Science, Ethics & Law.* New York, NY: Oxford University Press. Pp. 81–102.

Brody JL, Scherer DG, Annett RD, Pearson-Bish M. 2003. Voluntary assent in biomedical research with adolescents: A comparison of parent and adolescent views. *Ethics & Behavior* 13(1):79–95.

Brokowski C. 2003 (July 11). Testimony before the Committee on Clinical Research Involving Children. Washington, DC: Institute of Medicine.

Broome ME. 1999. Consent (assent) for research with pediatric patients. *Seminars in Oncology Nursing* 15(2):96–103.

Broome ME, Richards DJ. 2003. The influence of relationships on children's and adolescents' participation in research. *Nursing Research* 52(3):191–197.

Broome ME, Bates T, Lillis P, McGahee T. 1990. Children's medical fears, coping behaviors, and pain perceptions during a lumbar puncture. *Oncology Nursing Forum* 17(3):361–367.

Broome ME, Richards DJ, Hall JM. 2001. Children in research: The experience of ill children and adolescents. *Journal of Family Nursing* 7(1):32–49.

Broome ME, Kodish E, Geller G, Siminoff LA. 2003. Children in research: New perspectives and practices for informed consent. *IRB: Ethics & Human Research* 25(Supp 5):S20–S25.

Bruzzese JM, Fisher CB. 2003. Assessing and enhancing the research consent capacity of children and youth. *Applied Developmental Science* 7(1):13–26.

Bullinger M, Petersen C, Schmidt S, Baars R, Hatziagorou E, Koopman H, Vidalis A, Tsanakas J, Karagianni P, Hoare P, Atherton C, Phillips K, Simeoni MC, Clement A, Chaplin JE, Quittan M, Schuhfried O, Hachemian N, Thyen U, Muller-Godeffroy E, Ravens-Sieberer U. 2002. European paediatric health-related quality of life assessment: The DISABKIDS Group. *MAPI Research Institute Quality of Life Newsletter* 29:5–6. [Online]. Available: http://www.mapi-research-inst.com/pdf/art/QOL29_Bullinger%20.pdf [accessed March 11, 2004].

Burgess E, Singhal N, Amin H, McMillan DD, Devrome H. 2003. Consent for clinical research in the neonatal intensive care unit: A retrospective survey and a prospective study. *Archives of Disease in Childhood Fetal Neonatal Edition* 88(4):F280–F285.

Burman WJ, Reves RR, Cohn DL, Schooley RT. 2001. Breaking the camel's back: Multicenter clinical trials and local institutional review boards. *Annals of Internal Medicine* 134(2):152–157.

Burman W, Breese P, Weis S, Bock N, Bernardo J, Vernon A, the Tuberculosis Trials Consortium. 2003. The effects of local review on informed consent documents from a multicenter clinical trials consortium. *Controlled Clinical Trials* 24(3):245–255.

Caldwell PHY, Butow PN, Craig JC. 2003. Parents' attitudes to children's participation in randomized controlled trials. *Journal of Pediatrics* 142(5):554–559.

Callahan D. 2003. *The Research Imperative: What Price Better Health?* Berkeley, CA: University of California Press.

Campbell H, Surry SAM, Royle EM. 1998. A review of randomized controlled trials published in Archives of Disease in Childhood from 1982-1996. *Archives of Disease in Childhood* 79(2):192–197.

Capon N, Kuhn D. 1982. Can consumers calculate best buys? *Journal of Consumer Research* 8:449–453.

Carome MA. 2000 (November 3). Letter to Michael M. Gottesman re: Human research subject protections under Multiple Project Assurance (MPA) M-1000. Research project: Population differences in the insulin sensitivity, resting energy expenditure, and body composition of overweight children and children of overweight parents. [Online]. Available: http://ohrp.osophs.dhhs.gov/detrm_letrs/nov00a.pdf [accessed March 11, 2004].

Carome MA. 2003 (January 9). *Overview of OHRP Research Ethics Compliance Activities and Data Resources.* Presentation to the Committee on Clinical Research Involving Children. Washington, DC: Institute of Medicine.

Casarett D, Karlawish JHT, Sugarman J. 2000. Determining when quality improvement initiatives should be considered research: Proposed criteria and potential implications. *Journal of the American Medical Association* 283(17):2275–2280.

Cassileth BR, Lusk EJ, Miller DS, Hurwitz S. 1982. Attitudes toward clinical trials among patients and the public. *Journal of the American Medical Association* 248:968–970.

Castile R, Filbrun D, Flucke R, Franklin W, McCoy K. 2000. Adult-type pulmonary function tests in infants without respiratory disease. *Pediatric Pulmonology* 30(3):215–227.

CDC (Centers for Disease Control). 1982. Neonatal deaths associated with use of benzyl alcohol—United States. *Morbidity and Mortality Weekly Report* 31(22):290–291. [Online]. Available: http://www.cdc.gov/mmwr/preview/mmwrhtml/00001109.htm [accessed March 11, 2004].

CDC. 1999. Achievements in public health, 1900-1999. Impact of vaccines universally recommended for children—United States, 1990-1998. *Morbidity and Mortality Weekly
Report* 48(12):243–248. [Online]. Available: http://www.cdc.gov/mmwr/preview/
mmwrhtml/00056803.htm [accessed March 11, 2004].

CFF (Cystic Fibrosis Foundation). 2002. *Cystic Fibrosis Foundation Patient Registry 2002
Annual Data Report to the Center Directors*. Bethesda, MD: Cystic Fibrosis Foundation.

Charrow V. 1988. Readability vs. comprehensibility: A case study in improving a real document. In: Davison A, Green G, eds. *Linguistic Complexity and Text Comprehension*.
Hillsdale, NJ: Lawrence Erlbaum. Pp. 85–114.

Cheng JD, Hitt J, Koczwara B, Schulman KA, Burnett CB, Gaskin DJ, Rowland JH, Meropol
NJ. 2000. Impact of quality of life on patient expectations regarding phase I clinical
trials. *Journal of Clinical Oncology* 18(2):421–428.

Chi MTH, Ceci SJ. 1987. Content knowledge: Its role, representation, and restructuring in
memory development. In: Reese H, ed. *Advances in Child Development and Behavior*.
New York, NY: Academic Press. Pp. 93–141.

Chien YC, Lin C, Worthley J. 1996. Effect of framing on adolescents' decision making.
Perceptual and Motor Skills 83(3 Pt 1):811–819.

Children's Hospital Boston. No date. *A Family's Guide to Clinical Research*. Boston, MA:
Children's Hospital Boston.

Children's Hospital Boston. 2003. *Policies and Procedures for the Protection of Human
Research Subjects*. Boston, MA: Children's Hospital Boston.

Children's Hospital of Philadelphia. 2002. *An Introduction to Pediatric Clinical Research:
Help Lead the Way*. Philadelphia, PA: Children's Hospital of Philadelphia.

Choonara I, Conroy S. 2002. Unlicensed and off-label drug use in children: Implications for
safety. *Drug Safety* 25(1):1–5.

Churchill LR, Collins ML, King NM, Pemberton SG, Wailoo KA. 1998. Genetic research as
therapy: Implications of "gene therapy" for informed consent. *Journal of Law and
Medical Ethics* 26(1):38–47.

Churchill LR, Nelson DK, Henderson NMP, Davis AM, Leahey E, Wilfond BS. 2003. Assessing benefits in clinical research: Why diversity in benefit assessment can be risky. *IRB: A
Review of Human Subjects Research* 25(3):1.

CIOMS. 2002. *International Ethical Guidelines for Biomedical Research Involving Human
Subjects*. Geneva, Switzerland: CIOMS. [Online]. Available: http://www.cioms.ch/frame_
guidelines_nov_2002.htm [accessed March 11, 2004].

COG (Children's Oncology Group). No date. *Children's Oncology Group Home Page*.
[Online]. Available: http://www.childrensoncologygroup.org [accessed March 11, 2004].

COG. 2003 (July 9). *Statement on Clinical Research Involving Children*. Statement to the
Committee on Clinical Research Involving Children. Washington, DC: Institute of Medicine.

Cohn LD, Schydlower M, Foley J, Copeland RL. 1995. Adolescents' misinterpretation of
health risk probability expressions. *Pediatrics* 95(5):713–716.

Collins F. 2001. *The Human Genome Project*. Presentation at the National Human Research
Protections Advisory Committee Meeting, Bethesda, MD. Department of Health and
Human Services. [Online]. Available: http://ohrp.osophs.dhhs.gov/nhrpac/mtg04-01/
franciscollins.pdf [accessed March 11, 2004].

Conroy S, Choonara I, Impicciatore P, Mohn A, Arnell H, Rane A, Knoeppel C, Seyberth H,
Pandolfini C, Raffaelli MP, Rocchi F, Bonati M, Jong G, de Hoog M, van den Anker J,
on behalf of the European Network for Drug Investigation in Children. 2000. Survey of
unlicensed and off-label drug use in paediatric wards in European countries. *British
Medical Journal* 320(7227):79–82.

Corey M, Edwards L, Levison H, Knowles M. 1997. Longitudinal analysis of pulmonary function decline in patients with cystic fibrosis. *Journal of Pediatrics* 131(6):809–814.

Cousens P, Waters B, Said J, Stevens M. 1988. Cognitive effects of cranial irradiation in leukaemia: A survey and meta-analysis. *Journal of Child Psychology and Psychiatry, and Allied Disciplines* 29:839–852.

Cowdry R. 1997. Presentation at the Human Subjects Subcommittee Meeting, National Bioethics Advisory Commission. [Online]. Available: http://www.georgetown.edu/research/nrcbl/nbac/transcripts/1997/7-15-97.pdf [accessed March 11, 2004].

Coyne CA, Xu R, Raich P, Plomer K, Dignan M, Wenzel LB, Fairclough D, Habermann T, Schnell L, Quella S, Cella D. 2003. Randomized, controlled trial of an easy-to-read informed consent statement for clinical trial participation: A study of the Eastern Cooperative Oncology Group. *Journal of Clinical Oncology* 21(5):836–842.

Dahan E. 2000. Intraocular lens implantation in children. *Current Opinion in Ophthalmology* 11(1):51–55.

Daugherty CK, Ratain MJ, Grochowski E, Stocking C, Kodish E, Mick R, Siegler M. 1995. Perceptions of cancer patients and their physicians involved in phase I trials. *Journal of Clinical Oncology* 13(5):1062–1072.

Davis TC, Crouch MA, Wills G, Miller S, Abdehou DM. 1990. The gap between patient reading comprehension and the readability of patient education materials. *Journal of Family Practice* 31(5):533–538.

Davis TC, Mayeaux EJ, Fredrickson D, Bocchini JA, Jackson RH, Murphy PW. 1994. Reading ability of parents compared with reading level of pediatric patient education materials. *Pediatrics* 93(3):460–468.

Davis TC, Holcombe RF, Berkel HJ, Pramanik S, Divers SG. 1998. Informed consent for clinical trials: A comparative study of standard versus simplified forms. *Journal of National Cancer Institute* 90(9):668–674.

de Vane PJ. 2001 (March 21). Letter to Health Care Professional re: two recent changes to the Cordarone I.V. (amiodarone HCl) prescribing information. [Online]. Available: http://www.fda.gov/medwatch/safety/2001/cordarone_deardoc.pdf [accessed March 11, 2004].

Deatrick JA, Angst DB, Moore C. 2002. Parents' views of their children's participation in phase I oncology clinical trials. *Journal of Pediatric Oncology Nursing* 19(4):114-121.

Dembner A. 2001 (February 18). Drug research on children raises concerns. *Boston Globe*. P. 1.

Deyo RA, Cherkin DC, Weinstein J, Howe J, Ciol M, Mulley Jr AG. 2000. Involving patients in clinical decisions: Impact of an interactive video program on use of back surgery. *Medical Care* 38(9):959-969.

DHEW (Department of Health Education and Welfare). 1973a. *Final Report of the Tuskegee Syphilis Study Ad Hoc Advisory Panel*. Washington, DC: U.S. Government Printing Office. [Online]. Available: http://biotech.law.lsu.edu/cphl/history/reports/tuskegee/tuskegee.htm [March 11, 2004].

DHEW. 1973b. H.E.W. draft working document on experimentation with children. *Federal Register* 38:31746. [Online]. Available: http://www.bumc.bu.edu/www/sph/lw/pvl/book/Ch9.pdf [accessed March 11, 2004].

DHEW. 1974. H.E.W. proposed rules on experimentation with the institutionalized mentally disabled. *Federal Register* 39:30655–30656. [Online]. Available: http://www.bumc.bu.edu/www/sph/lw/pvl/book/Ch9.pdf [accessed March 11, 2004].

DHHS (Department of Health and Human Services). 1981. Final regulations amending basic HHS policy for the protection of human research subjects. *Federal Register* 46:8366.

DHHS. 1998. Protection of human subjects: Categories of research that may be reviewed by the institutional review board (IRB) through an expedited review procedure. *Federal Register* 63:60353.

DHHS. 2000. Office of Public Health and Science, and National Institutes of Health, Office of the Director. Statement of organization, functions, and delegations of authority. *Federal Register* 65:37136–37137. [Online]. Available: http://ohrp.osophs.dhhs.gov/references/fr.pdf [accessed March 11, 2004].

DHHS. 2001. *Protections for Children in Research: A Report to Congress in Accord with Section 1003 of P.L. 106–310, Children's Health Act of 2000.* Washington, DC: DHHS. [Online]. Available: http://ohrp.osophs.dhhs.gov/reports/ohrp5-02.pdf [March 11, 2004].

DHHS. 2002a. Proposed research protocol: Precursors to diabetes in Japanese American youth. *Federal Register* 67:77495.

DHHS. 2002b. Solicitation of public review and comment on research protocol: A multicenter, randomized dose response study of the safety, clinical and immune response of Dryvax administered to children 2 to 5 years of age. *Federal Register* 67:66403.

DHHS. 2003a. *HHS Identifies Drugs for Pediatric Testing and Announces FY 2003 and FY 2004 Funding.* [Online]. Available: http://www.hhs.gov/news/press/2003pres/20030121. html [accessed March 11, 2004].

DHHS. 2003b. Solicitation of public review and comment on research protocol: Sleep mechanism in children: Role of metabolism. *Federal Register* 68:35415–35416.

Dickert N, Grady C. 1999. What's the price of a research subject? Approaches to payment for research participation. *New England Journal of Medicine* 341(3):198–203.

Dickert N, Emanuel E, Grady C. 2002. Paying research subjects: An analysis of current policies. *Annals of Internal Medicine* 136(5):368–373.

Doolittle P. 1997. Vygotsky's zone of proximal development as a theoretical foundation for cooperative learning. *Journal on Excellence in College Teaching* 8(1):83–103.

Dorn LD, Susman EJ, Fletcher JC. 1995. Informed consent in children and adolescents: Age, maturation and psychological state. *Journal of Adolescent Health* 16(3):185–190.

Dresser R. 2001. *When Science Offers Salvation: Patient Advocacy and Research Ethics.* Oxford, United Kingdom: Oxford University Press.

Dresser R. 2003. Patient advocates in research: New possibilities, new problems. *Washington University Journal of Law and Policy* 11:237–248.

Driscoll DA. 2003. Polycystic ovary syndrome in adolescence. *Annals of the New York Academy of Sciences* 997:49–55.

Duffy TM. 1985. Readability formulas: What's the use? In: Duffy T, Waller R, eds. *Designing Usable Texts.* New York, NY: Academic Press. Pp. 113–143.

Duffy TM, Kabance P. 1982. Testing a readable writing approach to text revision. *Journal of Educational Psychology* 74(5):733–747.

ECRI. 2002. *Should I Enter a Clinical Trial. A Patient Reference Guide for Adults with Serious or Life-Threatening Illness.* Washington, DC: American Association of Heath Plans.

Edejer TT. 1999. North-South research partnerships: The ethics of carrying out research in developing countries. *British Medical Journal* 319(7207):438–441.

Edsall G. 1971. Experiments at Willowbrook. *Lancet* 298(7715):95.

Edwards A, Elwyn G, Covey J, Matthews E, Pill R. 2001. Presenting risk information—a review of the effects of "framing" and other manipulations on patient outcomes. *Journal of Health Communication* 6(1):61–82.

Edwards SJL, Lilford RJ, Hewison J. 1998. The ethics of randomised controlled trials from the perspectives of patients, the public, and healthcare professionals. *British Medical Journal* 317(7167):1209–1212.

Eisenberg N, Guthrie IK, Cumberland A, Murphy BC, Shepard SA, Zhou Q, Carlo G. 2002. Prosocial development in early adulthood: A longitudinal study. *Journal of Personality and Social Psychology* 82(6):993–1006.

Ellenberg SS, Braun MM. 2002. Monitoring the safety of vaccines: Assessing the risks. *Drug Safety* 25(3):145–152.

Ellenberg SS, Temple R. 2000. Placebo-controlled trials and active-control trials in the evaluation of new treatments: Part 2: Practical issues and specific cases. *Annals of Internal Medicine* 133(6):464–470.

Ellis GB, Lin MH. 1996 (October 31). Letter to Institutional Officials and Institutional Review Board (IRB) Chairs re: Informed Consent Requirements in Emergency Research. [Online]. Available: http://ohrp.osophs.dhhs.gov/humansubjects/guidance/hsdc97-01.htm [accessed March 11, 2004].

Emanuel EJ, Miller FG. 2001. The ethics of placebo-controlled trials—a middle ground. *New England Journal of Medicine* 345(12):915–919.

Emerson J, Rosenfeld M, McNamara S, Ramsey B, Gibson RL. 2002. Pseudomonas aeruginosa and other predictors of mortality and morbidity in young children with cystic fibrosis. *Pediatric Pulmonology* 34(2):91–100.

English A, Kenney KE. 2003. *State Minor Consent Laws: A Summary*. 2nd ed. Chapel Hill, NC: Center for Adolescent Health & the Law.

Faden R, Beauchamp T. 1986. *A History and Theory of Informed Consent*. New York, NY: Oxford University Press.

Fallowfield LJ, Jenkins V, Brennan C, Sawtell M, Moynihan C, Souhami RL. 1998. Attitudes of patients to randomised clinical trials of cancer therapy. *European Journal of Cancer* 34(10):1554–1559.

Fazzi E, Orcesi S, Telesca C, Ometto A, Rondini G , Lanzi G. 1997. Neurodevelopmental outcome in very low birth weight infants at 24 months and 5 to 7 years of age: Changing diagnosis. *Pediatric Neurology* 17(3):240–248.

FDA (Food and Drug Administration). 1979a. Prescription drug products: Patient labeling requirements. *Federal Register* 44:37434-37467.

FDA. 1979b. Protection of human subjects; proposed establishment of regulations. *Federal Register* 44:24106–24111.

FDA. 1991a. Protection of human subjects; informed consent; standards for institutional review boards for clinical investigations. *Federal Register* 56:28025. [Online]. Available: http://ohrp.osophs.dhhs.gov/references/comrulp4.pdf [accessed March 11, 2004].

FDA. 1991b. Withdrawal of certain pre-1986 proposed rules: Final action. *Federal Register* 56:67440.

FDA. 1994a. Specific requirements on content and format of labeling for human prescription drugs: Revision of "Pediatric Use" subsection in the labeling; final rule. *Federal Register* 59:64240. [Online]. Available: http://frwebgate3.access.gpo.gov/cgi-bin/waisgate.cgi? WAISdocID=4062924610+1+0+0&WAISaction=retrieve [accessed March 11, 2004].

FDA. 1994b. *Studies in Support of Special Populations: Geriatrics [ICH E7]*. Rockville, MD: FDA. [Online]. Available: http://www.fda.gov/cder/guidance/iche7.pdf [accessed March 11, 2004].

FDA. 1996a. *E6 Good Clinical Practice: Consolidated Guidance*. Rockville, MD: FDA. [Online]. Available: http://www.fda.gov/cder/guidance/959fnl.pdf [accessed March 11, 2004].

FDA. 1996b. Protection of human subjects. Informed consent. *Federal Register* 61:51498.

FDA. 1997. International conference on harmonisation: Good clinical practice: Consolidated guideline; Availability, Part II. *Federal Register* 62:25692–25709.

FDA. 1998a. *Guidance for Institutional Review Boards and Clinical Investigators, 1998 Update: Continuing Review after Study Approval*. Rockville, MD: FDA. [Online]. Available: http://www.fda.gov/oc/ohrt/irbs/review.html [accessed March 11, 2004].

FDA. 1998b. *Guidance for Institutional Review Boards and Clinical Investigators, 1998 Update: Cooperative Research.* Rockville, MD: FDA. [Online]. Available: http://www.fda.gov/oc/ohrt/irbs/research.html [accessed March 11, 2004].

FDA. 1998c. *Guidance for Institutional Review Boards and Clinical Investigators, 1998 Update: Non-Local IRB Review.* Rockville, MD: FDA. [Online]. Available: http://www.fda.gov/oc/ohrt/irbs/nonlocalreview.html [accessed March 11, 2004].

FDA. 1998d. *Guidance for Institutional Review Boards and Clinical Investigators, 1998 Update: Payment to Research Subjects.* Rockville, MD: FDA. [Online]. Available: http://www.fda.gov/oc/ohrt/irbs/toc4.html#payment [accessed March 11, 2004].

FDA. 1998e. Regulations requiring manufacturers to assess the safety and effectiveness of new drugs and biological products in pediatric patients; final rule. *Federal Register* 63:66631–66672. [Online]. Available: http://www.fda.gov/ohrms/dockets/ac/03/briefing/3927B1_05_1998%20Pediatric%20Rule.pdf [accessed March 11, 2004].

FDA. 2000a. Draft guidance for institutional review boards, clinical investigators, and sponsors: Exception from informed consent requirements for emergency research. *Federal Register* 65:16923. [Online]. Available: http://www.fda.gov/ora/compliance_ref/bimo/emrfinal.pdf [accessed March 11, 2004].

FDA. 2000b. *E11 Clinical Investigation of Medicinal Products in the Pediatric Population.* Rockville, MD: FDA. [Online]. Available: http://www.fda.gov/cber/gdlns/ichclinped.pdf [accessed March 11, 2004].

FDA. 2000c (March 7). *New Initiatives to Protect Participants in Gene Therapy Trials.* [Online]. Available: http://www.fda.gov/bbs/topics/NEWS/NEW00717.html [accessed March 11, 2004].

FDA. 2001a. *Acceptance of Foreign Clinical Studies.* Rockville, MD: FDA. [Online]. Available: http://www.fda.gov/cder/guidance/fstud.pdf [accessed March 11, 2004].

FDA. 2001b. Additional safeguards for children in clinical investigations of FDA-regulated products. *Federal Register* 66:20589-20600. [Online]. Available: http://www.fda.gov/OHRMS/DOCKETS/98fr/042401a.htm [accessed March 11, 2004].

FDA. 2001c. *Draft Guidance for Clinical Trial Sponsors on the Establishment and Operation of Clinical Trial Data Monitoring Committees.* Rockville, MD: FDA. [Online]. Available: http://www.fda.gov/cber/gdlns/clindatmon.pdf [accessed March 11, 2004].

FDA. 2001d. *E10 Choice of Control Group and Related Issues in Clinical Trials.* Rockville, MD: FDA. [Online]. Available: http://www.fda.gov/cder/guidance/4155fnl.pdf [accessed March 11, 2004].

FDA. 2002a (August 5). *FDA Backgrounder: Milestones in U.S. Food and Drug Law History.* [Online]. Available: http://www.fda.gov/opacom/backgrounders/miles.html [accessed March 11, 2004].

FDA. 2002b. Institutional review boards: Requiring sponsors and investigators to inform IRBs of any prior IRB reviews (proposed rules). *Federal Register* 67:10115–10116. [Online]. Available: http://www.fda.gov/OHRMS/DOCKETS/98fr/030602a.pdf [accessed March 11, 2004].

FDA. 2003a. Draft financial relationships and interests in research involving human subjects: Guidance for human subject protection. *Federal Register* 68:15456–15460.

FDA. 2003b. *Draft Guidance for Industry and FDA Staff: Premarket Assessment of Pediatric Medical Devices.* Rockville, MD: FDA. [Online]. Available: http://www.fda.gov/cdrh/mdufma/guidance/1220.pdf [accessed March 11, 2004].

FDA. 2003c. *Questions and Answers on Paxil (Paroxentine Hydrochloride).* [Online]. Available: http://www.fda.gov/cder/drug/infopage/paxil/paxilQ&A.htm#q3 [accessed March 11, 2004].

FDA. 2004 (February 6). *Pediatric Rule Labeling Changes.* [Online]. Available: http://www.fda.gov/cder/pediatric/labelchange.htm [accessed March 11, 2004].

Findling RL, McNamara NK, Gracious BL. 2000. Paediatric uses of atypical antipsychotics. *Expert Opinion on Pharmacotherapy* 1:935–945.

Fisher CB. 2003. A goodness-of-fit ethic for child assent to non-beneficial research. *American Journal of Bioethics* 3(4):27–28.

Fisher CB, Hoagwood K, Boyce C, Duster T, Frank DA, Grisso T, Levine RJ, Macklin R, Spencer MB, Takanishi R, Trimble JE, Zayas LH. 2002. Research ethics for mental health science involving ethnic minority children and youths. *American Psychologist* 57(12):1024–1040.

Flegel KM. 1997. Physicians, finder's fees and free, informed consent. *Canadian Medical Association Journal* 157(10):1373–1374.

FOPO (Federation of Pediatric Organizations). 1991. Statement on pediatric fellowship training. *Pediatrics* 87(2):265.

Forrow L, Taylor WC, Arnold RM. 1992. Absolutely relative: How research results are summarized can affect treatment decisions. *American Journal of Medicine* 92:121–124.

Frankenburg WK, Dodds J, Archer P, Shapiro H, Bresnick B. 1992. The Denver II: A major revision and restandardization of the Denver Developmental Screening Test. *Pediatrics* 89(1):91–97.

Freedman B. 1987. Equipoise and the ethics of clinical research. *New England Journal of Medicine* 317(3):141–145.

Freedman B, Weijer C, Glass KC. 1996. Placebo orthodoxy in clinical research, I: Empirical and methodological myths. *Journal of Law, Medicine & Ethics* 24(3):243–251.

Freiman JA, Chalmers TC, Smith H, Kuebler RR. 1986. The importance of beta, the type II error, and sample size in the design and interpretation of the randomized controlled trial: Survey of 71 "negative" trials. In: Bailar JCI, Mosteller F, eds. *Medical Uses of Statistics*. Boston, MA: New England Journal of Medicine Books. Pp. 357–374.

Fuchs HJ, Borowitz DS, Christiansen DH, Morris EM, Nash ML, Ramsey BW, Rosenstein BJ, Smith AL, Wohl ME, for the Pulmozyme Study Group. 1994. Effect of aerosolized recombinant human DNase on exacerbations of respiratory symptoms and on pulmonary function in patients with cystic fibrosis. *New England Journal of Medicine* 331(10): 637–642.

Gallin JI, Alling DW, Malech HL, Wesley R, Koziol D, Marciano B, Eisenstein EM, Turner ML, DeCarlo ES, Starling JM, Holland SM. 2003. Intraconazole to prevent fungal infections in chronic granulomatous disease. *New England Journal of Medicine* 348(24): 2416–2422.

Gallo AM. 2003. The fifth vital sign: Implementation of the Neonatal Infant Pain Scale. *The Journal of Obstetrics and Gynecology Neonatal Nursing* 32(3):199–206.

GAO (General Accounting Office). 1996. *Scientific Research: Continued Vigilance Critical to Protecting Human Subjects*. Washington, DC: GAO. [Online]. Available: http://frwebgate.access.gpo.gov/cgi-bin/useftp.cgi?IPaddress=162.140.64.21&filename=he96072.pdf&directory=/diskb/wais/data/gao [accessed March 11, 2004].

GAO. 2001. *Biomedical Research: HHS Direction Needed to Address Financial Conflicts of Interest*. Report to the Ranking Minority Member, Subcommittee on Public Health, Committee on Health, Education, Labor, and Pensions, U.S. Senate. [Online]. Available: http://www.gao.gov/new.items/d0289.pdf [accessed March 11, 2004].

GAO. 2003. Pediatric Drug Research. Food and Drug Administration Should More Efficiently Monitor Inclusion of Minority Children. *Report to the Committee on Health, Education, Labor, and Pensions, U.S. Senate, and the Committee on Energy and Commerce, House of Representatives*. Washington, DC: GAO.

Gappa M, Ranganathan SC, Stocks J. 2001. Lung function testing in infants with cystic fibrosis: Lessons from the past and future directions. *Pediatric Pulmonology* 32(3):228–245.

Garrison EG. 1991. Children's competence to participate in divorce custody decisionmaking. *Journal of Clinical Child Psychology* 20(1):78–87.

Gee L, Abbott SP, Conway JP, Etherington C, Webb AK. 2000. Development of a disease specific health related quality of life measure for adults and adolescents with cystic fibrosis. *Thorax* 55(11):946–954.

Geller G, Tambor ES, Bernhardt BA, Fraser G, Wissow LS. 2003. Informed consent for enrolling minors in genetic susceptibility research: A qualitative study of at-risk children's and parents' views about children's role in decision-making. *Journal of Adolescent Health* 32(4):260–271.

Gerteis M, Edgman-Levitan S, Daley J, Delbanco TL, eds. 1993. *Through the Patient's Eyes: Understanding and Promoting Patient-Centered Care.* San Francisco, CA: Jossey-Bass.

Gibson RL, Emerson J, McNamara S, Burns J, Rosenfeld M, Yunker A, Hamblett N, Accurso F, Dovey M, Hiatt P, Konstan MW, Moss R, Retsch-Bogart G, Wagener J, Waltz D, Wilmott R, Zeitlin PL, Ramsey B, Cystic Fibrosis Therapeutics Development Network Study Group. 2003. Significant microbiological effect of inhaled tobramycin in young children with cystic fibrosis. *American Journal of Respiratory Critical Care Medicine* 67(6):841–849.

Gigerenzer G. 1996. The psychology of good judgment: Frequency formats and simple algorithms. *Journal of Medical Decision Making* 16(3):273–280.

Gilman JT, Gal P. 1992. Pharmacokinetic and pharmacodynamic data collection in children and neonates. *Clinical Pharmacokinetics* 23(1):1–9.

Glantz LH. 1992. Influence of the Nuremberg Code on U.S. Statutes. In: Annas GL, Grodin MA, eds. *The Nazi Doctors and the Nuremburg Code: Human Rights in Human Experimentation.* New York, NY: Oxford University Press.

Glantz LH. 1994. The law of human experimentation with children. In: Grodin M, Glantz L, eds. *Children as Research Subjects: Science, Ethics, and Law.* New York, NY: Oxford University Press.

Goldby S. 1971. Experiments at the Willowbrook state school. *Lancet* 297(7702):749.

Goldman L. 1971. Was Dr. Krugman justified in giving children hepatitis? *Medical World News* 15:20–31.

Goldman L. 1973. The Willowbrook debate: Concluded? *World Medicine* 9(2):79–90.

Goldner JA. 2000. Dealing with conflicts of interest in biomedical research: IRB oversight as the next best solution to the abolitionist approach. *Journal of Law, Medicine & Ethics* 28(4):379–404.

Goldstein AO, Frasier P, Curtis P, Reid A, Kreher NE. 1996. Consent form readability in university-sponsored research. *Journal of Family Practice* 42(6):606–611.

Good WV. 2001. Cataract surgery in young children. *British Journal of Ophthalmology* 85(3):254.

Goodman LS, Gilman AG, Limbird LE, Hardman JG, eds. 2001. *Goodman & Gilman's the Pharmacological Basis of Therapeutics.* 10th ed. New York, NY: McGraw-Hill Professional.

Goold G, ed. 1923. Hippocrates. Epidemics I, section XI . In: *Hippocrates, Volume 1.* W.H.S. Jones translation. Cambridge, MA: Harvard University Press. P. 165.

Goss CH, Mayer-Hamblett N, Kronmal RA, Ramsey BW. 2002. The Cystic Fibrosis Therapeutics Development Network (CFTDN): A paradigm of a clinical trials network for genetic and orphan diseases. *Advanced Drug Delivery Reviews* 54(11):1505–1528.

Grisso T, Vierling L. 1978. Minors' consent to treatment: A developmental perspective. *Professional Psychology* 9:412–426.

Grodin MA. 1992. Historical origins of the Nuremberg Code. In: Annas GJ, Grodin MA, eds. *The Nazi Doctors and the Nuremburg Code: Human Rights in Human Experimentation.* New York, NY: Oxford University Press.

Grodin MA, Glantz LH. 1994. *Children as Research Subjects: Science, Ethics and Law*. New York, NY: Oxford University Press.

Grossman SA, Piantadosi S, Covahey C. 1994. Are informed consent forms that describe clinical oncology research protocols readable by most patients and their families? *Journal of Clinical Oncology* 12(10):2211–2215.

Grunbaum JA, LaBarthe D, Ayars C, Harrist R, Nichaman MZ. 1996. Recruitment and enrollment for Project Heartbeat: Achieving the goals of minority inclusion. *Ethnicity and Disease* 6:203–212.

Halim NS. 2000. Gene therapy institute faces uphill battle: Investigations may lead to better gene therapy trials. *The Scientist* 14(3):1.

Halpern-Felsher BL, Cauffman E. 2001. Costs and benefits of a decision: Decision-making competence in adolescents and adults. *Journal of Applied Developmental Psychology* 22:257–273.

Halsey NA. 2002. Letter to Office for Human Research Protections re: a multicenter, randomizes dose response study of the safety clinical and immune responses of Dryvax administered to children 2 to 5 years of age. [Online]. Available: http://ohrp.osophs.dhhs.gov/dpanel/halsey.pdf [accessed March 11, 2004].

Hammerschmidt DE. 2002 (October). Letter to the Office for Human Research Protections re: a multicenter, randomizes dose response study of the safety clinical and immune responses of Dryvax administered to children 2 to 5 years of age. [Online]. Available: http://ohrp.osophs.dhhs.gov/dpanel/hammerschmidt.pdf [accessed March 11, 2004].

Hammerschmidt DE, Keane MA. 1992. Institutional review board (IRB) review lacks impact on the readability of consent forms for research. *American Journal of the Medical Sciences* 304(6):348–351.

Hanif M, Mobarak MR, Ronan A, Rahman D, Donovan Jr JJ, Bennish ML. 1995. Fatal renal failure caused by diethylene glycol in paracetamol elixir: The Bangladesh epidemic. *British Medical Journal* 311(6997):88–91.

Harmon WE. 2003 (July 9). Statement on behalf of the American Society of Transplantation, Children's Hospital Boston, and the North American Pediatric Renal Transplant Cooperative Study to the Committee on Clinical Research Involving Children. Washington, DC: Institute of Medicine.

Harth SC, Thong YH. 1995. Parental perceptions and attitudes about informed consent in clinical research involving children. *Social Science and Medicine* 41(12):1647–1651.

Hayman RM, Taylor BJ, Peart NS, Galland BC, Sayers RM. 2001. Participation in research: Informed consent, motivation and influence. *Journal of Paediatrics and Child Health* 37(1):51–54.

Heinrich J. 2001. *Human Subjects Research: HHS Takes Steps to Strengthen Protections, But Concerns Remain. Hearing before the Senate Committee on Health, Education, Labor, and Pensions, Subcommittee on Public Health*. Washington, DC: Government Accounting Office. [Online]. Available: http://www.gao.gov/new.items/d01775t.pdf [accessed March 11, 2004].

Heller J. 1972. Syphilis victims in the U.S. study went untreated for 40 Years. *New York Times*. P. A8.

Henry B, Grosskopf C, Aussage P, de Fontbrune S, Goehrs J, the French CFQOL Study Group. 1997. Measuring quality of life in children with cystic fibrosis: The cystic fibrosis questionnaires. *Pediatric Pulmonolgy* 14:331.

Hillabrant W. 2002. Research in Indian country: Challenges and changes. Paper presented at the Symposium on Research and Evaluation Methodology. In: Davis J, Erickson J, Johnson S, Marshall C, Running Wolf P, Santiago R, eds. *Work Group on American Indian Research and Program Evaluation Methodology (AIRPEM), Symposium on Research and Evaluation Methodology: Lifespan Issues Related to American Indians/Alaska*

Natives With Disabilities. Flagstaff: Northern Arizona University, Institute for Human Development, Arizona University Center on Disabilities, American Indian Rehabilitation Research and Training Center. Pp. 19–31. [Online]. Available: http://www.nau.edu/~ihd/airrtc/pdfs/monograph.pdf [accessed March 11, 2004].

Hilts PJ. 2003. *Protecting America's Health: The FDA, Business, and One Hundred Years of Regulation.* New York, NY: Alfred A. Knopf.

Hinds PS, Birenbaum LK, Clarke-Steffen L, Quargnenti A, Kreissman S, Kazak A, Meyer W, Mulhern R, Pratt C, Wilimas J. 1996. Coming to terms: Parents' response to a first cancer recurrence in their child. *Nursing Research* 45(3):148-153.

Hirshon JM, Krugman SD, Witting MD, Furuno JP, Limcangco MR, Perisse AR, Rasch EK. 2002. Variability in institutional review board assessment of minimal-risk research. *Academic Emergency Medicine* 9(12):1417–1420.

Hockenberry-Eaton M, Barrera P, Brown M, Bottomley SJ, O'Neill JB. 1999. *Pain Management in Children with Cancer.* Houston, TX: Texas Cancer Council. [Online]. Available: http://www.childcancerpain.org/contents/childpainmgmt.pdf [accessed March 11, 2004].

Hoffman ML. 1990. Empathy and justice motivation. *Motivation & Emotion* 14:151–172.

Hohmann E. No date. *What Does the IRB Really Want? Part 2.* Inservices Given by the PHRC and HRO Staff: Partners Human Research Committee. [Online]. Available: http://healthcare.partners.org/hrcedweb/inserv.htm [accessed March 11, 2004].

Hopper KD, TenHave TR, Hartzel J. 1995. Informed consent forms for clinical and research imaging procedures: How much do patients understand? *American Journal of Roentgenology* 164(2):493–496.

Hopper KD, TenHave TR, Tully DA, Hall TE. 1998. The readability of currently used surgical/procedure consent forms in the United States. *Surgery* 123(5):496–503.

Hoppu K, Koskimies O, Holmberg C, Hirvisalo E. 1991. Pharmacokinetically determined cyclosporine dosage in young children. *Pediatric Nephrology* 5(1):1–4.

Hurley JC, Underwood MK. 2002. Children's understanding of their research rights before and after debriefing: Informed assent, confidentiality, and stopping participation. *Child Development* 73(1):132–143.

Hutchison C. 1998. Phase I trials in cancer patients: Participants' perceptions. *European Journal of Cancer Care* 7(1):15–22.

ICH (International Conference on Harmonisation). 1996. *Guideline for Good Clinical Practice: E6.* Geneva, Switzerland: ICH. [Online]. Available: http://www.ich.org/MediaServer.jser?@_ID=487&@_TYPE=MULTIMEDIA&@_TEMPLATE=616&@_MODE=GLB [accessed March 11, 2004].

ICH. 2000a. *Choice of Control Group and Related Issues in Clinical Trials: E10.* Geneva, Switzerland: ICH. [Online]. Available: http://www.ich.org/MediaServer.jser?@_ID=486&@_TYPE=MULTIMEDIA&@_TEMPLATE=616&@_MODE=GLB [accessed March 11, 2004].

ICH. 2000b. *Clinical Investigation of Medicinal Products in the Pediatric Population: E11.* Geneva, Switzerland: ICH. [Online]. Available: http://www.ich.org/MediaServer.jser?@_ID=487&@_TYPE=MULTIMEDIA&@_TEMPLATE=616&@_MODE=GLB [accessed March 11, 2004].

IHS (Indian Health Services). 2002 (February 19). *Indian Health Service Research Program: Area/Tribal IRB Chair.* [Online]. Available: http://www.ihs.gov/MedicalPrograms/Research/areairb.htm [accessed March 11, 2004].

Ingelfinger FJ. 1973. Ethics of experiments on children. *New England Journal of Medicine* 288(15):791–792.

Inhelder B, Piaget J. 1958. *The Growth of Logical Thinking from Childhood to Adolescence.* New York, NY: Basic Books.

IOM (Institute of Medicine). 1989. *The Responsible Conduct of Research in the Health Sciences*. Washington, DC: National Academy Press.

IOM. 1990. *Clinical Practice Guidelines: Directions for a New Program*. Washington, DC: National Academy Press.

IOM. 1994a. *Careers in Clinical Research: Obstacles and Opportunities*. Washington, DC: National Academy Press.

IOM. 1994b. Justice in Clinical Studies: Guiding Principles. In: *Women and Health Research: Ethical and Legal Issues of Including Women in Clinical Studies, Vol. I*. Washington, DC: National Academy Press.

IOM. 2000a. *Protecting Data Privacy in Health Services Research: Committee on the Role of Institutional Review Boards in Health Services Research Data Privacy Protection*. Washington, DC: National Academy Press.

IOM. 2000b. *Rational Therapeutics for Infants and Children: Workshop Summary*. Washington, DC: National Academy Press.

IOM. 2001. *Preserving Public Trust: Accreditation and Human Research Participant Protection Programs*. Washington, DC: National Academy Press.

IOM. 2003a. *Responsible Research: A Systems Approach to Protecting Research Participants*. Washington, DC: The National Academies Press.

IOM. 2003b. *When Children Die: Improving Palliative and End-of-Life Care for Children and Their Families*. Washington, DC: The National Academies Press.

IOM/NRC (National Research Council). 2002. *Integrity in Scientific Research: Creating an Environment That Promotes Responsible Conduct*. Washington, DC: National Academy Press.

IRBnet. 2003. *About the IRBnet*. [Online]. Available: https://www.irbnet.org/beta/public/about.jsp [accessed March 11, 2004].

Iyasu S. 2003. *One Year Post-Pediatric Exclusivity Postmarketing Adverse Event Review SERTRALINE (Zoloft)*. Presentation to the Pediatric Advisory Subcommittee of the Anti-Infective Drugs Advisory Committee, Gaithersburg, MD. Food and Drug Administration. [Online]. Available: http://www.fda.gov/cder/pediatric/presentation/ac6-03si/ped_files/frame.htm [accessed March 11, 2004].

James S, Lanman JT. 1976. History of oxygen therapy and retrolental fibroplasia. Prepared by the American Academy of Pediatrics, Committee on Fetus and Newborn with the collaboration of special consultants. *Pediatrics* 57(Suppl 2):591–642.

Janner M, Knill SE, Diem P, Zuppinger KA, Mullis PE. 1994. Persistent microalbuminuria in adolescents with type I (insulin-dependent) diabetes mellitus is associated to early rather than late puberty. Results of a prospective longitudinal study. *European Journal of Pediatrics* 153(6):403–408.

Janofsky J, Starfield B. 1981. Assessment of risk in research on children. *Journal of Pediatrics* 98(5):842–846.

JCAHO (Joint Commission on the Accreditation of Healthcare Organizations). 2003. *Root Cause Analysis in Health Care*. 2nd ed. Oak Brook Terrace, IL: Joint Commission Resources.

Jobe AH. 1993. Pulmonary surfactant therapy. *New England Journal of Medicine* 328:861–868.

Johnson BH, Jeppson ES, Redburn L. 1992. *Caring for Children and Families. Guidelines for Hospitals*. Bethesda, MD: Association for the Care of Children's Health.

Jones JH. 1992. *Bad Blood: The Tuskegee Experiment*. New York, NY: Free Press.

Jonsen AR. 1998a. *The Birth of Bioethics*. New York, NY: Oxford University Press.

Jonsen, AR. 1998b (July 14). *The Birth of the Belmont Report*. Presentation at the National Bioethics Advisory Committee meeting, Portland, OR. NBAC. [Online]. Available: http://www.georgetown.edu/research/nrcbl/nbac/transcripts/jul98/belmont.html [accessed March 11, 2004].

Jonsen AR, Siegler M, Winslade WJ. 1998. *Clinical Ethics: A Practical Approach to Ethical Decisions in Clinical Medicine.* 4th ed. New York, NY: McGraw-Hill Companies.

Kaitin KI, ed. 2003. Post-approval R&D raises total drug development costs to $897 million. *Tufts Center for the Study of Drug Development Impact Report 2003* 5(3). [Online]. Available: http://csdd.tufts.edu/NewsEvents/RecentNews.asp?newsid=29 [accessed March 11, 2004].

Karlawish JHT, Lantos J. 1997. Community equipoise and the architecture of clinical research. *Cambridge Quarterly of Healthcare Ethics* 6:385–396.

Kaser-Boyd N, Adelman HS, Turner L. 1985. Minor's ability to identify risks and benefits of therapy. *Professional Psychology: Research and Practice* 16(3):411–417.

Kearns GL, Winter HS. 2003. Proton pump inhibitors in pediatrics: Relevant pharmacokinetic and pharmacodynamics. *Journal of Pediatric Gastroenterology and Nutrition* 37(Supp 1):S52–S59.

Kerem E, Reisman J, Corey M, Canny GJ, Levison H. 1992. Prediction of mortality in patients with cystic fibrosis. *New England Journal of Medicine* 326(18):1187–1191.

King NMP. 2000. Defining and describing benefit appropriately in clinical trials. *The Journal of Law, Medicine & Ethics.* 28(4):332–343.

Kirsch I, Jungeblut A, Jenkins L, Kolstad A. 1993. *Adult Literacy in America: A First Look at the Results of the National Adult Literacy Survey.* Washington, DC: U.S. Department of Education.

Klaczynski PA, Gordon DH. 1996. Everyday statistical reasoning during adolescence and young adulthood: Motivational, general ability, and developmental influences. *Child Development* 67(6):2873–2891.

Klaczynski PA, Narasimham G. 1998. Development of scientific reasoning biases: Cognitive versus ego-protective explanations. *Developmental Psychology* 43(1):175–187.

Klaczynski PA, Robinson B. 2000. Personal theories, intellectual ability, and epistemological beliefs: Adult age differences in everyday reasoning biases. *Psychology and Aging* 15(3): 400–416.

Kodish E. 2003a. *Assent and Informed Parental Permission: Insights from the PIC.* Presentation to the Committee on Clinical Research Involving Children. Washington, DC: Institute of Medicine.

Kodish E. 2003b. Informed consent for pediatric research: Is it really possible? *Journal of Pediatrics* 142(2):89–90.

Kodish E. 2003c. Pediatric ethics and early-phase childhood cancer research: Conflicted goals and the prospect of benefit. *Accountability in Research* 10:17–25.

Kodish E, Pentz RD, Noll RB, Ruccione K, Buckley J, Lange BL. 1998. Informed consent in the Children Cancer Group: Results of preliminary research. *Cancer* 82(12):2467–2481.

Kodish E, Eder M, Noll RB, Ruccione K, Lange B, Angiolillo A, Pentz R, Zyzanski S, Siminoff LA, Drotar D. 2004. Communication of randomization in childhood leukemia trials. *Journal of the American Medical Association* 291(4):470–475.

Kopelman LM. 1989. When is the risk minimal enough for children to be research subjects? In: Kopelman L, Moskop J, eds. *Children and Health Care: Moral and Social Issues.* Moskop, Dordrecht, The Netherlands: Kluwer Academic Publishers. Pp. 89–99.

Kopelman LM. 2000. Children as research subjects: A dilemma. *The Journal of Medicine and Philosophy* 25(6):745–764.

Kopelman LM. In press. Minimal risk as an international ethical standard in research. *The Journal of Medicine and Philosophy.*

Kopelman LM, Murphy TF. In press. Ethical concerns about federal approval of risky pediatrics studies. *Pediatrics.*

Koski G. 2000 (December 4). Letter to OHRP Staff re: *Compliance Oversight Procedures.* [Online]. Available: http://ohrp.osophs.dhhs.gov/references/ohrpcomp.pdf [accessed March 11, 2004].

Koski G. 2001 (May 2). *Biomedical Research Progress: In Whose Interest?* Presentation at the Institute of Medicine Southern California Regional Meeting, University of Southern California Keck School of Medicine. Los Angeles: Institute of Medicine. Quoted in: Oliwenstein L. 2002. Media, public scrutinize clinical trials. *HSC Weekly* 8(13):1.

Koski G. 2002 (October 9). Letter to Honorable Tommy Thompson Secretary, United States Department of Health and Human Services. [Online]. Available: http://irb.mc.duke.edu/PDF/koskiLetter.pdf [accessed March 11, 2004].

Kowaleski J. 1997. *State Definitions and Reporting Requirements for Live Births, Fetal Deaths, and Induced Terminations of Pregnancy (1997 Revision).* Hyattsville, MD: National Center for Health Statistics. [Online]. Available: http://www.cdc.gov/nchs/data/itop97.pdf [accessed March 11, 2004].

Krechel SW, Bildner J. 1995. CRIES: A new neonatal postoperative pain measurement score. Initial testing of validity and reliability. *Paediatric Anaesthesia* 5(1):53–61.

Krugman S, Shapiro S. 1971. Letters to the Editor: Experiments at the Willowbrook State School. *Lancet* 297(7706):966–967.

Kupst MJ, Patenaude AF, Walco GA, Sterling C. 2003. Clinical trials in pediatric cancer: Parental perspectives on informed consent. *Journal of Pediatric Hematology/Oncology* 25(10):787–790.

Lambert GH, Kotake AN, Schoeller D. 1983. The CO_2 breath tests as monitors of the cytochrome P450 dependent mixed function monooxygenase system. *Progress in Clinical and Biological Research* 135:119–145.

Lambert GH, Schoeller DA, Kotake AN, Flores C, Hay D. 1986. The effect of age, gender, and sexual maturation on the caffeine breath test. *Developmental Pharmacology and Therapeutics* 9(6):375–388.

Langley JM, Halperin SA, Mills EL, Eastwood B. 1998. Parental willingness to enter a child in a controlled vaccine trial. *Medecine Clinique et Experimentale (Clinical and Investigative Medicine)* 21(1):12–16.

Lasagna L. 1994. Interview by Susan White-Junod and Jon Harkness (ACHRE), Transcript of Audio Recording (ACHRE Research Project Series, Interview Program Files, Ethics Oral History Project). Pp. 37–38. [Online]. Available: http://tis.eh.doe.gov/ohre/roadmap/achre/chap3_fn.html [accessed March 11, 2004].

Lascari AD. 1981. Editorial: Risk of research in children. *Journal of Pediatrics* 98:759–760.

Le Guennec JC, Billon B. 1987. Delay in caffeine elimination in breast-fed infants. *Pediatrics* 79(2):264–268.

Lederer SE. 1992. Orphans as guinea pigs: American children and medical experimenters, 1890-1930. In: Cooter R, ed. *The Name of the Child: Health and Welfare, 1880-1940.* London: Routledge. Pp. 96–123.

Lederer SE. 1995. *Subjected to Science: Human Experimentation in America Before the Second World War.* Baltimore, MD: Johns Hopkins University Press.

Lederer SE, Grodin MA. 1994. Historical overview: Pediatric experimentation. In: Grodin MA, Glantz LH, eds. *Children as Research Subjects: Science, Ethics and Law.* New York, NY: Oxford University Press.

Leiken S. 1993. The role of adolescents in decisions concerning their cancer treatment. *Cancer Supplement* 71(10):3342–3346.

Lepay D. 2003 (January 9). *Overview of FDA Research Ethics Compliance Activities and Data Resources.* Presentation to the Committee on Clinical Research Involving Children. Washington, DC: Institute of Medicine.

Levi R, Marsick R, Drotar D, Kodish E. 2000. Diagnosis, disclosure, and informed consent: Learning from parents of children with cancer. *Journal of Pediatric Hematology and Oncology* 22(1):3–12.

Levine RJ. 1999. The need to revise the Declaration of Helsinki. *New England Journal of Medicine* 341(7):531–534.

Levinsky N. 2002. Nonfinancial conflicts of interest in research. *New England Journal of Medicine* 347(10):759–761.

Lewis CC. 1981. How adolescents approach decisions: Changes over grades seven to twelve and policy implications. *Child Development* 52:538–544.

Lewis CE, Lewis MA, Ifekwunigue M. 1978. Informed consent by children and participation in an influenza trial. *American Journal of Public Health* 68(11):1079–1082.

Lidz CW, Appelbaum PS. 2002. The therapeutic misconception: Problems and solutions. *Medical Care* 40(9):V55–V63.

Lilly J. 2003 (July 11). Testimony before the Committee on Clinical Research Involving Children. Washington, DC: Institute of Medicine.

Lilly MT. 2000 (February 29). Statement at Congressional Policy Briefing on Quality Cancer Care, Washington, DC. American Society for Clinical Oncology. [Online]. Available: http://www.asco.org/ac/1,1003,_12-002166-00_18-0010746-00_19001074900_20002,00.asp?ArticleId=10746&ArticleBodyId=10749&ShowHead=&PageNo=1&cancer_type_id=&state= [accessed March 11, 2004].

Liou TG, Adler FR, Fitzsimmons SC, Cahill BC, Hibbs JR, Marshall BC. 2001. Predictive 5-year survivorship model of cystic fibrosis. *American Journal of Epidemiology* 153(4): 345–352.

Lippincott S. 2003 (July 11). Testimony before the Committee on Clinical Research Involving Children. Washington, DC: Institute of Medicine.

Liu L, Krailo M, Reaman GH, Bernstein L, Surveillance, Epidemiology and End Results Childhood Cancer Linkage Group. 2003. Childhood cancer patients' access to cooperative group cancer programs: A population-based study. *Cancer* 97(5):1339–1345.

Llewellyn-Thomas HA, McGreal MJ, Thiel EC. 1995. Cancer patients' decision making and trial-entry preferences: The effects of "framing" information about short-term toxicity and long-term survival. *Medical Decision Making* 15(1):4–12.

Lo B, Wolf LE, Berkeley A. 2000. Conflict-of-interest policies for investigators in clinical trials. *New England Journal of Medicine* 343(22):1616–1620.

Lowen R. 1995. Letter to ACHRE (Advisory Committee on Human Radiation Experiments) re: Discussion of the Ethics of Human Experimentation in the Medical and Scientific Literature. [Online]. Available: http://www.gwu.edu/~nsarchiv/radiation/dir/mstreet/commeet/meet13/brief13/tab_d/br13d3a.txt [accessed March 11, 2004].

Ludmerer KM. 1999. Instilling professionalism in medical education. *Journal of the American Medical Association* 282(9):881–882.

Lysaught MT. 1998. Commentary: Reconstruing genetic research as research. *Journal of Law, Medicine and Ethics* 26(1):48–54, 4.

Madsen SM, Holm S, Davidsen B, Munkholm P, Schlichting P, Riis P. 2000. Ethical aspects of clinical trials: The attitudes of participants in two non-cancer trials. *Journal of Internal Medicine* 248(6):463–474.

Malenka DJ, Baron JA, Johansen S, Wahrenberger JW, Ross JM. 1993. The framing effect of relative and absolute risk. *Journal of General Internal Medicine* 8(10):543–548.

Mammel KA, Kaplan DW. 1995. Research consent by adolescent minors and institutional review boards. *Journal of Adolescent Health* 17(5):323–330.

Man-Son-Hing M, O'Connor AM, Drake E, Biggs J, Hum V, Laupacis A. 2002. The effect of qualitative vs. quantitative presentation of probability estimates on patient decision-making: A randomized trial. *Health Expectations* 5(3):246–255.

Mann H, Djulbegovic B. 2003. Choosing a control intervention for a randomised clinical trial. *BMC Medical Research Methodology* 3(1):7–11.

Manworren RCB, Hynan LS. 2003. Clinical validation of FLACC: Preverbal patient pain scale. *Pediatric Nursing* 29(2):140–146.

Marshall MF. 2001 (August 13). Letter to Food and Drug Administration re: Comment on: Docket 00N-0074 April 24, 2001. Interim Rule: Additional Safeguards for Children in Clinical Investigations of FDA-Regulated Products. [Online]. Available: http://ohrp.osophs.dhhs.gov/nhrpac/mtg07-01/fda.pdf [accessed March 11, 2004].

Martin JA, Hamilton BE, Ventura SJ, Menacker F, Park MM, Sutton PD. 2002. Births: Final data for 2001. *National Vital Statistics Report* 51(2):1–3. [Online]. Available: http://www.cdc.gov/nchs/data/nvsr/nvsr51/nvsr51_02.pdf [accessed March 11, 2004].

Mason SA, Allmark PJ. 2000. Obtaining informed consent to neonatal randomized controlled trials: Interviews with parents and clinicians in the Euricon study. *Lancet* 356(9247): 2045–2051.

Mattson ME, Curb JD, McArdle R. 1985. Participation in a clinical trial: The patients' point of view. *Control Clinical Trials* 6(2):156–167.

Mazur DJ, Hickam DH. 1991. Patients' interpretations of probability terms. *Journal of General Internal Medicine* 6(3):237–240.

Mazur DJ, Merz JF. 1994. Patients' interpretations of verbal expressions of probability: Implications for securing informed consent to medical interventions. *Behavioral Sciences and the Law* 12(4):417–426.

McGettigan P, Sly K, O'Connell D, Hill S, Henry D. 1999. The effects of information framing on the practices of physicians. *Journal of General Internal Medicine* 14(10):633–642.

McGrath P. 2002. Beginning treatment for childhood acute lymphoblastic leukemia: Insights from the parents' perspective. *Oncology Nursing Forum* 29(6):988–996.

MCHB (Maternal and Child Health Bureau). 2003 (December). *Strategic Plan: FY 2003-2007*. [Online]. Available: http://mchb.hrsa.gov/about/stratplan03-07.htm [accessed January 27, 2004].

McIntyre MO. 2002 (September 10). Promise you'll tell me if it will hurt: A 7-year-old patient offers some rules for the grown-ups who work in hospitals. *Washington Post*. P. HE7.

McNeilly PJ. 2001 (October 3). Letter to Vice Dean for Research, Johns Hopkins University re: Human research subject protection under multiple project assurance. [Online]. Available: http://ohrp.osophs.dhhs.gov/detrm_letrs/oct01a.pdf [accessed March 11, 2004].

McWilliams R, Hoover-Fong J, Hamosh A, Beck S, Beaty T, Cutting G. 2003. Problematic variation in local institutional review of a multicenter genetic epidemiology study. *Journal of the American Medical Association* 290(3):360–366.

Meadows M. 2003. Drug research and children. *FDA Consumer Magazine* 37(12-17). [Online]. Available: http://www.fda.gov/fdac/features/2003/103_drugs.html [accessed January 27, 2004].

Meropol NJ, Weinfurt KP, Burnett CB, Balshem A, Benson AB III, Castel L, Corbett S, Diefenbach M, Gaskin D, Li Y, Manne S, Marshall J, Rowland JH, Slater E, Sulmasy DP, Van Echo D, Washington S, Schulman KA. 2003. Perceptions of patients and physicians regarding phase I cancer clinical trials: Implications for physician-patient communication. *Journal of Clinical Oncology* 21(13):2589–2596.

Merriam-Webster. 2003. *Merriam-Webster's Collegiate Dictionary*. 11th ed. Springfield, MA: Merriam-Webster, Inc.

Miller FG, Brody H. 2002. What makes placebo-controlled trials unethical? *American Journal of Bioethics* 2(2):3–9.

Millstein SG, Halpern-Felsher BL. 2001. Perceptions of risk and vulnerability in adolescent risk and vulnerability: Concepts and measurement. In: Institute of Medicine, National Research Council, eds. *Adolescent Risk and Vulnerability: Concepts and Measurement*. Washington, DC: National Academy Press.

Milne C. 2002. *How Have Pediatric Clinical Trials Influenced Practice: Past and Future*. Presentation at the Pediatric Anesthesiology Meeting, Society for Pediatric Anesthesia and American Academy of Pediatrics. [Online]. Available: http://www.pedsanesthesia. org/meetings/2002winter/syllabus/friday.pdf [accessed March 11, 2004].

Mofenson L. 2000. Perinatal exposure to zidovudine—Benefits and risks. *New England Journal of Medicine* 343(11):803–805.

Moher D, Dulberg CS, Wells GA. 1994. Statistical power, sample size, and their reporting in randomized controlled trials. *Journal of the American Medical Association* 272(2):122–124.

Morris AK, Sloutsky VM. 1998. Understanding of logical necessity: Developmental antecedents and cognitive consequences. *Child Development* 69(3):721–741.

Naar-King S, Ellis DA, Frey MA. 2004. *Assessing Children's Well-Being: A Handbook of Measures*. Mahwah, NJ: Erlbaum.

Nahata MC. 1992. Advances in paediatric pharmacotherapy. *Journal of Clinical Pharmacy and Therapeutics* 17(3):141–146.

Nahata MC. 1999. Lack of pediatric drug formulations. *Pediatrics* 104(3 Pt 2):607–609.

Nannis ED. 1991. Children's understanding of their participation in psychological research: Implication for issues of assent consent. *Canadian Journal of Behavioural Science* 23(2): 133–141.

NAS (National Academy of Sciences). 1992. *Responsible Science, Volume I: Ensuring the Integrity of the Research Process*. Washington, DC: National Academy Press.

NAS. 1995. *On Being a Scientist: Responsible Conduct in Research*. 2nd ed. Washington, DC: National Academy Press.

National Commission (National Commission for the Protection of Human Subjects of Biomedical and Behavioral Research). 1975. *Report and Recommendations: Research on the Fetus*. Washington, DC: U.S. Department of Commerce.

National Commission. 1976. *Report and Recommendations: Research Involving Prisoners*. Washington, DC: U.S. Department of Commerce. [Online]. Available: http://www.reb.ca/ assets/documents/NATCOM/doc4.pdf [accessed March 11, 2004].

National Commission. 1977. *Report and Recommendations: Research Involving Children*. Washington, DC: U.S. Government Printing Office.

National Commission. 1978a. *The Belmont Report: Ethical Principles and Guidelines for the Protection of Human Subjects of Research*. Washington, DC: U.S. Government Printing Office.

National Commission. 1978b. *Research Involving Those Institutionalized As Mentally Infirm: Report and Recommendations*. Washington, DC: U.S. Government Printing Office.

NBAC (National Bioethics Advisory Commission). 1998. *Research Involving Persons with Mental Disorders That May Affect Decisionmaking Capacity*. Bethesda, MD: NBAC. [Online]. Available: http://www.georgetown.edu/research/nrcbl/nbac/capacity/TOC.htm [accessed March 11, 2004].

NBAC. 1999. *Research Involving Human Biological Materials: Ethical Issues and Policy Guidance*. Bethesda, MD: NBAC.

NBAC. 2001a. *Ethical and Policy Issues in International Research: Clinical Trials in Developing Countries, Volume I*. Bethesda, MD: NBAC. [Online]. Available: http://www. georgetown.edu/research/nrcbl/nbac/clinical/Vol1.pdf [accessed March 11, 2004].

NBAC. 2001b. *Ethical and Policy Issues in Research Involving Human Participants.* Bethesda, MD: NBAC. [Online]. Available: http://www.georgetown.edu/research/nrcbl/nbac/human/overvol1.pdf [accessed March 11, 2004].

NCHS (National Center for Human Statistics). 2000. *Health, United States, 2000 with Adolescent Health Chartbook.* Hyattsville, MD: NCHS. [Online]. Available: http://www.cdc.gov/nchs/data/hus/hus00.pdf [accessed March 11, 2004].

NCI (National Cancer Institute). 1999. *Policy of the National Cancer Institute for Data and Safety Monitoring of Clinical Trials.* Bethesda, MD: National Institutes of Health. [Online]. Available: http://deainfo.nci.nih.gov/grantspolicies/datasafety.htm [accessed March 11, 2004].

NCI. 2001. *Simplification of Informed Consent Documents: Recommendations.* [Online]. Available: http://www.cancer.gov/clinical_trials/doc_header.aspx?viewid= 5fca4dc5-b6a7-4272-be96-b489f23022e5&docid=61f9435e-c529-42fa-81a5-fc6ecd30d42e [accessed March 11, 2004].

NCI. 2002a (July 8). *Data and Safety Monitoring Example Plans.* [Online]. Available: http://www.cancer.gov/ClinicalTrials/conducting/dsm-example-plans [accessed March 11, 2004].

NCI. 2002b (December 18). *Facts and Figures About Cancer Clinical Trials.* [Online]. Available: http://www.nci.nih.gov/clinicaltrials/facts-and-figures [accessed March 11, 2004].

NCI. 2003. *How Does the CIRB Process Work? (Detailed Version).* [Online]. Available: http://www.ncicirb.org/CIRB_HowWorks_Detailed.asp [accessed March 11, 2004].

Neergaard L. 2003 (June 19). FDA cites possible suicide link in Paxil. *AP Online.* [Online]. Available: http://www.intelihealth.com/IH/ihtPrint/EMIHC270/333/21291/365913.html?hide=t&k=basePrint [accessed March 11, 2004].

Nelson EC, Batalden PB, Ryer JC, eds. 1998. *Joint Commission Clinical Improvement Action Guide.* Oakbrook Terrace, IL: Joint Commission on Accreditation of Healthcare Organizations.

Nelson RM. 1999. Unpublished interview. Supported in part by grant K01 NS02151-06 from the National Institute of Neurological Disorders and Stroke.

Nelson RM. 2002 (June 4). Letter to Food and Drug Administration re: Docket No. 01N-0322. [Online]. Available: http://216.239.41.104/search?q=cache:PrcwZmrrZ0AJ: www.fda.gov/ohrms/dockets/dailys/02/Jun02/060602/01N-0322_emc-000018-01.doc+ %22irb+shopping%22+nelson&hl=en&ie=UTF-8 [accessed February 6, 2004].

Nelson RM. 2003. *Algorithm for Subpart D Analysis (45 CFR 46 and 21 CFR 50).* Presentation to the Pediatric Advisory Subcommittee Meeting on Current Epidemiology and Therapeutic Interventions Relevant to Hyperbilirubinemia in the Term and Near-Term Newborn, Food and Drug Administration. [Online]. Available: http://www.fda.gov/ohrms/dockets/ac/cder03.html#Anti-Infective [accessed March 11, 2004].

NHRPAC (National Human Research Protections Advisory Committee). 2001. *Children's Workgroup Report (Draft).* [Online]. Available: http://ohrp.osophs.dhhs.gov/nhrpac/mtg04-01/child-workgroup4-5-01.pdf [accessed March 11, 2004].

NHRPAC. 2002. *Clarifying Specific Portion of 45 CFR 46 Subpart D That Governs Children's Research.* [Online]. Available: http://ohrp.osophs.dhhs.gov/nhrpac/documents/nhrpac16.pdf [accessed March 11, 2004].

NICHD (National Institute of Child Health and Human Development). No date. *Pediatric AIDS Clinical Trials Group Interview: History/Background.* [Online]. Available: http://pactg.s-3.com/pinfo_history.htm [accessed March 11, 2004].

NICHD. 2002. *What Does the NICHD Do?* [Online]. Available: http://www. nichd.nih.gov/about/nichd_ does.cfm [accessed March 11, 2004].

NICHD. 2003 (April 30). *Research Panels.* [Online]. Available: http://www. nichd.nih.gov/crmc/pp/research_programs.htm [accessed March 11, 2004].

Nicoletti A. 2003. Teens, confidentiality, and HIPPA. *Journal of Pediatric and Adolescent Gynecology* 16(2):113–114.

NIDDK (National Institute of Diabetes and Digestive and Kidney Diseases). 2001. Research needs in pediatric kidney disease: 2000 and beyond. *Research Updates in Kidney and Urologic Health.* [Online]. Available: http://www.niddk.nih.gov/health/kidney/Research_Updates/win00-01/needs.htm [accessed March 11, 2004].

NIH (National Institutes of Health). 1994. NIH Guidelines on the inclusion of women and minorities as subjects in clinical research. *Federal Register* 59:11146–11151.

NIH. 1998a. *NIH Policy and Guidelines on the Inclusion of Children as Participants in Research Involving Human Subjects, March 6, 1998.* Bethesda, MD: NIH. [Online]. Available: http://grants.nih.gov/grants/guide/notice-files/not98-024.html [accessed March 11, 2004].

NIH. 1998b. *Policy for Data and Safety Monitoring.* Bethesda, MD: NIH. [Online]. Available: http://grants1.nih.gov/grants/guide/notice-files/not98-084.html [accessed January 13, 2004].

NIH. 2000a. Figure 6: NIH-2514-1- Consent to participate in a clinical research study. In: Khuu M, ed. *Protomechanics: A Guide to Preparing and Conducting a Clinical Research Study.* Bethesda, MD: NIH. [Online]. Available: http://www.cc.nih.gov/ccc/protomechanics/pdfs/figure_6.pdf [accessed March 11, 2004].

NIH. 2000b. *Revised Policy for IRB Review of Human Subjects Protocols in Grant Applications.* Bethesda, MD: NIH. [Online]. Available: http://grants.nih.gov/grants/guide/notice-files/NOT-OD-00-031.html [accessed March 11, 2004].

NIH. 2001. *NIH Grants Policy Statement (Rev. 03/01).* Bethesda, MD: NIH. [Online]. Available: http://grants2.nih.gov/grants/policy/nihgps_2001/nihgps_2001.pdf [accessed March 11, 2004].

NIH. 2002 (July 18). *Financial Conflict of Interest: Objectivity in Research.* [Online]. Available: http://grants1.nih.gov/grants/policy/coi/nih_review.htm [accessed March 11, 2004].

NIH. 2003a (July 21). *Certificates of Confidentiality: Background Information.* [Online]. Available: http://grants1.nih.gov/grants/policy/coc/background.htm [accessed March 11, 2004].

NIH. 2003b. *Multidisciplinary Clinical Research Career Development Programs.* [Online]. Available: http://grants2.nih.gov/grants/guide/rfa-files/RFA-RM-04-006.html [accessed March 11, 2004].

NIH. 2003c. *Protecting Personal Health Information in Research: Understanding the HIPAA Privacy Rule.* Bethesda, MD: NIH. [Online]. Available: http://privacyruleandresearch.nih.gov/pdf/HIPAA_Privacy_Rule_Booklet.pdf [accessed March 11, 2004].

NINR (National Institute of Nursing Research). 1993. *Priority Expert Panel Report: Vol 5 Health Promotion for Older Children and Adolescents 1993.* Bethesda, MD: National Institutes of Health.

Nisbett RE, Fong GT, Lehman DR, Cheng PW. 1987. Teaching reasoning. *Science* 238:623–631.

NLM (U.S. National Library of Medicine). 2002. *Smallpox: A Great and Terrible Scourge.* [Online]. Available: http://www.nlm.nih.gov/exhibition/smallpox/sp_vaccination.html [accessed March 11, 2004].

NRC (National Research Council). 2003. *Protecting Participants and Facilitating Social and Behavioral Sciences Research.* Washington, DC: The National Academies Press.

NRC/IOM (Institute of Medicine). 1999. Forum on adolescence. In: *Adolescent Development and the Biology of Puberty: Summary of a Workshop on New Research.* Washington, DC: The National Academies Press. [Online]. Available: http://books.nap.edu/catalog/9634.html [accessed March 11, 2004].

Nuremberg Code: Directives for human experimentation. 1949. In: *Trials of War Criminals Before the Nuremberg Military Tribunals Under Control Council Law No. 10, Vol. 2.* Washington, DC: U.S. Governmental Printing Office. Pp. 181–182. [Online]. Available: http://ohsr.od.nih.gov/nuremberg.php3 [accessed March 11, 2004].

O'Brien KL, Selanikio JD, Hecdivert C, Placide M, Louis M, Barr DB, Barr JR, Hospedales CJ, Lewis MJ, Schwartz B, Philen RM, St. Victor S, Espindola J, Needham LL, Denerville K, for the Acute Renal Failure Investigation Team. 1998. Epidemic of pediatric deaths from acute renal failure caused by diethylene glycol poisoning. *Journal of the American Medical Association* 279(15):1175–1180.

O'Connor AM, Rostom A, Fiset V, Tetroe J, Entwistle V, Llewellyn-Thomas H, Holmes-Rovner M, Barry M, Jones J. 1999. Decision aids for patients facing health treatment or screening decisions: Systematic review. *British Medical Journal* 319(7212):731–734.

OCR (Office of Civil Rights). 2000. *Policy Guidance on the Title VI Prohibition Against National Origin Discrimination as It Affects Persons with Limited English Proficiency.* Washington, DC: U.S. Department of Health and Human Services. [Online]. Available: http://cms.hhs.gov/states/letters/lepguide.pdf [accessed March 11, 2004].

Oglaff FR, Otto RK. 1991. Are research participants truly informed? Readability of informed consent forms used in research. *Ethics & Behavior* 1(4):239–252.

OHRP (Office for Human Research Protections). 2001. *Draft Interim Guidance: Financial Relationships in Clinical Research: Issues for Institutions, Clinical Investigators, and IRBs to Consider When Dealing With Issues or Financial Interest and Human Subject Protection.* Washington, DC: U.S. Department of Health and Human Services. [Online]. Available: http://ohrp.osophs.dhhs.gov/humansubjects/finreltn/finguid.htm [accessed March 11, 2004].

OHRP. 2002a. *Federalwide Assurance of Protection for Human Subjects.* Washington, DC: U.S. Department of Health and Human Services. [Online]. Available: http://ohrp.osophs.dhhs.gov/humansubjects/assurance/filasurt.htm [accessed March 11, 2004].

OHRP. 2002b. *Objectives and Overview of the OHRP Quality Improvement Program.* Washington, DC: U.S. Department of Health and Human Services. [Online]. Available: http://ohrp.osophs.dhhs.gov/humansubjects/qip/qipdesc.pdf [accessed March 11, 2004].

OHRP. 2002c. *OHRP Compliance Activities: Common Findings and Guidance Clickable Index.* [Online]. Available: http://ohrp.osophs.dhhs.gov/references/findings.pdf [accessed March 11, 2004].

OHRP. 2002d. *Quality Assurance Self-Assessment Tool.* [Online]. Available: http://ohrp.osophs.dhhs.gov/humansubjects/qip/qatoold.htm [accessed March 11, 2004].

OHRP. 2003. Amendment of statement of organization functions and delegations of authority for the Office for Human Research Protections. *Federal Register* 68:60392–60393. [Online]. Available: http://ohrp.osophs.dhhs.gov/references/reorgfr.pdf [accessed March 11, 2004].

OIG (Office of Inspector General). 1998a. *Institutional Review Boards: A Time for Reform.* Washington, DC: U.S. Department of Health and Human Services. [Online]. Available: http://www.researchroundtable.com/pdfiles/time_reform.pdf [accessed March 11, 2004].

OIG. 1998b. *Institutional Review Boards: The Emergence of Independent Boards.* Washington, DC: U.S. Department of Health and Human Services. [Online]. Available: http://www.researchroundtable.com/pdfiles/irbemergence.pdf [accessed March 11, 2004].

OIG. 1998c. *Institutional Review Boards: Their Role in Reviewing Approved Research.* Washington, DC: U.S. Department of Health and Human Services. [Online]. Available: http://oig.hhs.gov/oei/reports/oei-01-97-00190.pdf [accessed March 11, 2004].

OIG. 2000a. *Protecting Human Research Subjects: Status of Recommendations.* Washington, DC: U.S. Department of Health and Human Services. [Online]. Available: http://www.researchroundtable.com/pdfiles/protecting_human.pdf [accessed March 11, 2004].

OIG. 2000b. *Recruiting Human Subjects: Pressures in Industry-Sponsored Clinical Research.* Washington, DC: U.S. Department of Health and Human Services. [Online]. Available: http://www.researchroundtable.com/pdfiles/a459.pdf [accessed March 11, 2004].

OIG. 2001. *The Globalization of Clinical Trials: A Growing Challenge in Protecting Human Subjects.* Washington, DC: U.S. Department of Health and Human Services. [Online]. Available: http://oig.hhs.gov/oei/reports/oei-01-00-00190.pdf [accessed March 11, 2004].

Olechnowicz JQ, Eder M, Simon C, Zyzanski S, Kodish E. 2002. Assent observed: Children's involvement in leukemia treatment and research discussions. *Pediatrics* 109(5):806–814.

Ondrusek N, Abramovitch R, Pencharz P, Koren G. 1998. Empirical examination of the ability of children to consent to clinical research. *Journal of Medical Ethics (London)* 24(3):158–165.

OPRR (Office for Protection from Research Risk). 1993. *Protecting Human Research Subjects: Institutional Review Board Guidebook.* Washington, DC: U.S. Government Printing Office. [Online]. Available: http://ohrp.osophs.dhhs.gov/irb/irb_chapter3.htm [accessed March 11, 2004].

Paasche-Orlow MK, Taylor HA, Brancati FL. 2003. Readability standards for informed-consent forms as compared with actual readability. *New England Journal of Medicine* 348(8):721–726.

Pandey SK, Wilson ME, Trivedi RH, Izak AM, Macky TA, Werner LM, Apple DJ. 2001. Pediatric cataract surgery and intraocular lens implantation: Current techniques, complications, and management. *International Ophthalmology Clinics* 41(3):175–196.

Pattee S. 2003. Testimony on behalf of the Cystic Fibrosis Foundation before the Committee on Clinical Research Involving Children. Washington, DC: Institute of Medicine.

Pattishall EN. 1990. Negative clinical trials in cystic fibrosis research. *Pediatrics* 85(3):277–281.

Pellegrino ED. 1992. Character and the ethical conduct of research. *Accountability in Research* 2(1):1–11.

Peppercorn JM, Weeks JC, Cook EF, Joffe S. 2004. Comparison of outcomes in cancer patients treated within and outside clinical trials: Conceptual framework and structured review. *Lancet* 363:263–270.

Perkins J, Simon H, Cheng F, Olson K, Vera Y. 1998. *Ensuring Linguistic Access in Health Care Settings: Legal Rights and Responsibilities.* Los Angeles, CA: National Health Law Program.

Peterson JW, Sterling YM. 1999. Research involving African Americans: Implications for family nursing research. *Journal of Child and Family Nursing* 2(3):162–170.

PHRP (Partnership for Human Research Protection). 2003. Statement to the Committee on Clinical Research Involving Children. Washington, DC: Institute of Medicine.

Piaget J, Inhelder B. 1969. *The Psychology of the Child.* New York, NY: Basic Books.

Pina LM. 1997. Center IDs top 10 drugs used off-label in out-patient setting. *The Pike* 3(1):6–7. [Online]. Available: http://www.fda.gov/cder/pike/jan97.pdf [accessed March 11, 2004].

Pletsch PK, Stevens PE. 2001. Children in research: Informed consent and critical factors affecting mothers. *Journal of Family Nursing* 7(1):50–70.

PPRU (Pediatric Pharmacy Research Unit Network). No date. *Sites: 13 Pioneer Pediatric Sites Throughout the U.S.* [Online]. Available: http://www.ppru.org [accessed March 11, 2004].

President's Commission (President's Commission for the Study of Ethical Problems in Medicine and Biomedical and Behavioral Research). 1981. *Protecting Human Subjects: The Adequacy and Uniformity of Federal Rules and Their Implementation.* Washington, DC: U.S. Government Printing Office.

Pui C, Sandlund JT, Pei D, Rivera GK, Howard SC, Ribeiro RC, Rubnitz JE, Razzouk BI, Hudson MM, Cheng C, Raimondi SC, Behm FG, Downing JR, Relling MV, Evans WE. 2003. Results of therapy for acute lymphoblastic leukemia in black and white children. *Journal of the American Medical Association* 290(15):2001–2007.

Pyke-Grimm KA, Degner L, Small A, Mueller B. 1999. Preferences for participation in treatment decision making and information needs of parents of children with cancer: A pilot study. *Journal of Pediatric Oncology Nursing* 16(1):13–24.

Quintana H, Keshavan M. 1995. Case study: Risperidone in children and adolescents with schizophrenia. *Journal of the American Academy of Child and Adolescent Psychiatry* 34(10):1292–1296.

Quittner AL, Sweeny SH, Watrous M, Munzenberger P, Bearss K, Gibson Nitza A, Fisher L, Henry B. 2000. Translation and linguistic validation of a disease-specific quality of life measure for cystic fibrosis. *Journal of Pediatric Physiology* 25(6):403–414.

Ramsey BW. 2003. Unpublished paper. *Examples of Multicenter Phase I Clinical Trials Conducted Through the Cystic Fibrosis Therapeutics Development Network Between 2001 and 2003.* Seattle, WA: Cystic Fibrosis Research Center, University of Washington.

Ramsey BW, Boat TF. 1994. Outcome measures for clinical trials in cystic fibrosis; summary of a Cystic Fibrosis Foundation Consensus Conference. *Journal of Pediatrics* 124:177–192.

Ramsey BW, Pepe MS, Quan JM, Otto KL, Montgomery AB, Williams-Warren J, Vasiljev-K M, Borowitz D, Bowman CM, Marshall BC, Marshall S, Smith AL, for the Cystic Fibrosis Inhaled Tobramyacin Study Group. 1999. Intermittent administration of inhaled tobramycin in patients with cystic fibrosis. *New England Journal of Medicine* 340(1):23–30.

Ramsey P. 1970. *The Patient as Person: Explorations in Medical Ethics.* New Haven, CT: Yale University Press.

Ramsey P. 1977. Children as research subjects: A reply. *Hastings Center Report* 7(2):40–42.

Ransohoff DF, Harris RP. 1997. Lessons from the mammography screening controversy: Can we improve the debate? *Annals of Internal Medicine* 127(11):1029–1034.

Reed MD, Gal P. 2004. Principles of drug therapy. In: Berhman R, Kliegman R, Jenson H, eds. *Nelson Textbook of Pediatrics.* 17th ed. Philadelphia, PA: WB Sanders.

Ries LAG, Smith MA, Gurney JG, Linet M, Tamra T, Young JL, Bunin GR, eds. 1999. *Cancer Incidence and Survival among Children and Adolescents: United States SEER Program 1975-1995, National Cancer Institute, SEER Program.* Bethesda, MD: National Institutes of Health. [Online]. Available: http://seer.cancer.gov/publications/childhood/ [accessed March 11, 2004].

Ries LAG, Eisner MP, Kosary CL, Hankey BF, Miller BA, Clegg L, Mariotto A, Fay MP, Feuer E J, Edwards BK, eds. 2003. Childhood cancer by site incidence, survival and mortality. In: *SEER Cancer Statistics Review, 1975-2000.* Bethesda, MD: National Cancer Institute. [Online]. Available: http://seer.cancer.gov/csr/1975_2000 [accessed March 11, 2004].

Rivera R, Reed JS, Menius D. 1992. Evaluating the readability of informed consent forms used in contraceptive clinical trials. *International Journal of Gynaecology and Obstetrics* 38(3):227–230.

Roberts R, Rodriguez W, Murphy D, Crescenzi T. 2003. Pediatric drug labeling: Improving the safety and efficacy of pediatric therapies. *Journal of American Medical Association* 290(7):905–911.

Rogers AS, Schwartz DF, Weissman G, English A, Adolescent Medicine HIV/AIDS Research Network. 1999. A case study in adolescent participation in clinical research: Eleven clinical sites, one common protocol, and eleven IRBs. *IRB: A Review of Human Subjects Research* 21(1):6–10.

Roman DD, Sperduto PW. 1995. Neuropsychological effects of cranial radiation: Current knowledge and future directions. *International Journal of Radiation, Oncology, Biology, and Physics* 31:983–998.

Rosella JD. 1994. Review of adolescent coping research: Representation of key demographic variables and methodological approaches to assessment. *Issues in Mental Health Nursing* 15(5):483–485.

Ross LF. 1998. *Children, Families and Health Care Decision Making.* New York, NY: Oxford University Press.

Rossi WC, Reynolds W, Nelson RM. 2003. Child assent and parental permission in pediatric research. *Theoretical Medicine* 24(2):131–148.

Rothman KJ, Michels KB. 1994. The continuing unethical use of placebo controls. *New England Journal of Medicine* 331(6):394–398.

Rothman AJ, Salovey P. 1997. Shaping perceptions to motivate healthy behavior: The role of message framing. *Psychological Bulletin* 121:3–19.

Rothman AJ, Salovey P, Antone C, Keough K, Martin CD. 1993. The influence of message framing on intentions to perform health behaviors. *Journal of Experimental Social Psychology* 29:408–433.

Rothmier JD, Lasley MV, Shapiro GG. 2003. Factors influencing parental consent in pediatric clinical research. *Pediatrics* 111(5):1037–1041.

Ruccione K, Kramer RF, Moore IK, Perin G. 1991. Informed consent for treatment of childhood cancer: Factors affecting parents' decision making. *Journal of Pediatric Oncology Nursing* 8(3):112–121.

Rutkow IM. 1998. Beaumont and St. Martin: A blast from the past. *Archives of Surgery* 133:1259.

Sackett DL. 2000. Equipoise, a term whose time (if it ever came) has surely gone. *Canadian Medical Association Journal* 163(7):835–836. [Online]. Available: http://www.cmaj.ca/cgi/content/full/163/7/835?ijkey=4b1a3c08c63ec062b261aab49e49482f7abc9830&keytype2=tf_ipsecsha [accessed March 11, 2004].

Sagan L. 1994 (November 17). Interview by Javitt G, White-Junod S, Thomas S, and Kruger J (ACHRE Research Project Series, Interview Program File, Ethics Oral History Project), transcript of audio recording. P. 13–14.

Salgo v. Stanford Jr. (*Olga Salgo, as Administratrix etc. Respondent v. Leland Stanford Jr. University Board of Trustees et al.*). 1957. 154 Cal., App. 2d 560 (Cal. Dist. Ct. App. 57).

SAM (Society for Adolescent Medicine). 1995. Guidelines for adolescent health research. *Journal of Adolescent Health* 17(5): 264–269.

Sander N. 2003 (July 9). Statement on Behalf of the Allergy & Asthma Network/Mothers of Asthmatics to the Committee on Clinical Research Involving Children. Washington, DC: Institute of Medicine.

Sarnblad S, Kroon M, Aman J. 2003. Metformin as additional therapy in adolescents with poorly controlled type 1 diabetes: Randomised placebo-controlled trial with aspects on insulin sensitivity. *European Journal of Endocrinology* 149(4):323–329.

Sateren W, Trimble E, Abrams J, Brawley O, Breen N, Ford L, McCabe M, Kaplan R, Smith M, Ungerleider R, Christian M. 2002. How sociodemographics, presence of oncology specialists, and hospital cancer programs affect accrual to cancer treatment trials. *Journal of Clinical Oncology* 20(8):2109–2117.

Schachter AD, Meyers KE, Spaneas LD, Palmer JA, Salmanullah M, Baluarte J, Brayman KL, Harmon WE. 2004. Short Sirolimus half-life in pediatric renal transplant recipients on a calcineurin inhibitor-free protocol. *Pediatric Transplantation* 8(2):171–177.

Scherer DG. 1991. The capacities of minors to exercise voluntariness in medical treatment decisions. *Law and Human Behavior* 15:431–449.

Scherer DG, Reppucci ND. 1988. Adolescents' capacities to provide voluntary informed consent: The effect of parental influence and medical dilemmas. *Law and Human Behaviour* 12(2):123–141.

Schultz CJ, Konopelska-Bahu T, Dalton RN, Carroll TA, Stratton I, Gale EA, Neil A, Dunger DB. 1999. Microalbuminuria prevalence varies with age, sex, and puberty in children with type 1 diabetes followed from diagnosis in a longitudinal study. Oxford Regional Prospective Study Group. *Diabetes Care* 22(3):495–502.

Schuster M. 2000. Well child care. In: McGlynn E, Damberg C, Kerr E, Schuster M, eds. *Quality of Care for Children and Adolescents: A Review of Selected Clinical Conditions and Quality Indicators*. Santa Monica, CA: Rand Corporation. [Online]. Available: http://www.rand.org/publications/MR/MR1283/mr1283.ch22.pdf [accessed March 11, 2004].

Schutta KM, Burnett CB. 2000. Factors that influence a patient's decision to participate in a phase I cancer clinical trial. *Oncology Nursing Forum* 27(9):1435–1438.

Scott ES, Reppucci ND, Woolard JL. 1995. Evaluating adolescent decision making in legal contexts. *Law and Human Behavior* 19:221–244.

Segall MH, Dasen PR, Berry JW, Poartinga GH. 1999. *Human Development in Global Perspective*. Boston, MA: Allyn & Bacon.

Shah S, Whittle A, Wilfond B, Gensler G, Wendler D. 2004. How do institutional review boards apply the federal risk and benefit standards for pediatric research? *Journal of the American Medical Association* 291(4):476–482.

Sharav VH. 2003. Children in clinical research: A conflict of moral values. *American Journal of Bioethics* 3(1): InFocus. [Online]. Available: http://bioethics.net/in_focus/sharav.pdf [accessed March 11, 2004].

Shelton TL, Jeppson ES, Johnson BH. 1987. *Family-Centered Care for Children with Special Health Care Needs*. Bethesda, MD: Association for the Care of Children's Health.

Shirkey HC. 1968. Editorial comment: Therapeutic orphans. *Journal of Pediatrics* 72(1):119–120.

Shochat SJ, Fremgen AM, Murphy SB, Hutchinson C, Donaldson SS, Haase GM, Provisor AJ, Clive-Bumpus RE, Winchester DP. 2001. Childhood cancer: Patterns of protocol participation in a national survey. *American Cancer Journal for Clinicians* 51(2):119–130. [Online]. Available: http://caonline.amcancersoc.org/cgi/reprint/51/2/119.pdf [accessed March 11, 2004].

Shore RE, Woodard E, Hildreth N, Dvoretsky P, Hempelmann L, Pasternack B. 1985. Thyroid tumors following thymus irradiation. *Journal of the National Cancer Institute* 74(6):1177–1184.

Shore RE, Hildreth N, Dvoretsky P, Andresen E, Moseson M, Pasternack B. 1993. Thyroid cancer among persons given X-ray treatment in infancy for an enlarged thymus gland. *American Journal of Epidemiology* 137(10):1068–1080.

Shrier I. 2001. Uncertainty about clinical equipoise. *Canadian Medical Association Journal* 164(13):1831.

Siegler M. 2002. Training doctors for professionalism: Some lessons from teaching clinical medical ethics. *The Mount Sinai Journal of Medicine* 69(6):404–409. [Online]. Available: http://www.mssm.edu/msjournal/69/v69_6_page404_409.pdf [accessed January 27, 2004].

Siegler RS. 1991. *Children's Thinking*. Englewood Cliffs, NJ: Prentice Hall.

Sikand A, Schubiner H, Simpson PM. 1997. Parent and adolescent perceived need for parental consent involving research with minors. *Archives of Pediatrics and Adolescent Medicine* 151(6):603–607.

Silverman H, Hull SC, Sugarman J. 2001. Variability among institutional review boards' decisions within the context of a multicenter trial. *Critical Care Medicine* 29(2):235–241.

Silverman WA. 1977. The lesson of retrolental fibroplasias. *Scientific America* 236:100–107.

Simon C, Eder M, Raiz P, Zyzanski S, Pentz R, Kodish ED. 2001. Informed consent for pediatric leukemia research: Clinician perspectives. *Cancer* 92(3):691–700.

Simon C, Zyzanski SJ, Eder M, Raiz P, Kodish ED, Siminoff LA. 2003. Groups potentially at risk for making poorly informed decisions about entry into clinical trials for childhood cancer. *Journal of Clinical Oncology* 21(11):2173–2178.

Simone JV. 2003. Childhood leukemia—successes and challenges for survivors. *New England Journal of Medicine* 349(7):627–628.

Singhal N, Oberle K, Burgess E, Huber-Okrainec J. 2002. Parents' perceptions of research with newborns. *Journal of Perinatology* 22(1):57–63.

Smith KW, Avis NE, Assmann SF. 1999. Distinguishing between quality of life and health status in quality of life research: A meta-analysis. *Quality of Life Research* 8:447–459.

Snowdon C, Garcia J, Elbourne D. 1997. Making sense of randomization: Responses of parents of critically ill babies to random allocation of treatment in a clinical trial. *Social Science Medicine* 45(9):1337–1355.

Somers S. 2003. *Q & A: Interpreters for Home Health Care.* [Online]. Available: http://www.healthlaw.org/pubs/200307.qanda.html [accessed March 11, 2004].

Sourkes BM. 1995. *Armfuls of Time: The Psychological Experience of the Child with a Life-Threatening Illness.* Pittsburgh, PA: University of Pittsburgh Press.

SPR and APS (Society for Pediatric Research and American Pediatric Society). 2003. *Participation and Protection of Children in Clinical Research.* Paper presented to the Committee on Clinical Research Involving Children. Washington, DC: Institute of Medicine.

Stair TO, Reed CR, Radeos MS, Koski G, Camargo CA, on behalf of the Multicenter Airway Research Collaboration (MARC) Investigators. 2001. Variation in institutional review board responses to a standard protocol for a multicenter clinical trial. *Academic Emergency Medicine* 8(6):636–641. [Online]. Available: http://healthcare.partners.org/marc/articles/Stair_2001.pdf [accessed March 11, 2004].

Stanovich KE, West RF. 2000. Individual differences in reasoning: Implications for the rationality debate? *Behavioral and Brain Sciences* 23(5):645–665, discussion 665–726.

Stedman T. 2000. *Stedman's Medical Dictionary.* 27th ed. Baltimore, MD: Lippincott Williams & Wilkins.

Steinberg L, Cauffman E. 1996. Maturity of judgment in adolescence: Psychosocial factors in adolescent decision making. *Law and Human Behavior* 20(3):249–272.

Steinbrook R. 2002. Testing medications in children. *New England Journal of Medicine* 110(2):364–370.

Stiffman AR, Striley CW, Brown E, Limb G, Ostmann E. 2002. *American Indian Adolescents, Addictions, Trauma, and HIV Risk.* Paper presented at the 130th Annual Meeting and Exposition of the American Public Health Association, San Francisco, CA. American Public Health Association. [Online]. Available: http://apha.confex.com/apha/130am/techprogram/paper_43748.htm [accessed March 11, 2004].

Stith-Coleman I. 1994. *Protection of Human Subjects in Research. CRS Report to Congress.* Washington, DC: U.S. Government Printing Office. [Online]. Available: http://www.gwu.edu/~nsarchiv/radiation/dir/mstreet/commeet/meet2/brief2/tab_i/br2i1d.txt [accessed March 11, 2004].

Stolberg SG. 1999 (December 9). F.D.A. officials fault Penn team in gene therapy death. *New York Times*. P. A22. [Online]. Available: http://www.nytimes.com/library/national/science/health/120999hth-gene-therapy.html [accessed March 11, 2004].

Susman EJ, Dorn LD, Fletcher JC. 1992. Participation in biomedical research: The consent process as viewed by children, adolescents, young adults, and physicians. *Journal of Pediatrics* 121(4):547–552.

Sutherland HJ, Lockwood GA, Tritchler DL, Sem F, Brooks L, Till JE. 1991. Communicating probabilistic information to cancer patients: Is there "noise" on the line? *Social Science and Medicine* 32(6):725–731.

Tait AR, Voepel-Lewis T, Siewert M, Malviya S. 1998. Factors that influence parents' decisions to consent to their child's participation in clinical anesthesia research. *Anesthesia and Analgesia* 86(1):50–53.

Tait AR, Voepel-Lewis T, Munro HM, Malviya S. 2001. Parents' preferences for participation in decisions made regarding their child's anaesthetic care. *Paediatric Anaesthesia* 11(3):283–290.

Tait AR, Voepel-Lewis T, Robinson A, Malviya S. 2002. Priorities for disclosure of the elements of informed consent for research: A comparison between parents and investigators. *Paediatric Anaesthesia* 12(4):332–336.

Tait AR, Voepel-Lewis T, Malviya S. 2003a. Do they understand? (part I): Parental consent for children participating in clinical anesthesia and surgery research. *Anesthesiology* 98(3):603–608.

Tait AR, Voepel-Lewis T, Malviya S. 2003b. Do they understand? (part II): Assent of children participating in clinical anesthesia and surgery research. *Anesthesiology* 98(3):609–614.

Tanner JM. 1962. *Growth of Adolescents*. Oxford, United Kingdom: Blackwell Scientific Publications.

Tarnowski KJ, Allen DM, Mayhall C, Kelly PA. 1990. Readability of pediatric biomedical research informed consent forms. *Pediatrics* 85(1):58–62.

Taylor KM, Bezjak A, Hunter R, Fraser S. 1998. Informed consent for clinical trials: Is simpler better? *Journal of the National Cancer Institute* 90(9):644–645.

TDN (Therapeutics Development Network). 2003. Guidelines for reimbursement to study subjects. In: *Manual of Operations*. Bethesda, MD: Cystic Fibrosis Foundation. P. F-2.

Tejeda HA, Green SB, Trimble EL, Ford L, High JL, Ungerleider RS, Friedman MA, Brawley OW. 1996. Representation of African-Americans, Hispanics, and Whites in National Cancer Institute cancer treatment trials. *Journal of the National Cancer Institute* 88(12): 812–816. [Online]. Available: http://jncicancerspectrum.oupjournals.org/cgi/reprint/jnci;88/12/812.pdf [accessed March 11, 2004].

Thompson L. 2000a. Human gene therapy: Harsh lessons, high hopes. *FDA Consumer* 34(5). [Online]. Available: http://www.fda.gov/fdac/features/2000/500_gene. html [accessed March 11, 2004].

Thompson RA. 2000b. Appendix C: Protecting the health services research data of minors. In: Institute of Medicine. *Protecting Data Privacy in Health Services Research*. Washington, DC: National Academy Press. [Online]. Available: http://www.nap.edu/html/data_privacy/appC.html [accessed March 11, 2004].

Thorndike RL, Hagen EP, Sattler JM. 1986. *Stanford-Binet Intelligence Scale*. 4th ed. Chicago, IL: Riverside Publishing.

Travers SH, Jeffers BW, Bloch CA, Hill JO, Eckel RH. 1995. Gender and Tanner stage differences in body composition and insulin sensitivity in early pubertal children. *Journal of Clinical Endocrinology and Metabolism* 80(1):172–178.

Tri-Council (Medical Research Council of Canada, the Natural Sciences and Engineering Research Council of Canada, and the Social Sciences and Humanities Research Council of Canada). 1998. *Tri-Council Policy Statement: Ethical Conduct for Research Involving Humans.* Ottawa, Ontario, Canada: Minister of Supply and Services.

Truog RD, Robinson W, Randolph A, Morris A. 1999. Is informed consent always necessary for randomized, controlled trials? *New England Journal of Medicine* 340(10):804–807.

Turner S, Nunn AJ, Fielding K, Choonara I. 1999. Adverse drug reactions to unlicensed and off-label drugs on paediatric wards: A prospective study. *Acta Paediatrica* 88(9):965–968.

Ubel PA. 2002. Is information always a good thing? Helping patients make "good" decisions. *Medical Care* 40(9 Supp):V39–V44.

UCLA (University of California Los Angeles). 1997. *Investigator's Manual for the Protection of Human Subjects.* Los Angeles, CA: UCLA. [Online]. Available: http://www.oprs.ucla.edu/human/hspcmanual/hspc497c.pdf [accessed March 11, 2004].

UNC (University of North Carolina, Chapel Hill). 2003. *About UNC CERTs.* [Online]. Available: http://www.sph.unc.edu/health-outcomes/certs/about2.htm [accessed March 11, 2004].

UNCHR (United Nations Commission on Human Rights). 1976. *International Covenant on Civil and Political Right, G.A. Res. 2200A (XXI), 21 U.N. GAOR Supp.* (No. 16) at 52, U.N. Doc. A/6316 (1966), 999 U.N.T.S. 171. [Online]. Available: http://www.unhchr.ch/html/menu3/b/a_ccpr.htm [accessed March 11, 2004].

U.S. Congress. 1995. *Department of Labor, Health and Human Services, and Education, and Related Agencies Appropriation Bill, 1996.* H.R. Report No. 209. Washington, DC: U.S. Congress. [Online]. Available: http://thomas.loc.gov/cgi-bin/cpquery/T?&report=hr209&dbname=cp104& [accessed March 11, 2004].

USDA (Department of Agriculture, Department of Energy, National Aeronautics and Space Administration, Department of Commerce, Consumer Product Safety Commission, International Development Cooperation Agency, Agency for International Development, Department of Housing and Urban Development, Department of Justice, Department of Defense, Department of Education, Department of Veterans Affairs, Environmental Protection Agency, Department of Health and Human Services, National Science Foundation, Department of Transportation). 1991. Federal policy for the protection of human subjects. *Federal Register* 56:28003.

USPSTF (U.S. Preventive Services Task Force). 1995. *Guide to Clinical Preventive Services.* 2nd ed. Baltimore, MD: Lippincott Williams & Wilkins.

U.S. Surgeon General. 1966. *U.S. Surgeon General Policy Statement: "Clinical Research and Investigation Involving Human Beings," Surgeon General, Public Health Service to the Heads of the Institutions Conducting Research With Public Health Service Grants.* Washington, DC: U.S. Surgeon General (Public Health Service).

Van Stuijvenberg M, Suur MJ, de Vos S, Tjiang GCH, Steyerberg EW, Derksen-Lusen G, Moll HA. 1998. Informed consent, parental awareness, and reasons for participating in a randomized controlled study. *Archives of Disease in Childhood* 79:120–125.

Varni, JW. 2003. *The PedsQL 4.0 Measurement Model for the Pediatric Quality of Life Inventory version 4.0.* [Online]. Available: http://www.pedsql.org/pedsql2.html [accessed March 11, 2004].

Vaughn A. 2003. Testimony before the Committee on Clinical Research Involving Children. Washington, DC: Institute of Medicine.

Vedantam S. 2004 (January 29). Antidepressant makers withhold data on children. *Washington Post.* P. A1.

Villarrruel A. 1999. Culturally competent nursing research: Are we there yet? *Journal of Child and Family Nursing* 2(2):82–91.

Volk RJ, Spann SJ, Cass AR, Hawley ST. 2003. Patient education for informed decision making about prostate cancer screening: A randomized controlled trial with 1-year follow-up. *Annals of Family Medicine* 1(1):22–28.

Vollman J, Winau R. 1996. Informed consent in human experimentation before the Nuremburg Code. *British Medical Journal* 313(7070):1445–1447.

Vygotsky LS. 1978. *Mind in Society: The Development of Higher Psychological Processes.* Cambridge, MA: Harvard University Press.

Wax PM. 1995. Elixirs, diluents, and the passage of the 1938 Federal Food, Drug and Cosmetic Act. *Annals of Internal Medicine* 122(6):456–461. [Online]. Available: http://www.annals.org/cgi/content/full/122/6/456 [accessed March 4, 2004].

Wechsler D. 1989. *Wechsler Preschool and Primary Scale of Intelligence Revised.* New York, NY: The Psychological Corporation.

Wechsler D. 1991. *Wechsler Intelligence Scale for Children.* 3rd ed. New York, NY: The Psychological Corporation.

Weijer C. 2001. The ethical analysis of risks and potential benefits in human subjects research: History, theory, and implications for U.S. regulation. In: National Bioethics Advisory Commission. *Ethical and Policy Issues in Research Involving Human Participants, Vol. II.* Besthesda, MD: NBAC.

Weijer C, Shapiro SH, Glass KC. 2000. Clinical equipoise and not the uncertainty principle is the moral underpinning of the randomised controlled trial. *British Medical Journal* 321(7263):756–758.

Weinfurt KP, Castel LD, Li Y, Sulmasy DP, Balshem AM, Benson 3rd A, Burnett CB, Gaskin DJ, Marshall JL, Slater EF, Schulman KA, Meropol NJ. 2003. The correlation between patient characteristics and expectations of benefit from phase I clinical trials. *Cancer* 98(1):166–175.

Weir RF. 2000. The ongoing debate about stored tissue samples. In: National Bioethics Advisory Commission. *Research Involving Human Biological Materials: Ethical Issues and Policy Guidance, Vol. II. Commissioned Papers.* Rockville, MD: National Bioethics Advisory Commitssion. [Online]. Available: http://www.georgetown.edu/research/nrcbl/nbac/hbmII.pdf [accessed March 11, 2004].

Weir RF, Horton JR. 1995. Genetic research, adolescents, and informed consent. *Theoretical Medicine* 16(4):347–373.

Weir RF, Peters C. 1997. Affirming the decisions adolescents make about life and death. *Hastings Center Report* 27(6):29–40.

Weise KL, Smith ML, Maschke KJ, Copeland HL. 2002. National practices regarding payment to research subjects for participating in pediatric research. *Pediatrics* 110(3):577–582.

Weiss CF, Glazko AJ, Weston JK. 1960. Chloramphenicol in the newborn infant: A physiologic explanation of its toxicity when given in excessive doses. *New England Journal of Medicine* 262:787–794.

Weiss R, Nelson D. 2000 (March 4). FDA lists violations by gene therapy director at U-Penn. *Washington Post.* P. A4.

Weithorn LA, Campbell SB. 1982. The competency of children and adolescents to make informed treatment decisions. *Child Development* 53(6):1589–1598.

Welton AJ, Vickers MR, Cooper JA, Meade TW, Marteau TM. 1999. Is recruitment more difficult with a placebo arm in randomized controlled trials? A quasirandomised, interview based study. *British Medical Journal* 318(7191):1114–1117.

Wendler D. 2003 (January 9). *The Ethics of Pediatric Research.* Presentation to the Committee on Clinical Research Involving Children. Washington, DC: Institute of Medicine.

Wendler D, Rackoff JE, Emanuel EJ, Grady C. 2002. The ethics of paying for children's participation in research. *Journal of Pediatrics* 141(2):166–171.

Wertz DC, Fanos JH, Reilly PR. 1994. Genetic testing for children and adolescents. Who decides? *Journal of the American Medical Association* 272(11):875–881.

White LJ, Jones JS, Felton CW, Pool LC. 1996. Informed consent for medical research: Common discrepancies and readability. *Academic Emergency Medicine* 3(8):745–750.

White M. 2003 (July 9). Statement on behalf of the Asthma and Allergy Network/Mothers of Asthmatics to the Committee on Clinical Research Involving Children. Washington, DC: Institute of Medicine.

White MT, Gamm J. 2002. Informed consent for research on stored blood and tissue samples: A survey of institutional review board practices. *Accountability in Research* 9(1):1–16.

Wilcox M, Schroer S. 1994. The perspective of patients with vascular disease on participation in clinical trials. *Journal of Vascular Nursing* 12(4):112–116.

Wilson JT. 1975. Pragmatic assessment of medicines available for young children and pregnant or breast-feeding women. In: Morselli P, Garattini S, Sereni F, eds. *Basic and Therapeutic Aspects of Perinatal Pharmacology.* New York, NY: Raven Press. Pp. 411–421.

WMA (World Medical Association). 1964. Declaration of Helsinki. In: Annas G, Glantz L, Katz B. *Informed Consent to Human Experimentation: The Subject's Dilemma.* Appendix II. New York, NY: Harper Information. P. 281. [Online]. Available: http://www.bumc.bu.edu/www/sph/lw/pvl/book/Ch9.pdf [accessed March 11, 2004].

WMA. 2002. *World Medical Association Declaration of Helsinki: Ethical Principles for Medical Research Involving Human Subjects.* Document 17.C. Washington, DC: WMA. [Online]. Available: http://www.wma.net/e/policy/pdf/17c.pdf [accessed March 11, 2004].

Wong D, Baker C. 1988. Pain in children: Comparison of assessment scales. *Pediatric Nursing* 14(4):9–17.

Yasui L. 2003 (July 11). Testimony before the Committee on Clinical Research Involving Children. Washington, DC: Institute of Medicine.

Yoder LH, O'Rourke TJ, Etnyre A, Spears DT, Brown T. 1997. Expectations and experiences of patients with cancer participating in phase I clinical trials. *Oncology Nursing Forum* 24(5):891–896.

Yuval R, Halon DA, Merdler A, Khader N, Karkabi B, Uziel K, Lewis B. 2000. Patient comprehension and reaction to participating in a double blind randomized clinical trial (ISIS-4) in acute myocardial infarction. *Archives of Internal Medicine* 160(8):1142–1146.

Zupancic JAF, Gillie P, Streiner DL, Watts JL, Schmidt B. 1997. Determinants of parental authorization for involvement of newborn infants in clinical trials. *Pediatrics* 99(1):1–6. [Online]. Available: http://pediatrics.aappublications.org/cgi/reprint/99/1/e6.pdf [accessed March 11, 2004].

APPENDICES

A

STUDY ORIGINS AND ACTIVITIES

The Best Pharmaceuticals for Children Act of 2002 (P.L. 107-109) called for the Institute of Medicine (IOM) to conduct a study of research involving children. The report was to review federal regulations, reports, and research and to make recommendations about desirable practices in ethical research involving children. IOM appointed a committee of 14 experts to oversee the study. Its task was to develop a report that specifically examined

- the appropriateness of the federal regulations for children of different ages and maturity levels;
- the interpretation of regulatory criteria for approving research involving children, including the concept of "minimal risk";
- the processes for securing parent's and children's agreement to a child's participation in research;
- the expectations and comprehension of children and parents about

what it means to participate in research and how research differs from medical treatment;;

- the appropriateness of payment to a child, parent, guardian, or legally authorized representative for the child's participation in research;
- the compliance with and enforcement of federal regulations; and
- the roles and responsibilities of institutional review boards (IRBs) in reviewing research involving children.

The committee met five times between January 2003 and November 2003. It commissioned a background paper, included as Appendix B of this report, to review state laws relating to children's agreement to medical care and research participation. The committee conducted four public meetings, including a 1-day meeting to hear the views of family support and advocacy organizations and health care groups (with written statements invited from additional organizations). The committee also met for a half day with parents and adolescents who had personal experiences with studies involving children. The agendas and participants for the public meetings are included in this appendix.

INSTITUTE OF MEDICINE
COMMITTEE ON CLINICAL RESEARCH INVOLVING CHILDREN
Room 101, The Keck Center, National Academy of Sciences
500 Fifth Street NW, Washington, DC
January 9, 2003

1:00   Welcome and Introductions

1:10   Overview of OHRP research ethics compliance activities and data resources
       Michael Carome, M.D., Associate Director for Regulatory Affairs
       Director, Division of Compliance Oversight,
       Office for Human Research Protections
       U.S. Department of Health and Human Services

       FDA's oversight of clinical research
       David Lepay, M.D., Ph.D., Senior Advisor for Clinical Science
       Office of the Commissioner
       Food and Drug Administration

2:40   Break

3:00   Survey of IRB chairs on issues related to children
       David Wendler, Ph.D., Head, Unit on Vulnerable Populations
       Department of Clinical Bioethics
       National Institutes of Health

3:45   **Work of National Human Research Protections Advisory Committee**
       Alan Fleischman, M.D., Senior Vice President
       New York Academy of Medicine

4:15   **National Institute of Child Health and Human Development perspectives and activities**
       Duane Alexander, M.D., Director
       National Institute of Child Health and Human Development

4:45   **Proposed IOM/National Research Council (NRC) study: Housing interventions involving children**
       Jane Ross, Ph.D., Acting Director
       IOM/NRC Board on Children Youth and Families

5:00   Opportunity for Public Comment

5:15   Adjourn

* * *

INSTITUTE OF MEDICINE
COMMITTEE ON CLINICAL RESEARCH INVOLVING CHILDREN
Huntington Room, Arnold and Mabel Beckman Center,
National Academy of Sciences
100 Academy Drive, Irvine, California
March 15, 2003

8:30   Welcome and Introductions
        Richard E. Behrman, M.D., J.D., IOM Committee Chair
        Executive Chair, Federation of Pediatric Organizations,
            Education Steering Committee

8:40   **Panel 1: Minimal Risk and the NRHPAC Working Group Report**
        Robert Nelson, M.D., IOM Committee Member
        Associate Professor of Anesthesia & Pediatrics, University of
            Pennsylvania
        Chair, Committees for the Protection of Human Subjects
        The Children's Hospital of Philadelphia

        Thomas G. Keens, M.D., Professor of Medicine
        University of Southern California School of Medicine
        Chair, Children's Hospital Los Angeles Institutional Review
            Board

9:45   **Panel 2: Pediatric Research and 45 CFR 46.407**
        Ernest Prentice, Ph.D., Vice Chancellor for Academic Affairs and
            Regulatory Compliance
        University of Nebraska Medical School
        Chair, Secretary's Advisory Committee on Human Research
            Protections,
        U.S. Department of Health and Human Services

        Stewart A. Laidlaw, Ph.D., Director, Office of Compliance and
            Regulatory Affairs
        Harbor-UCLA Research and Education Institute
        Adjunct Associate Professor of Medicine
        University of California, Los Angeles

Susan Partridge, B.S.N., M.B.A., Assistant Professor of Pediatrics
Division of Pediatric Infectious Diseases, Department of
    Pediatrics
Harbor-UCLA Medical Center
Member, Harbor-UCLA Internal Review Board

Leslie K. Ball, M.D., Medical Officer [by telephone]
Office for Human Research Protections
U.S. Department of Health and Human Services

11:00   Break

11:20   Panel 3: Selected Issues in Longitudinal Research
John Landsverk, Ph.D., Director
Child and Adolescent Services Research Center
San Diego

Benjamin Wilfond, M.D.
Cochair, Ethics Working Group, National Children's Study
Department of Clinical Bioethics
National Human Genome Research Institute
National Institutes of Health

12:45   Comments

Adjourn

* * *

INSTITUTE OF MEDICINE
COMMITTEE ON CLINICAL RESEARCH INVOLVING CHILDREN
Lecture Room, National Academy of Sciences
2101 Constitution Avenue NW/2100 C Street NW, Washington, DC
July 9, 2003

8:45   Welcome and Introductions
Richard E. Behrman, M.D., J.D., Chair, IOM Committee on
    Clinical Research Involving Children

8:55   **Panel 1**

American Academy of Pediatrics (AAP)
David J. Schonfeld, M.D.
Member, AAP Committee on Pediatric Research
Yale University School of Medicine

Society for Pediatric Research
Christine A. Gleason, M.D.
University of Washington, Seattle

Association of Medical School Pediatric Department Chairs
George J. Dover, M.D.
Johns Hopkins University School of Medicine

9:35   **Panel 2**

Children's Oncology Group (COG)
Gregory H. Reaman, M.D.
Chair, COG
The George Washington University and Children's National
   Medical Center

The Pediatric AIDS Clinical Trials Group (PACTG)
Stephen A. Spector, M.D.
PACTG Group Chair, Executive Committee
University of California, San Diego, School of Medicine

Allergy & Asthma Network, Mothers of Asthmatics
Nancy Sander
President and Founder

Martha White, M.D.
Founding Board Member

10:15   **Break**

10:50   **Panel 3**

Children's Clinical Research Institute, The Children's Hospital of Philadelphia
Mark S. Schreiner, M.D.
Senior Medical Director

American Society of Transplantation
William E. Harmon, M.D.
Immediate Past President, American Society of Transplantation
Director of the Division of Nephrology, Children's Hospital
    Boston
Chair, North American Pediatric Renal Transplant Cooperative
    Study

11:20   Panel 4

Public Citizen, Health Research Group
Peter Lurie, M.D., M.P.H.
Deputy Director

Citizens for Responsible Care and Research
Paul Gelsinger
Vice President

Adil E. Shamoo, Ph.D.
Founder
Editor-in-Chief, *Accountability in Research*

11:50   Break

1:00   Panel 5

Genetic Alliance
Mary Ann Wilson
Consumer Staff Representative

**Children and Adults with Attention-Deficit/Hyperactivity
Disorder (CHADD)**
Phyllis Anne Teeter Ellison, Ed.D.
Immediate Past Chair, CHADD Professional Advisory Board
Chair, CHADD Editorial Advisory Board
University of Wisconsin, Milwaukee

Cystic Fibrosis Foundation
Suzanne R. Pattee, J.D.
Vice President of Public Policy & Patient Affairs

1:40   Panel 6

        Applied Research Ethics National Association/PRIMR
        Leonard H. Glantz, J.D.
        Board Chair, PRIMR
        Boston University School of Public Health

        **Association for the Accreditation of Human Research Protection
        Programs, Inc.**
        Marjorie A. Speers, Ph.D.
        Executive Director

        Partnership for Human Research Protection
        Jessica Briefer French
        Assistant Vice President

2:20   **Break**

2:40   **Issues in Research in Pediatric Psychology and Psychiatry**
        Anthony Spirito, Ph.D.
        Brown University Medical School

        Philip C. Kendall, Ph.D., ABPP
        Temple University

        Laurence L. Greenhill, M.D.
        New York State Psychiatric Institute

3:50   **Research on Children's Comprehension of Research Participation**
        Eric D. Kodish, M.D.
        Rainbow Babies and Children's Hospital

        Myra Bluebond-Langner, Ph.D.
        Rutgers University, Camden, New Jersey

5:00   **Public Comment**

Adjourn

The following organization submitted written statements.
        NIH Neonatal Network
        Pediatric Pharmacology Research Unit Network

Society for Adolescent Medicine
Society for Developmental and Behavioral Pediatrics
Society for Research in Child Development
The Children's Cause
Alliance for Human Research Protection
Association of American Medical Colleges
Juvenile Diabetes Research Foundation
(National Association of Children's Hospitals and Related
Institutions endorsed the statement of the American Academy of
Pediatrics)

* * *

INSTITUTE OF MEDICINE
Committee on Clinical Research Involving Children
Lecture Room, National Academy of Sciences
2101 Constitution Avenue NW/2100 C Street NW, Washington, DC
10:00 a.m. - 12:15 p.m., July 11, 2003

Parents

Joan Lippincott
Maureen and Joseph Lilly
Lise Yasui
Andrell Vaughn

Research Participants

Carolyn Brokowski
Sarah Lippincott

B

STATE REGULATION OF MEDICAL RESEARCH WITH CHILDREN AND ADOLESCENTS: AN OVERVIEW AND ANALYSIS

Amy T. Campbell, J.D., M.Bioethics

Research with children and adolescents is increasingly recognized as vital to promote the health of our youth, both current and future. The conduct of such research requires access to children and adolescents both to enhance the scientific validity of research with relevance to these populations and, as a matter of justice, to ensure that children and adolescents enjoy the benefits of research.

Children and adolescents are considered—both in law and in ethics—"vulnerable" populations deserving special protections. These protections enable society to reach a reasonable balance between protecting the safety of children and adolescents from research risks and promoting their inclusion in studies to benefit them and future generations.

Special federal regulations provide guidance to child and adolescent heath care researchers. One section of these regulations (Subpart A of 45 CFR Part 46 for the U.S. Department of Health and Human Services) provides for basic human subject protections and is known as the "Common Rule" for its application to most research conducted, supported, or otherwise regulated by 17 federal agencies [1]. Additional protections (Subpart D of 45 CFR 46), which apply specifically to children, have been adopted by the U.S. Department of Health and Human Services [2], the Food and Drug Administration (FDA) (except for Section 46.408(c), which pertains to the waiver of parental permission), the U.S. Department of Education, the Central Intelligence Agency, and the Social Security Administration. Additional regulations issued by the U.S. Department of Education under the Protection of Pupil Rights Amendment govern social research conducted in school settings or otherwise related to education matters [3] (Table B.1; all tables are located in Addendum B1). The language of the federal regulations is frequently adopted as institutional review board (IRB) policy [4], with a likely result that most research, irrespective of the funding source, is reviewed—at least as an initial matter—according to the parameters of the federal guidelines.

Notably, with respect to several issues, the federal research regulations rely on state laws to provide relevant definitions or other elements essential to interpretation and application of the regulations. For example, the regulations define "children" as those persons who have "not attained the legal age for consent to treatments or procedures involved in the research, *under the applicable law of the jurisdiction in which the research will be conducted*" (emphasis added) [5]. Similarly, "guardian" means "an individual who is authorized under applicable state or local law to consent on behalf of a child to general medical care" [6].

Thus, it is critical that researchers, IRB members, and others engaged in or affected by the research process understand how state laws might affect research with children and adolescents. Relevant inquiries include the following issues: age of majority, emancipation status, the "mature minor" rule and other specific provisions related to age of consent for general medical care, and/or specific conditions (e.g., substance abuse disorders or emotional disturbances).

An overview of state laws related to these issues follows. Also addressed are state laws, regulations, or policies specific to children in state custody (e.g., children in foster care or detention facilities), when such laws, regulations, or policies are available.[1] These guidelines are of particular importance in that they apply to those children who likely have unique medical or psychosocial issues distinct from those of the general population

---

[1]A separate project conducted under the auspices of the University of Rochester Medical Center is also pending. That project will survey IRBs at major academic medical centers in each state for further input as to state and local policies, guidance, etc., related to research with children and adolescents. Results from that study will be analyzed and published at a later date in a separate report.

of children.[2] In light of these particular issues, targeted research is needed to focus on these specific concerns; however, special protections are justifiably attached to vulnerable ("at-risk") children.[3] A brief analysis incorporating relevant case law follows the overview to highlight the ways in which states do—or do not—regulate research with these specific populations. Directions for state guidance are also provided.

SUMMARY OF STATE LAWS RELEVANT TO MEDICAL AND BEHAVIORAL RESEARCH WITH CHILDREN AND ADOLESCENTS

Age of Majority

As a first issue, the age of majority in each state is important, as it sets forth the age above which Subpart D of the federal regulations, in addition to any special state protections, do not apply. That is, it is important to know what each state defines as the age of majority, since those who are above the age of majority should not be subject to Subpart D. Most states set the age of majority at 18 years, meaning that—for legal purposes—children are those individuals who have not yet reached the age of 18 (Table B.2).[4] This is a fairly easy "bright-line" standard of which to be aware. However, for purposes of determining the ability of children—most likely adolescents—to assent, and even consent, to research participation, it is important to go beyond these "majority" statutes to focus on other consent-related provisions.

It is also worth noting that this is a legal definition and, hence, is not necessarily indicative of the maturity level, decisional capacity, or cognitive abilities of youth. In fact, several commentators call for greater attention to this matter and clarity in the law to accord adolescents greater respect vis-

---

[2]In fact, statistics indicate that children in foster care often end up in out-of-home placements because of parental neglect and/or abuse, substance abuse, the disproportionate impact of poverty, human immunodeficiency virus infection/AIDS, and similar problems [7].

[3]These protections are typically state specific and are often not formalized in policy but, rather, are handled on a case-by-case basis and are dependent on a variety of factors, such as the risks-benefits of the study, the age ranges of the children, the presence or availability of parents, and treatment alternatives outside of research.

[4]State statutes, administrative regulations, case law, and other written policies were identified through searches of Lexis/Nexis (a legal database) and were affirmed through reference to ClinLaw (a Thompson Publishing Group-sponsored database containing information on clinical laws) and the advice of other experts. As this is a complicated area of the law, a great deal of it exists at an "informal" (less "explicit") level, and as adolescent maturity is an ever-changing concept, this review and the accompanying tables are not meant to be relied upon as exhaustive studies of the law; rather, they offer insights into the myriad of ways in which states may approach—or choose not to approach—these issues.

à-vis their decisional capacities and need for confidentiality in medical care and research [8]. Furthermore, it is important to recognize that while this sets out a bright-line distinction between legal attainment of "competence" in medical decision making (as an adult), who is or is not a "child" for purposes of federal research regulation references state laws (but not specifically the age of majority) on this matter. The latter, in turn, set forth conditions under which certain "minors" might be able to make medical decisions on their own on the basis of certain life events or in certain medical scenarios. Hence, they might be "minors" according to a bright-line test but are not subject to federal research regulations as "children" when state law is applied.

In the sections that follow, which discuss emancipation, the mature minor rule, and minor consent to treatment provisions, it should be emphasized that state laws have relevance in two different ways: the application of the definition of "children" and the waiver of parental permission to medical treatment and in other contexts. That is, certain state laws place a minor outside the definition of children (which would seemingly make Subpart D of the federal regulations inapplicable); other state law provisions support the waiver of parental permission (which would be much more context sensitive and which may or may not reasonably extend to research-related decisions).

Emancipated Minors

As noted earlier, certain life events remove minors from the purview of child or adolescent medical regulation. That is, the age of majority may not be met, but emancipation frees the former "child" from parental custody and control. Typical conditions that states use to establish emancipation are marriage [9], military service [10], or court order [11] (Table B.3).

The concept of emancipation arose in common law (court-developed law) and has only more recently been explicitly addressed in statutes.[5] The "classical" definition of emancipation under the common law could be summarized thusly: emancipation occurs when a minor voluntarily lives independently of his or her parents (whether by marriage, military service, or the establishment of financial independence), the latter who, in turn, make no attempt at ongoing control or care of their child. In turn, it does not seem to make sense to treat "children" who meet the common-law definition of emancipated minors as being under parental authority [12].

---

[5]Of note, this early impetus to define emancipation was driven by the desire to allow minors to enter contracts and own property and to relieve emancipated minors from the duty to turn over their wages to their parents.

More recently, states have begun to supplant the common law with statutory refinements on the concept, including a focus on a broadened range of emancipation effects, including, for example, an ability to consent to medical treatment [13]. However, not every state has an emancipation statute; moreover, some that do continue to apply the concept rather narrowly, for example, to allow certain contract rights [14]. Additionally, many statutes list only certain emancipation effects. For example, some statutes establishing criteria and procedures for emancipation explicitly allow for consent to medical care; others do not [15].[6]

Furthermore, despite early developments in common law from which "emancipation" emerged (i.e., a focus on rights to contract, own property, and retain wages), few state courts have recently addressed the issue with respect to an "expanded" view of the effects of emancipation [16]. Thus, unfortunately for the researcher searching for uniformity, the picture is far from clear. For the purposes of this review, however, emancipation, whatever the causal event, is taken to mean that the child becomes an adult in the eyes of the state; that is, all rules governing parental custody or control are severed, which could include parental permission for research participation, to the extent that states follow a broader range of emancipation effects. Moreover, in this appendix, only those individuals considered adults for all purposes under state law are included in the category "emancipated minors."

Mature Minors

Although emancipation in effect turns the "child" into an "adult" for the purposes of state law, other events may occur as a result of which the child or adolescent may be seen as sufficiently mature to make (certain) health care decisions [17]. In turn, the latter falls into two distinct categories: the "mature minor" rule (which is derived from common law and which has specific meaning and scope) and law that allows exceptions to the requirements of parental permission because of the types of services sought or the status of the minor. Moreover, it should be noted that the distinction between emancipation and mature minor status is unfortunately far from clear or uniform, especially as time has progressed and the two concepts have become more intertwined and complex.[7]

General lay audiences often confuse the concepts of emancipation and

---

[6]This does not imply that consent to other issues is barred; rather, it simply means that legislative action has only explicitly addressed certain situations that it finds imperative.

[7]Compare Tables B.3 and B.4 for areas of overlap.

maturity; for legal purposes, however, they are not the same. For the purposes of this appendix, and in accord with the general sentiments from common law, "mature minors" are typically defined as children who are seen as "sufficiently" mature (a subjective decision, made on a case-by-case basis) with the capacity to understand the risks and consequences of certain decisions and, hence, who have the ability to make those decisions, including, at times, decisions relating to medical treatment (Table B.4).[8] The historical development of the "mature minor" doctrine in common law supports a distinction from emancipation, inasmuch as the former doctrine is of more recent vintage conferring more context-sensitive consent rights in children, for example, to consent to certain medical treatments.[9]

Age of Consent for Medical Care

Some youth, who are still technically "minors" under state law, are allowed to consent to general medical treatment under specific state statutory provisions [19]. For example, several states allow minors to make medical decisions when they hold sufficient capacity to understand the nature of the treatment [20]. A few states have set age limits younger than 18 years at which they allow minors to provide general consent for health care, such as 14 years (Alabama) [21], 15 years (California, Oregon) [22], and 16 years (South Carolina) [23]. Other states (e.g., Colorado, Indiana, and Maine) allow earlier consent to health care or treatment on the basis of certain events that indicate that the minor has sufficient decisional capacity, such as living separately and apart from the parents [24]. It is worth noting again, however, that statutes delineating conditions of sufficient decisional capacity should be distinguished from "emancipation" status. Emancipation represents a "legal" transition to adulthood in the eyes of the state, whereas decisional maturity represents a context-specific ability to consent in certain instances.[10]

---

[8]As commented upon by the American Law Institute, a prominent legal authority, in its *Restatement (Second) of Torts*, a minor's consent should be effective if he or she is "capable of appreciating the nature, extent and probable consequences of the conduct consented to [e.g., medical treatment]," even if parental consent is "not obtained or is expressly refused" [18].

[9]This distinction (i.e., event versus context-sensitive maturity and the setting in which the decision is made) is followed in this paper.

[10]Again, however, it should be emphasized that the concept of "emancipation" in states is far from clear. For the purposes of this appendix, emancipation is seen as a transition to adulthood in state law, but researchers would need to consult experts in their own states for guidance on the bounds of emancipation in the respective states.

Age of Consent Under Certain Circumstances

In addition, all states explicitly authorize minors to provide consent to health care when the decisions are related to certain disorders or types of care. That is, for purposes of consenting to specific health care services, these minors may be explicitly allowed—by statute—consent authority [25]. It is important to note, however, that this does not mean that such minors cannot consent in other situations; rather, for public policy reasons, states have, at times, chosen to specifically address minors' decisional capacity in certain situations to promote health-seeking behavior [26].[11] Examples include consent for mental health treatment, substance abuse treatment, treatment for human immunodeficiency virus (HIV) infection or acquired immune deficiency syndrome (AIDS), testing or treatment for sexually transmitted diseases (STDs), and family planning services (Table B.5).

These conditions, in essence, allow individuals who are technically minors to make their own health care decisions under specific conditions. At issue, however, is the extent to which treatment-related consent, whether in general medical settings or for specific conditions, translates to the research setting.

Research-Specific Legislation

Few states have any regulations that apply specifically to research with children and adolescents [27]. Moreover, those statutes that address research with youth do so only under confined circumstances [28]. Thus, although federal regulations reference state law, state law—as specifically applied in the research setting—is a relative vacuum in terms of the regulation of research with children and adolescents.

This uncertainty and frequent silence on the matter leaves researchers and IRBs in a position to make a best guess as to whether state laws related to treatment also apply to research, although there are good reasons to believe that they do apply, at least in certain situations [29]. Arguments have been put forward that such laws should apply, at least to the extent that research relates to specific conditions for which consent to treatment laws apply, for example, mental health and STDs [30]. For example, if a study sought to investigate the behavioral mechanisms at play in adolescents' decisions to seek out treatment for an STD, a state that allows adolescents to consent to treatment for an STD should also allow for consent to research in connection with that STD. The argument might proceed

---

[11]Again, this does not mean that other areas of consent are prohibited; instead, they exist in the "gray zone" of prudent ("reasonable") responses to the facts of a given case.

that the legislative intent behind consent to treatment—to promote individual and public health while preserving confidentiality—should similarly apply to research.

Moreover, it is important to note that where the law is silent on the issue (e.g., the applicability of treatment consent by minors to research consent), silence does not imply impermissibility. In fact, it could be argued that actions are permissible unless they are specifically restricted by the courts or legislative actions [31].

> As a general principle, however, judicial development of the common law is not arrested by piece-meal legislative adoption of specific statutory exceptions to a general common law rule. . . . One of the great attributes of Anglo-American common law has been the flexibility demonstrated by the case by case judicial development of the principles and rules of the common law to adapt to the emerging conditions of society; this flexibility permits the law to remain relevant and reasonable, preventing "mindless obedience to [a] precept [that] can confound the search for truth and foster an attitude of contempt" [32].

Alternatively, of course, it should be noted that there is an important distinction between research and treatment. The former seeks to build generalizable knowledge without a focus on individual benefit, whereas the latter focuses on individual well-being. Accordingly, inasmuch as their intents vary, so too might the legal protections for children and adolescents attached to research versus treatment justifiably vary. Federal regulations also note that "assent," the child's "affirmative agreement to participate in research," is required when IRBs determine that children are capable of such, thus leaving much to the IRB's discretion [33]. This imprecision in federal regulations has not been addressed by the states [34].

Finally, it is also worth clarifying the distinction between emancipation and mature minor status, a distinction not always clearly made in state law.[12] In general, emancipation (in this appendix) confers broader "adult" status to youth in all aspects of their lives, whereas the attainment of "mature minor" status is more narrowly construed in terms of the sort of health care consent authority that it confers. These differences might similarly affect the reach of regulations on research with minors, or at least the requirements to consent to research. "Emancipated minors," to whose lives events have conferred—in the eyes of the state—legal adulthood, should be able to consent to research as adults.[13] "Mature minors," on the other

---

[12]See discussion infra, pp. 323–325.

[13]This still leaves the question, however, of how a researcher or IRB should reach the conclusion that a minor is emancipated. Arguably, at a minimum, minors who satisfy the common law criteria for emancipation or who have been emancipated by a court should be considered emancipated.

hand, are likely more limited in what they can and cannot consent to in treatment and in research.

Unfortunately, there is thus a great deal of uncertainty as to the extent of state regulations and the applicability of existing state regulations with respect to medical research with children and adolescents. Perhaps this should be unsurprising given the particularly recent nature of calls to enhance the base of research with populations of this age [35]. Whatever the case, states have for the most part seen fit to follow federal regulations in this area to date [36]. Whether the increasing demands for research with children and adolescents, coupled with advances in understanding of child and especially adolescent capacity and maturity, will affect states' perceived need for further regulation remains to be seen. However, it would not be surprising if the conduct of more research in the absence of clear authority led to litigation, not unlike that witnessed in Maryland [37]. Before the discussion turns to case law, however, it is also important to touch upon a certain subset of the child and adolescent population: children in state custody.

Research-Specific Regulations: Children Under State Custody

Of special concern to researchers and policy makers are regulations pertaining to children in state custody, for example, children in foster care, juvenile delinquents, and wards of the state. These children fall under state control under the doctrine of *parens patriae*, the concept that the states assume a "parental" role to protect children when biological parents are not able to do so, such as in instances of child neglect or abuse or when children enter the juvenile detention system.

As the primary "authority" figure for these children, the state therefore typically assumes a custodial role for children that may extend to health care decision-making. The federal child-specific regulations contain a section explicitly addressing research with "wards of the state" [38]. Research with such children is permissible only if it relates to their status as wards or if it is conducted in settings in which a majority of the children involved as subjects are not wards [39]. Examples of the former might include research specifically related to issues facing children in foster care subsequent to child abuse; the latter might pertain to school-based research in which wards of the state are in a minority.

The federal regulations further require that special advocates—not state-appointed guardians—be appointed for each child [40]. These regulations are in addition to the more general federal regulations, which require IRBs to weigh the risks and benefits of *any* studies with *any* child populations, to ensure that IRBs do not allow high-risk (greater than a "minor increase over minimal risk") studies unless they have a prospect of directly benefiting the participants. Of interest is the extent to which states expand on federal guidance, inasmuch as they are the custodians primarily concerned with the welfare of children.

A further distinction is whether parental ties have been terminated, that is, if the child is simply in temporary custody of the state (state as custodian) or if the child is in a permanent out-of-home placement (state as legal guardian) because parental rights were terminated. If ties are not terminated, states likely defer to the authority of the parents over their child's medical care, especially if the treatment is considered optional. If the state deems treatment to be necessary, however, and the parent refuses permission, the state could override the decision and provide its own authorization for treatment pursuant to parental neglect or abuse laws [41]. (This appendix refers generally to parental permission according to federal regulatory language, but some of the statutes and court decisions refer to parental consent, and that language is retained when individual statutes or court decisions are cited.)

The general tendency, however, is to defer to parental rights and, to the extent possible, involve parents in decision making when it is feasible and in the best interest of the child, as well as in keeping with constitutional law around parental rights [42]. It is likely that research participation decisions would follow a similar process, although deference to parental authority is even more likely unless the research is deemed of direct benefit and minimal risk.

A review of state law, regulation, and case law related to this research suggests that little formal guidance is available. To clarify this, commissioners of each state's child welfare or social services department were recently contacted for further information on state and local policies or other guidance related to research with children under state custody. On the basis of the feedback received, it appears that there is little guidance in this area beyond federal research regulations or state consent to treatment laws that generally apply to children and adolescents (Table B.6). In fact, there seems to be a general lack of familiarity with and training in research issues generally, and research ethics specifically, among state agency personnel.

Applicable policies, when such policies exist, tend to track federal regulations on research with children generally. They also typically apply different standards to research with various levels of risk and to research conducted by agency employees (e.g., state or local department of social services case workers) compared with the standards that they apply to research conducted by external researchers [43]. Other states choose not to apply special rules, relying on federal regulations and IRB review by relevant institutions (presumably, the home institutions of external researchers) [44].

Moreover, when policies do exist, they often restrict the research methods used with these populations—such as research with pharmaceuticals or the use of placebos—inasmuch as the "in-custody" child and adolescent population is seen as particularly vulnerable [45]. The extent to which these policies—or the general lack thereof—affect research with children under state custody is an important empirical question deserving further study. (See Addendum B2 for a discussion of two hypothetical studies proposing to perform research with children in state custody and how states might approach such proposals.)

CASE LAW

Case Example

Researchers at a prominent institute affiliated with an academic medical center propose to study the effects of various types of lead abatement on a group of already affected and at-risk children from an urban inner-city environment. The rental properties in the community at issue will be classified into five groups: the members of the first three groups live in homes experiencing various levels of lead abatement ("intervention" groups), and the members of the last two groups are the controls (the members of one control group live in homes that were previously fully abated and the members of the other control group live in homes built without lead paint). Landlords will be recruited, and those who agree to offer their properties for participation in the research will be encouraged, if not required, to rent to tenants with young children. Research investigators will also assist landlords to take advantage of loan programs supporting abatement.

The study would last 2 years, over which time the researchers would measure and compare the short- and long-term effects of the various abatement methods to reduce lead levels in dust and children's blood. The stated purpose is to see if the less expensive means of lead abatement adequately protect the children's health. That is, the hope is that children's health is safeguarded, while the availability of low-rent housing in inner cities is maintained.

Parents who permit their child's participation would be informed immediately if their child's blood level was elevated; lead levels in the dust would also be provided periodically. Lead Registry Surveillance statistics released in 1999 show that although the number of children with elevated blood lead levels (EBLs) and lead poisoning declined during the latter part of the 1990s, the levels were disproportionately concentrated in the study site (urban region). Significantly, although 6.3 percent of children tested statewide had EBLs and 0.9 percent had lead poisoning, the proportions at the study site (urban area) were 16.7 and 2.6 percent, respectively [46]. Furthermore, the researchers estimated that the chosen study site targeted children in the highest risk communities for EBLs and lead poisoning [47].

Additionally, an annual state report supports claims that during the years leading up to the study (when the study was designed), up to 95 percent of the homes in the study site had lead hazards [48].

The academic medical center's IRB approves the study, and with funding from the Environmental Protection Agency and state agencies, the research proceeds. After the study ends, two families sue the research institute for negligence, alleging untimely notice of EBLs, placing their children at unnecessary risk, in addition to a failure to meet standards of adequate parental informed permission.

The case proceeds to trial, with the lower court agreeing with the defendant that no legal duty exists between the researcher and the subject (summary judgment). The case is appealed and is taken to before the state's highest (appellate) court. How might it respond to the facts of this case?

Illustrative States

Maryland

Few cases directly address state treatment of research with children and adolescents. Perhaps the most compelling and recent case is that described in the "case example" above, which highlights the facts of a recent Maryland case, *Grimes v. Kennedy Krieger Institute, Inc.* [49]. In its decision on this case, the Court of Appeals of Maryland (the state's highest court) decided that a "legal duty normally exists between researcher and subject," by virtue of the "special relationship" between them and arising out of contract law (the "contract" being the informed consent and permission form signed by the parents, who received compensation for their child's participation) [50]. Finding that a duty could exist, the case was remanded to the trial court for a factual determination whether a duty did in fact exist in this case, whether that duty was breached, and if such breach was the proximate cause of damages (standard requirements of action in negligence) [51].

Of particular note was the court's decision to go beyond the issue of negligence to find that, under state law, parental authority to permit their children to participate in research does not extend to nontherapeutic research that carries with it the risk of harm to the health of the child [52].[14] In so deciding, the court referenced the history of abuse in research: from Nazi experiments (e.g., typhus experiments with concentration camp inmates) to the Tuskegee study (syphilis studies) and the Jewish Chronic

---

[14]Instead of referring to nontherapeutic research, many refer to research that does not present the prospect of direct benefit, as explained in Chapter 1.

Disease Hospital Study (cancer study without consent) [53]. The court was particularly troubled by the economically disadvantaged condition of the children and families in this case [54]. As the court stated:

> The determination of whether a duty exists under Maryland law is the ultimate function of various policy considerations as adopted by the Legislature, or, if it has not spoken, as it has not in respect to this situation, by Maryland courts. . . . We do not feel that it serves proper public policy concerns to permit children to be placed in situations of potential harm, during nontherapeutic procedures, even if parents, or other surrogates, consent [55].

That is, the court interpreted Maryland law as not allowing parental consent (permission) for greater than minimal risk, "nontherapeutic" research in the first instance (e.g., when a "reasonable parent" would not allow such) [56]. Similarly, research was found to be impermissible without valid informed consent [57].

The merits of this decision are beyond the scope of this paper. However, its ramifications are important for future researchers in Maryland and to the extent that it has received national scrutiny across the country. The case has received much press, especially in research, research subject advocate, and legal circles, which quite likely will translate to related case and state law developments [58]. It will be interesting to see if other courts, in Maryland and beyond, follow the appellate court's lead and further delineate those conditions under which research with children, including at-risk, sick, or healthy children, is permissible [59]. It will also be interesting to see how states respond to challenges to define "risk," "therapeutic," and "nontherapeutic," as well as the limits of "assent" and parental "permission" in relation to research with youth.

As noted in the preceding sections, state legislatures and executive agencies have, to date, had little to say about research in general and even less about research with children and adolescents. This case might serve to create ferment in state legislative bodies and within child-serving agencies to craft policies, guidelines, and even statutes to address research issues. Of note, however, is the fact that as of this writing (August 2003), the Maryland legislature has not passed legislation specifically responding to concerns raised by the *Grimes* decision. After the initial Court of Appeals decision, many believed that Johns Hopkins University and the University of Maryland would push for legislation to address the extent or limits of parental authority to permit research with their children, and a legislative committee hearing was scheduled to talk about what was seen as the crippling effect of the decision on research involving children.

However, after a subsequent clarification by the court in its denial of the Kennedy Krieger Institute's motion for reconsideration (in which it clarified its intent as to the meaning of "any risk" as per the bounds of parental authority), the universities backed off, deciding that the ruling would not dramatically alter their respective research portfolios [60]. The legislative committee hearing was conducted in October 2001, but its focus shifted from the *Grimes* case to the "regulatory gap" created by the limits of federal regulation and the unregulated status of non-federally funded, non-FDA research. To address this, a bill was enacted in 2002 [61]. Interestingly, however, no further legislative attention has been paid to the issues in the *Grimes* case itself [62].

On the basis of case-specific inactivity in the state legislature to date, how might Maryland trial courts respond? The Court of Appeals remanded the *Grimes* case back to the trial court for a decision as to the factual merits of claims of liability (by the researchers) and damages. In addition, the court also stated that a determination of "therapeutic" versus "non-therapeutic" research was for factual development on remand.

> By "any risk," we meant [in original decision] any articulable risk beyond the minimal kind of risk that is inherent in any endeavor. The context of the statement was a non-therapeutic study that promises no medical benefit to the child whatever, so that any balance between risk and benefit is necessarily negative. As we indicated, the determination of whether the study in question offered some benefit, and therefore could be regarded as therapeutic in nature, or involved more than minimal risk is open for further factual development on remand [63].

The lower court's decision is still pending. What is less an issue for the specific parties, but a big issue for future researchers, is the appellate court's decision to extend its holding to the bounds of the consent (permission) authority of parents on behalf of their children. This legal holding is not before the trial court. Thus, the lower court is left to decide if—in this instance—the research was therapeutic or not, was minimal or not, or was conducted with "at-risk" or healthy children.

Although it is likely that the case will be settled, if it proceeds to trial, the lower court could conclude that the research in this matter is "nontherapeutic" (i.e., there is insufficient evidence in the record that the researchers contemplated medically benefiting the "healthy" child subjects). Given the strong language of the high court's decision, such an approach would not be out of the question. Inasmuch as the appellate court's decision provided a litany of reasons—in quite dramatic language—for protecting children from overzealousness in research, researchers might now be a bit more hesitant when proposing studies with children in Maryland, especially when the children come from disadvantaged backgrounds, the risks are uncertain, and the notion of "benefits" is a stretch.

The relative silence thus far should not be seen as a defeat for those who would seize upon the arguments used by the Maryland Court of Appeals; rather, it might well be the quiet before the storm. The case continues to be discussed in research meetings and is still cited by research subject advocates [64]. Thus, the issues raised by the court are still "in the air" and might very well surface in other decisions and on the agendas of other states' legislatures. What might such cases look like in other states, based on their statutory and case law climates to date?

New York

Apply the same facts in the case example cited above to New York: where might its courts fall? New York is generally a conservative state with respect to research with "vulnerable subjects," especially with persons with mental impairments.[15] New York law generally designates parents or guardians as "legally authorized representatives" able to consent to (provide permission for) research with their minor children [66]; however, for persons residing in mental health treatment facilities, agencies take over decision-making authority. Furthermore, New York has in place an active mental health legal advocate structure that affects treatment decisions with mentally and developmentally challenged individuals, which also likely translates to research settings.

New York is also the only other known state, beyond Maryland, to address nontherapeutic research with vulnerable populations. In *T.D. v. New York State Office of Mental Health* [67], New York's trial court ruled that the state's Office of Mental Health (OMH) overstepped its bounds by issuing regulations pertinent to research with persons incapable of giving consent, including children. On appeal, the Appellate Division, First Department, affirmed this decision, but also went on to discuss constitutional and common law defects in the OMH regulations [68]. Of specific concern were regulations for consent to greater-than-minimal-risk nontherapeutic (or only possibly therapeutic) research with children and adults unable to give or withhold consent. Of note, the appellate level court went beyond the scope of the earlier ruling to condemn this research, much like the *Grimes* court did.

Although the court focused on non-federally funded research with children and adults residing in state-run mental health facilities, the court's language appears to go far beyond this specific population to include all

---

[15]Query whether this stems from a prime example of research abuse within its own borders: the Willowbrook scandal [65]. It stands to reason that states which have experienced the ill effects, including bad press, of research cases are more likely to respond with protective statutory and common law approaches.

human subjects of questionable capacity, whose interests should be protected even at the expense of some research [69]. With respect to children, the court took issue with the fact that persons other than parents or guardians could provide consent (permission) for participation of children in "greater than minimal risk nontherapeutic research" [70]. Furthermore, the court did not simply condemn allowing nonparents to make decisions; the court also addressed the limits of parental authority, in ways similar to the *Grimes* decision.

> We are not dealing here with parental choice among reasonable treatment alternatives, but with a decision to subject the child to nontherapeutic treatments and procedures that may cause harmful permanent or fatal side effects. It follows therefore that a parent or guardian, let alone another adult who may be a member of the child's family, may not consent to have a child submit to painful and/or potentially life-threatening research procedures that hold no prospect of benefit for the child and that may have the same result as a denial of necessary medical treatment [71].

The court was not moved by federal regulations that might allow such research, instead setting forth a standard for New York's approach to research with minors of certain categories of risk and benefit. And, as in *Grimes*, the court was critical of the IRB's discretion in applying research protection [72].

Finally, of import for research with children under state custody, the court also critiqued the IRB's discretion in allowing waiver of parental consent (permission) when the latter is not a "reasonable requirement to protect the patients (for example, abused and neglected children)" [73]. The court's argument clarifies that consent (permission) authority for these subjects lies with the local commissioner of health (as in the treatment context) [74]. Moreover, it is also noteworthy for specifically referencing treatment-related law in a research case. That is, pursuant to the court's reasoning, this decision might provide support for an argument that treatment statutes, at least insofar as they address who can consent (provide permission) on behalf of minors, could also apply in research milieus [75].

Taken together with the *Grimes* case, these arguments point toward a highly "restrictive" environment on the continuum of permissibility of research with children and adolescents as regulated by the states, at least insofar as research exceeds minimal-risk standards without the prospect for direct benefit. Each court interpreted state law as restricting the ability to do nontherapeutic, greater-than-minimal-risk research with children. Furthermore, each did so by explicitly acknowledging the need for state protection, notwithstanding federal regulations or cases in which such regulations do not apply (non-federally funded research), especially when such research is tied to commercial interests [76].

Each decision also provides convenient language to support claims that research with a child that is not clearly minimal risk or therapeutic is best avoided—ethically and legally. In addition, each decision inserts the necessity for judicial review into the research process. "Science cannot be permitted to be the sole judge of the appropriateness of such research methods on human subjects, especially in respect to children" [77]. States with particularly activist courts might also subject researchers to judicial interpretations of permissible research and the limits thereof.

However, what about states without similar case laws dealing with research with vulnerable subjects? It is worth noting that most states do not have a body of state law on this issue, especially in relation to children and adolescents. Therefore, the general trend among state court decisions vis-à-vis medical treatment for children and adolescents might have some bearing on the issue, at least to the extent that they provide useful arguments—and possible comfort levels—for researchers.

Massachusetts

Consider, for example, Massachusetts, a state with recent case law addressing minors' ability to consent to or refuse medical treatment. In a noteworthy case, the Appeals Court of Massachusetts held that a 17-year-old female patient should have been able to voice her own interests in deciding against a blood transfusion, "where she apparently had the testimonial capacity to answer questions. . . . Only after evaluating this evidence in light of her maturity could the judge properly determine her best interests" [78].

The court so held the decision on the basis of "well-settled" state law that would apply a three-part balancing test for treatment decisions with unemancipated minors: the child's best interests, the parents' interests, and the state's interests [79]. Moreover, the best interests criteria parallel those used in substituted judgment cases, which would include the "patient's expressed preferences, if any" [80]. The court also noted that the state's legislature affirmed considering a minor's "maturity" in relation to enunciating her own interests by enacting law to allow an abortion without parental consent (permission) if the judge deems the minor "mature enough to make an informed decision" [81]. The court indicates that, at least in certain situations and with "minors" of a certain age or maturity level, the typical "best-interests" standard applied to treatment decisions should also include reference to what the minor him- or herself thinks.

Tennessee

The Tennessee Supreme Court has also recognized the common law "mature minor exception" by adopting the "Rule of Sevens" [82]. This common law rule of capacity holds that (1) a minor under the age of 7 years lacks capacity; (2) a minor between 7 and 14 years of age is presumed not to have capacity, but that assumption can be rebutted (the burden is on the minor arguing that he or she has capacity); and (3) a minor aged 14 years and over is presumed to have capacity (the burden is on the one arguing against capacity) [83]. It further held that the mature minor exception is part of Tennessee's common law to be applied on a case-by-case basis (i.e., not a bright-line test) and that such consent by a minor, when validly given (as it was in this case), freed the physician complying with such consent (again, in this case) from battery charges [84].[16]

Summary

Of course, there is no explicit reason to believe that reasoning similar to that described above would apply to a decision whether or not to allow a minor to consent to participation in a research protocol. In fact, it should be noted that many cases upholding a minor's consent based on "maturity" did so when the minor was near 18 years of age. Thus, for younger children, for decisions related to riskier research, and with stronger parental disagreement, there may be a less permissive attitude toward minor consent [85]. Nor is there reason to believe that nontherapeutic research would not fall to a similar fate as in New York and Maryland, wherein no matter the willingness to agree to research participation—by the parent or the minor— some research might be invalid per se. Yet, for states where there is greater silence or "leniency" as to research in state courts or legislatures and where strong case law exists to promote mature minor treatment decision making, the same principles could arguably extend to research decisions, at least inasmuch as research specifically relates to areas in which minor consent is allowed, for example, for STD treatment [86].

FUTURE DIRECTIONS:
UNIFORM STATE GUIDELINES AND NATIONAL DISCUSSION

In sum, where do the review and analysis presented above leave the research community? On the basis of a review of state law—statutory and case law—on this point (research with children and adolescents), there is little to go by in terms of the permissibility of and limits of such research. Moreover, even where case law does exist, arguments exist to preclude research with *certain* minors in *certain* situations, particularly if such children are deemed to be especially vulnerable (e.g., impoverished or suffering from emotional disturbances).

---

[16]See further discussion of the "mature minor" doctrine infra, pp. 324–326.

This is not to say that research will not or may not proceed. Rather, researchers are wise to review state law in the myriad of places where it might be found (e.g., health, public welfare, education, corrections, and social services codes). They should also judge the climates of their local and state courts and legislatures to determine the legal stance likely to be adopted in relation to research with children that goes beyond minimal risk and that is quite likely of no direct benefit. Researchers might also be well advised to seek agency approval for research with children in or at risk of being under state custody and also to develop research protocols with greater community input, particularly those members of the community from which subjects or families are likely to be drawn [87].

States, too, could respond to this uncertain climate by clarifying the bounds of what is and is not permissible in research with children and adolescents, while doing so in accord with laws that increasingly recognize "mature" status for certain medical decisions. States might be wise to do so proactively rather than wait for the "hard case" that could lead to "bad law."

A possible and advisable approach would be for a national body representing state governments, for example, the National Governors Association or the National Conference of State Legislatures, to convene a national group of key stakeholders and experts to develop state guidelines for research with children and adolescents. As state-based guidelines and not national law, the purpose would not be to mandate compliance by states or researchers within those states. Given the nascent nature of state regulation in this area in general, it seems premature to develop a model law.

However, the process of developing national guidelines might serve to foster a broader dialogue about the limits that society accepts for research with children and adolescents. In this fashion, guidelines could be used to develop a consensus on "best practices" in research with children and adolescents. In addition, their development might influence the research agenda itself, to promote additional studies that would support the empirical basis behind the guidelines, as well as an empirical base that could influence later revisions to the guidelines [88]. So, too, would it invite greater stakeholder input into the process of setting limits, inclusive of not only researchers and state officials but also potential subjects, families, advocacy groups, and representatives of groups or institutions affected by the variety of situations or locations in which such research might take place (e.g., schools). Although states have generally chosen, when they do address the issue, to track federal regulations, especially when describing the risk-benefit calculations for IRB reviews, federal regulations only extend to federally funded research; furthermore, they leave much to IRB discretion. These are areas where state-level dialogue could be especially beneficial.

Perhaps nothing will come of the recent court actions in New York and Maryland; in fact, as of this writing, the Maryland legislature declined to specifically address the facts of the *Grimes* case. Yet, as the impetus behind research with children and adolescents builds [89] and an increasingly vigilant and media-savvy subject advocate network grows [90], it seems likely that litigation could ensue. So, too, might litigation be prompted by new privacy regulations as applied in research settings [91]. In consideration of such regulations, might it be wise for states to address this issue proactively to clarify the landscape out of an ethical sense of obligation, a legal sense of duty, and a pragmatic response to the growing media "buzz"? Additionally, might it also be wise for states to set forth guidance more uniformly and to learn from each other's experiences, in recognition of the growing "multistate" nature of research? Such guidance could, for example, address more precisely what is meant by "emancipated minor" and "mature minor" on the one hand and "greater than minimal risk" and "nontherapeutic research" on the other [92].

It is likely that separate guidance would be needed for research with children and adolescents generally and research with children under state custody specifically, as the latter sit in unique circumstances in relation to the state's protection and oversight of their care. Yet, whether the guidelines address one, two, or even three situations (e.g., a third situation applying to "sensitive" research, such as studies related to sexual promiscuity among adolescents), it is arguably better to provide clarifying guidance before the research endeavor with children develops a force of its own or breaks down in the face of a few unfortunate research endeavors or before research guidelines split between guidelines for government-funded research and guidelines for industry-funded research. The future of the state response is unclear. The future, however, likely includes more, not less, research with children and adolescents and, hence, will raise more research-related issues, concerns that states could begin to address now in a systematic and empirically testable fashion.

ACKNOWLEDGMENTS

This review and analysis was funded by the Institute of Medicine. I wish to acknowledge the assistance of the Family Violence Clinic at the State University of New York at Buffalo School of Law, in particular, Shannon O'Keefe, clinic student, and Catherine Cerulli, faculty member. Thanks also to Abigail English and numerous child welfare representatives for sharing their ideas and resources. Finally, I owe a special thanks to Angela Roddey Holder for reviewing this paper and, most importantly, for her ongoing support and mentorship.

TABLE B.1 State Education-Related Provisions for Research with
Children and Adolescents (in School Settings) [a]

State	Provision	Statute
Alabama	None identified	
Alaska	None identified	
Arizona	None identified	
Arkansas	None identified	
California	School records may be released with written parental consent	Calif. Educ. Code § 49075
Colorado	None identified	
Connecticut	None identified	
Delaware	None identified	
District of Columbia	None identified	
Florida	School records may be released with written parental consent	Fla. Stat. Ann. § 228.093
Georgia	None identified	
Hawaii	None identified	
Idaho	None identified	
Illinois	School records may be released with dated, written parental consent	105 Ill. Comp. Stat. Ann. § 10/6
Indiana	Student may not be required to participate without prior consent of student or prior written consent of parent	Ind. Code Ann. § 20-10.1-4-15
Iowa	None identified	
Kansas	School records may not be released without parental consent	Kans. Stat. Ann. § 72-6214
Kentucky	School records may be released with parental consent or eligible student consent	Ky. Rev. Stat. Ann. § 160.720
Louisiana	None identified	
Maine	None identified	
Maryland	None identified	
Massachusetts	None identified	
Michigan	School records cannot be revealed by witness in court without parental consent	Mich. Comp. Laws Ann. § 600.2165
Minnesota	None identified	
Mississippi	None identified	
Missouri	School records cannot be released without written parental consent	Mo. Rev. Stat. § 167.020
Montana	School officials will notify sender that records cannot be released without written parental consent	Mont. Rev. Code § 20-1-213
Nebraska	None identified	
Nevada	School records will not be released without written parental consent	Nev. Rev. Stat: Ann. § 392.029

TABLE B.1 Continued

State	Provision	Statute
New Hampshire	None identified	
New Jersey	None identified	
New Mexico	None identified	
New York	None identified	
North Carolina	None identified	
North Dakota	None identified	
Ohio	Information other than directory information is not released without written parental consent	Ohio Rev. Code Ann. § 3319.321(B)
Oklahoma	None identified	
Oregon	None identified	
Pennsylvania	None identified	
Rhode Island	None identified	
South Carolina	None identified	
South Dakota	None identified	
Tennessee	Student records are not available without parental consent	Tenn. Code Ann. § 10-7-504(4)
Texas	None identified	
Utah	Parental consent required	Utah Code Ann. § 53A-13-302(1)(a)-(h)
Vermont	None identified	
Virginia	Records may be released to student or student's parent before obtaining consent	Va. Code Ann. § 22.1287(A)(1)
Washington	None identified	
West Virginia	None identified	
Wisconsin	Student or student's parent may be shown records upon request	Wis. Stat. Ann. § 118.125(2)
Wyoming	None identified	

*a*The U.S. Department of Education also regulates the release of certain of information from student records (34 CFR Part 99).

TABLE B.2 Age of Majority

State	Age of Majority	Statute
Alabama	19	Code of Ala. § 26-1-1
Alaska	18	Alaska Stat. § 25.20.010
Arizona	18	Ariz. Rev. Stat. § 14-1201
Arkansas	18	Ark. Code Ann. § 20-13-104
California	18	Cal. Probate Code § 3901
Colorado	18	Colo. Rev. Stat. § 13-22-103
Connecticut	18	Conn. Gen. Stat. Ann. § 19a-575a
Delaware	18	1 Del. Code § 701
District of Columbia	18	Code of D.C. Regs. §§ 22-6-600, 22-6-699
Florida	18	Fla. Stat. Ann. § 743.01
Georgia	18	O.C.G.A. §§ 31-9-2, 31-9-7
Hawaii	18	Haw. Rev. Stat. Ann. § 577-1
Idaho	18	Idaho Code § 32-101
Illinois	18	410 Illinois Comp. Stat. 210/1
Indiana	18	Ind. Code Ann. § 16-8-2-5
Iowa	18	Iowa Code § 234.1
Kansas	18	Kans. Admin. Regs. § 30-6-52
Kentucky	18	Ky. Rev. Stat. Ann. § 2.015
Louisiana	18	La. Rev. Stat. § 40:1299.56
Maine	18	1 Maine Rev. Stat. Ann. §§ 72,73; 22 Maine Rev. Stat. Ann. § 1501
Maryland	18	Md. Code Ann. Art. 1, § 24
Massachusetts	18	112 Mass. Gen. Laws Ann. § 12F
Michigan	18	M.S.A. §§ 25.244 (52), 14.15 (1105)
Minnesota	18	Minn. Code §§ 144.341-144.347
Mississippi	21	Miss. Code Ann. § 1-3-27[a]
Missouri	18	Mo. Rev. Stat. § 431.061
Montana	18	Mont. Rev. Code Ann. § 41-1-101
Nebraska	19	Nebr. Rev. Stat. Ann. § 43-2101
Nevada	18	Nev. Rev. Stat. Ann. § 129.030
New Hampshire	18	N.H. Rev. Stat. Ann. §§ 21:44, 21-B:1
New Jersey	18	N.J. Stat. § 9:17B-4
New Mexico	18	N.M. Stat. Ann. § 28-6-1
New York	18	N.Y. Dom. Rel. Law § 2
North Carolina	18	N.C. Gen. Stat. §§ 58-3-215, 48A-1, 48A-2
North Dakota	18	N.D. Cent. Code §§ 14-10-01, 14-10-17.1
Ohio	18	Ohio Rev. Code Ann. § 3109.01
Oklahoma	18	10 Okla. Stat. § 91
Oregon	18	Oreg. Rev. Stat. § 109.510
Pennsylvania	18	35 Pa. Stat. § 10101
Rhode Island	18	R.I. Gen. Laws § 23-4.6-1
South Carolina	18	S.C. Code Ann. § 15-1-320; S.C. Code of Laws § 20-7-30
South Dakota	18	S.D. Codified Laws §§ 26-1-1-1, 29A-5-102
Tennessee	18	Tenn. Code Ann. § 1-3-113
Texas	18	Tex. Rev. Civ. Stat. § 313.004

TABLE B.2 Continued

State	Age of Majority	Statute
Utah	18	Utah Code Ann. § 78-14-5
Vermont	18	1 Vt. Stat. Ann. § 173
Virginia	18	Va. Code Ann. § 1-13.42
Washington	18	Rev. Code Wash. § 26.28.010
West Virginia	18	W.V. Code §§ 2-2-10, 2-3-1
Wisconsin	18	Wis. Stat. § 115.807
Wyoming	18	Wyo. Stat. § 14-1-101

*a*Miss. Code Ann. § 41-41-3 states that "adult" means anyone 18+ for the purposes of consent to surgical or medical treatment procedures.

TABLE B.3 Emancipation Conditions

State	Conditions	Statute
Alabama	Married or divorced	Code of Ala. § 22-17A-1
	Court order	Code of Ala. § 22-17A-1
Alaska	Court order	Alaska Stat. § 09.55.590
Arizona	Veteran	Ariz. Rev. Stat. Ann. § 44-131
	Married	Op. Atty. Gen. No. 69-27
	Military service	Op. Atty. Gen. No. 69-27
Arkansas	Court order	Ark. Code Ann. § 9-26-104
California	Married	Calif. Fam. Code § 7002
	Active duty in armed forces	Calif. Fam. Code § 7002
	Court order	Calif. Fam. Code § 7002
Colorado	Over age 15 and has demonstrated independence from parents	Colo. Rev. Stat. § 19-1-103
Connecticut	Married	Conn. Gen. Stat. Ann. § 46b-150b
	Active duty in armed forces	Conn. Gen. Stat. Ann. § 46b-150b
	Living separate and apart from parents	Conn. Gen. Stat. Ann. § 46b-150b
	Court order	Conn. Gen. Stat. Ann. § 46b-150b
	Veteran	Conn. Gen. Stat. Ann. § 369-759
Delaware	Court order	1 Del. Code Ann. § 701
District of Columbia	a	
Florida	Married	Fla. Stat. Ann. § 743.01
	Court order	Fla. Stat. Ann. § 743.015
Georgia	Married	O.C.G.A. § 19-3-30
Hawaii	Married	Hawaii Rev. Stat. Ann. § 577-25
	Veteran or veteran's spouse	Hawaii Rev. Stat. Ann. § 577-2
Idaho	Married	Idaho Code § 32-101
Illinois	Court order	750 Ill. Comp. Stat. Ann. 30/1
Indiana	a	
Iowa	Veteran	Iowa Code § 599.5
Kansas	Court order	Kans. Stat. Ann. § 38-109
Kentucky	a	
Louisiana	Married	La. Civil Code Art. § 379-384
	Court order	La. Civil Code Art. § 385
Maine	a	

TABLE B.3 Continued

State	Conditions	Statute
Maryland	Married: individual may buy or sell property if spouse is of age	Md. Code Ann., Est. & Tr. Art. 13 §503 (a)
	Age 15 can contract regarding insurance	Md. Code Ann., Est. & Tr. Art. 13 §503 (c)
	Individuals in the military can enter into real estate transactions	Md. Code Ann., Est. & Tr. Art. 13 §503 (b)
Massachusetts	Married	201 Mass. Gen. Laws Ann. § 5
Michigan	Married	Mich. Comp. Laws § 551.251
	Court order	Mich. Comp. Laws § 722.4
Minnesota	*a*	
Mississippi	Married for divorce and custody claims	Miss. Code Ann. § 93-19-11
Missouri	Married for real estate if spouse of age	Mo. Rev. Stat. § 442.040
Montana	Married	Mont. Rev. Code Ann. § 40-6-234
Nebraska	Married	Nebr. Rev. Stat. Ann. § 43-2101
	Self-supporting and apart from parents	*Accent Serv. v. Ebsen*, 306 N.W.2d 575 (1981)
Nevada	Court order	Nev. Rev. Stat. Ann. § 129.080
	Veteran or spouse	Nev. Rev. Stat. Ann. § 129.020
New Hampshire	Emancipated in another state	R.S.A. 21-B:2
New Jersey	Married	N.J. Stat. § 2C:25-19
	Military service	N.J. Stat. § 2C:25-19
	Has child or is pregnant	N.J. Stat. § 2C:25-19
	Court order	N.J. Stat. § 2C:25-19
New Mexico	Marriage, death, adoption as well as death, resignation or removal of guardian	N.M. Stat. Ann. § 45-5-210
	Court order	N.M. Stat. Ann. § 24-7A-6.1
	In military	N.M. Stat. Ann. § 32A-21-5
New York	*a*	
North Carolina	Court order	N.C. Gen. Stat. § 7B-3500
North Dakota	Married	N.D. Cent. Code § 14-09-20
Ohio	Court order	Ohio Rev. Code Ann. § 2111.18.1
Oklahoma	Court order	Okla. Stat. Ann. Tit.10, 10
	Married	Okla. Stat. Ann. Tit. 10, 91

Continued

TABLE B.3 Continued

State	Conditions	Statute
Oregon	Married	Oreg. Rev. Stat. § 109.555
	Parental decree	Oreg. Rev. Stat. § 109.510
	Court order	Oreg. Rev. Stat. § 109.510
Pennsylvania	Married	55 Pa. Code 145.62
	Age 16+, living independently	55 Pa. Code 145.62
	Age 16+, orphan	55 Pa. Code 145.62
Rhode Island	[a]	
South Carolina	[a]	
South Dakota	Married	S.D. Codified Laws § 25-5-24
	Age 16+; no longer dependent and with parents' consent/ acquiescence; managing own financial affairs	S.D. Codified Laws § 25-5-26
	Military	S.D. Codified Laws § 25-5-24
	Court order (age 16+)	S.D. Codified Laws § 25-5-19, 25-5-26
Tennessee	[a]	
Texas	Age 16 or 17 and living apart from parent and self-supporting	Tex. Fam. Code Ann. § 31.01
Utah	Married	Utah Code Ann. § 15-2-1
Vermont	Married	12 V.S.A. § 7151
	On active military duty	12 V.S.A. § 7151
	Court order	12 V.S.A. § 7155
Virginia	Court order	Va. Code Ann. § 16.1-331
Washington	Court order	Rev. Code Wash. § 13.64
West Virginia	Married	W.Va. Code § 49-7-27
	Court order	W.Va. Code § 49-7-27
Wisconsin	Married	Wis. Stat. § 48.375
	Previously given birth	Wis. Stat. § 48.375
	Freed from care, custody, and control of parents	Wis. Stat. § 48.375
Wyoming	Married	Wyo. Stat. § 14-1-201
	In military	Wyo. Stat. § 14-1-201
	Court order	Wyo. Stat. § 14-1-203

[a]No applicable law identified through search strategy performed for the overview purposes of this appendix as explained in footnote 4 to the text.

TABLE B.4 Mature Minor Provisions

State	Mature Minor Status Events for Consenting to Health Care	Statute
Alabama	Pregnant	Code of Ala. § 22-8-4
	Married	Code of Ala. § 22-8-4
	Minor parent (may consent to child's and own medical treatment)	Code of Ala. § 22-8-5
	High school graduate	Code of Ala. § 22-8-4
	Age 14+	Code of Ala. § 22-8-4
Alaska	Minor parent (may consent to child's medical treatment)	Alaska Stat. § 25.20.025
	Living apart from parents and managing own financial affairs	Alaska Stat. § 25.20.025
	If parent cannot be contacted or withholds consent	Alaska Stat. § 25.20.025
Arizona	Married or divorced	Ariz. Rev. Stat. § 44-132
	Emancipated	Ariz. Rev. Stat. § 44-132
	Living apart from parents/homeless	Ariz. Rev. Stat. § 44-132
Arkansas	Married	Ark. Code Ann. § 20-9-602
	Unemancipated if of sufficient intelligence to appreciate consequences of medical treatment	Ark. Code Ann. § 20-9-602
	Pregnant	Ark. Code Ann. § 20-9-602
	Minor parent (may consent to child's medical treatment)	Ark. Code Ann. § 20-9-602
	Incarcerated	Ark. Code Ann. § 20-9-602
California	Pregnant	Calif. Fam. Code § 6925
	Age 15 years old and living apart from parents and managing own financial affairs	Calif. Fam. Code § 6922
Colorado	Married	Colo. Rev. Stat. § 13-22-103
	Minor parent (may consent to child's medical treatment)	Colo. Rev. Stat. § 13-22-103
	Living apart from parents and managing own financial affairs	Colo. Rev. Stat. § 13-22-103
Connecticut	Minor parent (may consent to child's medical treatment)	Conn. Gen. Stat. Ann. § 19a-285
Delaware	Married	13 Del. Code § 707
	Pregnant (related to pregnancy)	13 Del. Code § 708
	Minor parent (may consent to child's medical treatment)	13 Del. Code § 707
District of Columbia	Minor parent (may consent to child's medical treatment)	D.C.C. § 16-4901

TABLE B.4 Continued

State	Mature Minor Status Events for Consenting to Health Care	Statute
Florida	Age 16+ with court order	Fla. Stat. Ann. § 743.065
	Pregnant (if related to pregnancy)	Fla. Stat. Ann. § 743.065
	Minor parent (may consent to child's medical treatment)	Fla. Stat. Ann. § 743.065
Georgia	Married	O.C.G.A. § 31-9-2
	Pregnant (if related to pregnancy, pregnancy prevention, or childbirth)	O.C.G.A. § 31-9-2
	Minor parent (may consent to child's medical treatment)	O.C.G.A. § 31-9-2
Hawaii	Pregnant	Hawaii Rev. Stat. Ann. § 577A-2
Idaho	Minor parent (may consent to child's medical treatment)	Idaho Code § 39-4303
	Minor of ordinary intelligence and awareness to comprehend need for, nature of, and risks in medical care	Idaho Code § 39-4302
Illinois	Married	410 Ill. Comp. Stat. Ann. 210/1
	Pregnant	410 Ill. Comp. Stat. Ann. 210/1
	Minor parent (may consent to child's and own medical treatment)	410 Ill. Comp. Stat. Ann. 210/1 and 410 Ill. Comp. Stat. Ann. 210/2
Indiana	Married	Ind. Code Ann. § 16-36-1-3
	Emancipated	Ind. Code Ann. § 16-36-1-3
	Age 14+ and independent/living apart from parents and managing own affairs	Ind. Code Ann. § 16-36-1-3
	Military service	Ind. Code Ann. § 16-36-1-3
Iowa	Married	Iowa Code § 234.1
	Juvenile if tried and convicted as adult	Iowa Code § 599.1
Kansas	Married and age 16+	Kans. Stat. Ann. § 38-101
	Pregnant	Kans. Stat. Ann. § 38-123
	Minor parent (may consent to child's medical treatment)	Kans. Stat. Ann. § 38-122
	Emancipated minor through court order	Kans. Admin. Regs. § 30-6-52
	Age 16+ and no parent immediately available	Kans. Stat. Ann. § 38-123b

TABLE B.4 Continued

State	Mature Minor Status Events for Consenting to Health Care	Statute
Kentucky	Married	Ky. Rev. Stat. Ann. § 214.185
	Emancipated minor	Ky. Rev. Stat. Ann. § 214.185
	Pregnant	Ky. Rev. Stat. Ann. § 214.185
	Minor parent (may consent to child's and own medical treatment)	Ky. Rev. Stat. Ann. § 214.185
	Children with disabilities, age 21+	Ky. Rev. Stat. Ann. § 2.015
Louisiana	Minor parent (may consent to child's medical treatment and for pain or distress during labor)	La. Rev. Stat. § 40:1299.53
	Emancipation with court approval	La. Civil Code Art. 305
Maine	Married	22 Maine Rev. Stat. Ann. § 1503
	Living apart from parents and independent of support for at least 60 days	22 Maine Rev. Stat. Ann. § 1503
	Military service	22 Maine Rev. Stat. Ann. § 1503
	Emancipated by court order	15 Maine Rev. Stat. Ann. § 3506-A
Maryland	Married	Md. Code Ann. Health-Gen. I § 20-102
	Pregnant	Md. Code Ann. Health-Gen. I § 20-102
	Minor parent	Md. Code Ann. Health-Gen. I § 20-102
Massachusetts	Married	112 Mass. Gen. Laws Ann. § 12F
	Pregnant	112 Mass. Gen. Laws Ann. § 12F
	Minor parent (may consent for child's and own medical treatment)	112 Mass. Gen. Laws Ann. § 12F
	Living apart from parents	112 Mass. Gen. Laws Ann. § 12F
	Military service	112 Mass. Gen. Laws Ann. § 12F
Michigan	Pregnant (for prenatal and pregnancy related services)	M.S.A. § 333.9132
	Minor parent (may consent for child's medical treatment)	M.S.A. § 333.9132

Continued

TABLE B.4 Continued

State	Mature Minor Status Events for Consenting to Health Care	Statute
Minnesota	Married	Minn. Code § 144.342
	Borne a child	Minn. Code § 144.343
	Minor parent (may consent for child's and own medical treatment)	Minn. Code § 144.342
	Living apart from parents and maintains personal financial affairs	Minn. Code § 144.341
Mississippi	Married	Miss. Code Ann. § 41-41-3
	Pregnant (in connection with pregnancy)	Miss. Code Ann. § 41-41-3
	Minor parent (may consent for child's medical treatment)	Miss. Code Ann. § 41-41-3
Missouri	Married	Mo. Rev. Stat. § 431.061
	Pregnant (for self)	Mo. Rev. Stat. § 431.061
	Minor parent (may consent for child's and own medical treatment)	Mo. Rev. Stat. § 431.061
Montana	Married	Mont. Rev. Code Ann. § 41-1-404(1)(a)
	Emancipated	Mont. Rev. Code Ann. § 41-1-404(1)
	Pregnant	Mont. Rev. Code Ann. § 41-1-404(1)(c)
	Minor parent (may consent to child's and own medical treatment)	Mont. Rev. Code Ann. § 41-1-402
	Living apart from parents and self-supporting	Mont. Rev. Code Ann. § 41-1-402(1)(b)
	High school graduate	Mont. Rev. Code Ann. § 41-1-404(1)(a)
Nebraska	Emancipated if self-supporting and apart from parents	*Accent Serv. v. Ebsen*, 306 N.W.2d 575 (1981)
Nevada	Married	Nev. Rev. Stat. Ann. § 129.030
	Emancipated	Nev. Rev. Stat. Ann. § 129.010
	Living apart from parents for at least 4 months	Nev. Rev. Stat. Ann. § 129.030
	Borne a child	Nev. Rev. Stat. Ann. § 129.030
New Hampshire	*a*	
New Jersey	Married	N.J. Stat. § 9:17A-1
	Pregnant (on own behalf or for child)	N.J. Stat. § 9:17A-1
	Minor parent (may consent for child's medical treatment)	N.J. Stat. § 9:17A-1
	Military service	N.J. Stat. § 55:14L-2

TABLE B.4 Continued

State	Mature Minor Status Events for Consenting to Health Care	Statute
New Mexico	Married	N.M. Stat. Ann. § 32A-21
	Emancipated if age 16+ and married, by court order or in military	N.M. Stat. Ann. §§ 24-7A-1, 24-7A-6.1, 32A-21-5
	Living apart from parents	N.M. Stat. Ann. § 32A-21
New York	Married	N.Y. Pub. Health Law § 2504(1)
	Pregnant (related to prenatal care)	N.Y. Pub. Health Law § 2504(3)
	Minor parent (may consent for child's and own medical treatment)	N.Y. Pub. Health Law § 2504
North Carolina	Married	N.C. Gen. Stat. § 7A-726
	Emancipated	N.C. Gen. Stat. § 32A-29
	Pregnant (for self or child)	N.C. Gen. Stat. § 90-21.5
North Dakota	*a*	
Ohio	*a*	
Oklahoma	Married	63 Okla. Stat. Ann. § 2602(A)(1)
	Emancipated	63 Okla. Stat. Ann. § 2602(A)
	Pregnant	63 Okla. Stat. Ann. § 2602(A)(3)
	Minor parent (may consent for child's and own medical care)	63 Okla. Stat. Ann. § 2602
	Living apart from parents and not supported by them	63 Okla. Stat. Ann. § 2602(A)(2)
	Military service	63 Okla. Stat. Ann. § 2601
Oregon	Married	Oreg. Rev. Stat. § 109.520
	Age 15+	Oreg. Rev. Stat. § 109.640
	Living apart from parents	Oreg. Rev. Stat. § 109.627
Pennsylvania	Married	35 Pa. Stat. Ann. § 10101
	Pregnant (or has been pregnant)	35 Pa. Stat. Ann. § 10103
	Minor parent (may consent for child's and own medical care)	35 Pa. Stat. Ann. § 10102
	High school graduate	35 Pa. Stat. Ann. § 10101
Rhode Island	Married	R.I. Gen. Laws § 23-4.6-1
	Age 16+ if a "routine emergency"	R.I. Gen. Laws § 23-4.6-1
	Minor parent (may consent for child's medical care)	R.I. Gen. Laws § 23-4.6-1

Continued

TABLE B.4 Continued

State	Mature Minor Status Events for Consenting to Health Care	Statute
South Carolina	Married or spouse of married minor	S.C. Code Ann. § 20-7-270
	Minor parent (may consent for child's medical care)	S.C. Code Ann. § 20-7-300
	Age 16+ (other than for operations, unless necessary for the health or life of the minor)	S.C. Code Ann. § 20-7-280
South Dakota	Legally emancipated (age 16+)	S.D. Codified Laws §§ 25-5-25, 25-5-26
Tennessee	Pregnant	Tenn. Code Ann. § 63-6-223
	Minor parent (may consent for child's medical care)	Tenn. Code Ann. § 63-6-229
Texas	Pregnant (related to pregnancy)	Tex. Fam. Code Ann. § 32.003(a)(4)
	Minor parent (may consent for child's medical care)	Tex. Fam. Code Ann. § 32.003(a)(6)
	Living apart from parents and managing own affairs and age 16+	Tex. Fam. Code Ann. § 32.003(a)(2)
	Military service	Tex. Fam. Code Ann. § 32.003(a)(1)
Utah	Married	Utah Code Ann. § 78-14-5(4)(b)
	Pregnant	Utah Code Ann. § 78-14-5(4)(f)
	Minor parent (may consent for child's medical care)	Utah Code Ann. § 78-14-5(4)
Vermont	*a*	
Virginia	Married	Va. Code Ann. § 16.1-333(I)
	Emancipated (active military duty or separate from parents)	Va. Code Ann. § 16.1-333
	Pregnant (for self/child related to delivery and minor parent for child)	Va. Code Ann. § 54.1-2969(D)(2)
Washington	Married	Rev. Code Wash. § 26.28.020
	Minor parent (may consent for child's medical care)	Rev. Code Wash. § 26.28.015(5)
West Virginia	Mature minor, emancipated minor	W.Va. Code §§ 16-30-3, 16-30-6, 49-7-27
	Pregnant	W.Va. Code § 16-29-1(b)
Wisconsin	Minor parent (may consent for child's and own medical care)	Wis. Stat. § 48.375(2)(e)
	Living apart from parents	Wis. Stat. § 48.375(2)(e)
Wyoming	*a*	

*a*No applicable law identified through search strategy performed for the overview purposes of this appendix as explained in footnote 4 to the text.

TABLE B.5 FOLLOWS

TABLE B.5 Minor Consent for Certain Conditions/Disorders

State	Condition or Disorder	Age	Statute
Alabama	STD testing/treatment	12+	Code of Ala. § 22-8-6, 22-11A-19
	Alcohol or drug abuse treatment	Any minor	Code of Ala. § 22-8-6
	Emergency care when delay would result in increased risk to life	Any minor	Code of Ala. § 22-8-3
Alaska	STD testing/treatment	Any minor	Alaska Stat. § 25.20.025
	Family planning	Any minor	Alaska Stat. § 25.20.025
Arizona	Alcohol or drug abuse treatment	12+	Ariz. Rev. Stat. § 44-133.01
Arkansas	STD testing/treatment	Any minor	Ark. Code Ann. § 20-16-508
	Family planning	Any minor	Ark. Code Ann. § 20-16-304
	Blood donation	17+	Ark. Code Ann. § 20-27-301
	Medical treatment in prison	Any minor	Ark. Code Ann. § 20-9-602
California	STD testing/treatment, infectious diseases	12+	Calif. Fam. Code § 6926
	HIV testing/treatment	12+	Calif. Health & Safety Code § 121020
	Family planning	Any minor	Calif. Fam. Code § 6925
	Alcohol or drug abuse treatment	12+	Calif. Fam. Code § 6929
	Mental health care	12+	Calif. Fam. Code § 6924
Colorado	HIV or STD testing/treatment	Any minor (if less than 16, parent may be informed)	Colo. Rev. Stat. § 25-4-402
	Family planning	Any minor	Colo. Rev. Stat. § 13-22-105
	Alcohol or drug abuse treatment	Any minor	Colo. Rev. Stat. § 13-22-105

State	Service	Consent	Citation
Connecticut	STD testing/treatment	Any minor	Conn. Gen. Stat. Ann. § 19a-216
	HIV testing/treatment	Any minor (parental consent for treatment unless notice adversely affects treatment)	Conn. Gen. Stat. Ann. §§ 19a-582, 19a-598
	Alcohol or drug abuse treatment	Any minor	Conn. Gen. Stat. Ann. § 17a-688
	Blood donation	17+	Conn. Gen. Stat. Ann. § 19a-285a
	Mental health care	14+ (parental notice within 5 days)	Conn. Gen. Stat. Ann. § 17a-79
Delaware	STD testing/treatment	12+	13 Del. Code Ann. § 708
	HIV testing	12+	13 Del. Code Ann. § 708
	Family planning	12+	13 Del. Code Ann. § 708
	Alcohol or drug abuse treatment	12+	13 Del. Code Ann. § 707
	Blood donation	17+	13 Del. Code Ann. § 709
Florida	STD testing/treatment	Any minor	Fla. Stat. Ann. § 384.30
	Family planning	Any minor	Fla. Stat. Ann. § 381.0051
	Medical treatment in prison	Any minor	Fla. Stat. Ann. § 743.066
Georgia	STD testing/treatment	Any minor (physician's discretion whether or not to provide information to parents)	O.C.G.A. § 31-17-7
	Family planning	Any minor	O.C.G.A. § 31-9-2
	Alcohol or drug abuse treatment	Any minor	O.C.G.A. § 37-7-8
Hawaii	STD testing/treatment	Any minor	Hawaii Rev. Stat. Ann. § 577A-2
	Family planning	Any minor	Hawaii Rev. Stat. Ann. § 577A-2
	Alcohol or drug abuse treatment	Any minor	Hawaii Rev. Stat. Ann. § 577-26

Continued

TABLE B.5 Continued

State	Condition or Disorder	Age	Statute
Idaho	STD and reportable diseases testing/treatment	14+	Idaho Code § 39-3801
	HIV testing/treatment	14+	Idaho Code § 39-609
	Family planning	Any minor	Idaho Code § 18-603
	Alcohol or drug abuse treatment	16+	Idaho Code § 37-3102
Illinois	STD testing/treatment	12+	410 Ill. Comp. Stat. Ann. 210/4
	HIV testing/treatment	12+	410 Ill. Comp. Stat. Ann. 210/4
	Family planning	Any minor	325 Ill. Comp. Stat. Ann. 10/1
	Alcohol or drug abuse treatment	12+	410 Ill. Comp. Stat. Ann. 210/4
Indiana	STD testing/treatment (if the individual has been or is suspected of having been exposed)	Any minor	Ind. Code Ann. § 16-36-1-3
	Alcohol or drug abuse treatment	Any minor	Ind. Code Ann. § 12-23-12-1
	Blood donation	17+	Ind. Code Ann. § 16-36-1-3
Iowa	STD testing/treatment	Any minor	Iowa Code § 141.22
	HIV testing/treatment	Any minor	Iowa Code § 141.22
	Family planning	Any minor	Iowa Code § 141.22
	Alcohol or drug abuse treatment	Any minor	Iowa Code § 125.33
	Medical treatment in prison	Any minor	Iowa Code § 599.1
Kansas	STD testing/treatment	Any minor (physicians may inform parent/guardian if it is most beneficial to minor)	Kans. Stat. Ann. § 65-2892
Kentucky	STD testing/treatment	Any minor	Ky. Rev. Stat. Ann. § 214.185
	HIV testing/treatment	Any minor	Ky. Rev. Stat. Ann. § 214.185
	Family planning	Any minor	Ky. Rev. Stat. Ann. § 214.185

State	Service	Minor covered	Citation
	Alcohol or drug abuse treatment	Any minor	Ky. Rev. Stat. Ann. § 222.441
	Mental health treatment	16+	Ky. Rev. Stat. Ann. §§ 214.185, 645.030
Louisiana	STD testing/treatment (if minor believes he or she is infected with illness)	Any minor (may inform parent/guardian over minor's objection)	La. Rev. Stat. §§ 40:1065.1, 40:1095
	Alcohol or drug abuse treatment	Any minor	La. Rev. Stat. § 40:1096
	Blood donation	17+	La. Rev. Stat. § 40:1097
Maine	STD testing/treatment	Any minor	22 Maine Rev. Stat. Ann. § 1823
	Family planning	Minor parent, married, or physician's judgment of harm without services	22 Maine Rev. Stat. Ann. § 1908
	Alcohol or drug abuse treatment	Any minor	22 Maine Rev. Stat. Ann. § 1823
Maryland	STD testing/treatment	Any minor	Md. Code Ann., Health-Gen I, 20-102
	Family planning	Any minor	Md. Code Ann., Health-Gen I, 20-102
	Alcohol or drug abuse treatment	Any minor	Md. Code Ann., Health-Gen I, 20-102
	Mental health treatment	16+	Md. Code Ann., Health-Gen I, 20-104
Massachusetts	Testing/treatment for STDs or other "dangerous diseases"	Any minor	112 Mass. Gen. Laws Ann. § 12F
Michigan	STD testing/treatment	Any minor	M.S.A. § 333.5127
	HIV testing/treatment	Any minor	M.S.A. § 333.5127
	Alcohol or drug abuse treatment	Any minor	M.S.A. § 333.6121
	Medical treatment in prison	Any minor	M.S.A. § 722.4
	Mental health treatment (excluding use of psychotropic drugs)	14+	M.S.A. § 14.800 (707)
Minnesota	STD testing/treatment	Any minor	Minn. Code § 144.343
	Alcohol or drug abuse treatment	Any minor (may inform parents if failure would "jeopardize minor's health")	Minn. Code § 144.343

Continued

TABLE B.5 Continued

State	Condition or Disorder	Age	Statute
Mississippi	STD testing/treatment	Any minor	Miss. Code Ann. § 41-41-13
	Family planning	Any minor	Miss. Code Ann. § 41-42-7
	Alcohol or drug abuse treatment	15+	Miss. Code Ann. §41-41-14
	Blood donation	17+	Miss. Code Ann. § 41-41-15
Missouri	STD testing/treatment	Any minor	Mo. Rev. Stat. § 431.061
	Alcohol or drug abuse treatment	Any minor	Mo. Rev. Stat. § 431.061
Montana	STD testing/treatment	Any minor	Mont. Rev. Code Ann. § 41-1-402(1)(c)
	HIV testing/treatment	Any minor	Mont. Rev. Code Ann. § 50-16-1007(8)
	Alcohol or drug abuse treatment (limited to treatment of those conditions)	Any minor	Mont. Rev. Code Ann. § 41-1-402(1)(c)
Nebraska	STD testing/treatment	Any minor	Nebr. Rev. Stat. Ann. § 71-504
	Alcohol or drug abuse treatment	Any minor	Nebr. Rev. Stat. Ann. § 71-5041
Nevada	STD testing/treatment	Any minor	Nev. Rev. Stat. Ann. § 129.060
	Family planning	Any minor	Nev. Rev. Stat. Ann. § 430A.180
	Alcohol or drug abuse treatment	Any minor	Nev. Rev. Stat. Ann. § 129.050
New Hampshire	STD testing/treatment	14+	N.H. Rev. Stat. Ann. § 141-C:18(II)
	HIV testing/treatment (physician may inform parent/guardian)	Any minor	N.H. Rev. Stat. Ann. § 141-F:5
	Alcohol or drug abuse treatment	14+	N.H. Rev. Stat. Ann. § 318-B:12-a
	Blood donation	17+	N.H. Rev. Stat. Ann. § 571-C:1
	Medical treatment in prison	Any minor	N.H. Rev. Stat. Ann. § 141-F:5(IV)
New Jersey	STD testing/treatment (parents may be informed without minor consent)	Any minor	N.J. Stat. § 9:17A-4
	Alcohol or drug abuse treatment	Any minor	N.J. Stat. § 9:17A-4

	Emergency care when minor has been sexually assaulted (must notify parent/guardian unless not in "best interest")	Any minor	N.J. Stat. § 9:17A-4
	Blood donation	18+	N.J. Stat. § 9:17A-6
New Mexico	STD testing/treatment	Any minor	N.M. Stat. Ann. § 24-1-9
	HIV testing/treatment	Any minor	N.M. Stat. Ann. § 24-2B-3
	Family planning	Any minor	N.M. Stat. Ann. § 24-8-5
New York	STD testing/treatment	Any minor	N.Y. Pub. Health Law § 2305(2)
	HIV testing/treatment	Any minor	N.Y. Pub. Health Law § 2782
	Family planning	Any minor	N.Y. Soc. Serv. Law § 465(3)
	Alcohol or drug abuse treatment	Any minor	N.Y. Mental Hyg. Law § 21.11(a)
	Mental health care	18+, emancipated, has child, or 16+ and parents not available	N.Y. Mental Hyg. Law § 22.11, 33.21
North Carolina	STD testing/treatment	Any minor	N.C. Gen. Stat. § 90-21.5(a)(I)
	HIV testing/treatment	Any minor	N.C. Gen. Stat. §§ 90-21.5(a)(I), 130A-148
	Family planning	Any minor	N.C. Gen. Stat. § 90-21.5(a)
	Alcohol or drug abuse treatment	Any minor	N.C. Gen. Stat. §§ 122C-221(a), 90-21.5(a) (iii)
	Emotional disturbance	Any minor	N.C. Gen. Stat. § 90-21.5(a)(iv)
North Dakota	STD testing/treatment	14+	N.D. Cent. Code § 14-10-17
	HIV testing/treatment	Any minor	N.D. Cent. Code § 23-07.5-05
	Alcohol or drug abuse treatment	14+	N.D. Cent. Code § 14-10-17

Continued

TABLE B.5 Continued

State	Condition or Disorder	Age	Statute
Ohio	STD testing/treatment	Any minor	Ohio Rev. Code Ann. § 3709.241
	HIV testing	Any minor	Ohio Rev. Code Ann. § 3701.242(B)
	Alcohol or drug abuse treatment	Any minor	Ohio Rev. Code Ann. § 3719.012(A),(C)
	Blood donation	17+	Ohio Rev. Code Ann. § 2108.21
	Medical treatment in prison	Any minor	Ohio Rev. Code Ann. § 5120.172
	Health care subject to Department of Mental Health	18+	Ohio Admin. Code § 5122-28-05(A)(4)
	Mental health services (for limited time, except for use of medications)	14+	Ohio Admin. Code § 5122-27-05(B), Ohio Rev. Code Ann. § 5122.04
Oklahoma	STD testing/treatment	Any minor	63 Okla. Stat. Ann. § 2602(3)
	HIV testing	Any minor	63 Okla. Stat. Ann. §§ 2602(3),1-532.1
	Alcohol or drug abuse treatment	Any minor	63 Okla. Stat. Ann. § 2602(A)(3)
Oregon	STD testing/treatment	Any minor	Oreg. Rev. Stat. § 109.610(1)
	HIV testing/treatment	Any minor	Oreg. Rev. Stat. § 433.04(5)
	Family planning	Any minor	Oreg. Rev. Stat. § 109.640
	Alcohol or drug abuse treatment	14+	Oreg. Rev. Stat. § 109.675
	Blood donation	16+	Oreg. Rev. Stat. § 109.670
	Mental health care	14+	Oreg. Rev. Stat. § 109.675
Pennsylvania	STD testing/treatment	Any minor	35 Pa. Stat. Ann. § 10103; 35 Pa. Stat. Ann. § 521.14a
	HIV testing/treatment	Any minor	35 Pa. Stat. Ann. § 10103
	Alcohol or drug abuse treatment	Any minor	71 Pa. Stat. Ann. § 1690.112
	Blood donation	Any minor	35 Pa. Stat. Ann. § 10001
Rhode Island	STD testing/treatment	Any minor	R.I. Gen. Laws § 23-11-11
	HIV testing/treatment	Any minor	R.I. Gen. Laws §§ 23-6-17, 23-8-1.1
	Alcohol or drug abuse treatment	Any minor	R.I. Gen. Laws § 14-5-4

State	Topic	Age	Citation
	Blood donation	17+	R.I. Gen. Laws § 23-4.5-1
	Medical treatment in prison	Any minor	R.I. Gen. Laws § 11-37-17
South Carolina	Alcohol or drug abuse treatment	16+	S.C. Code Ann. § 44-52-20
South Dakota	STD testing/treatment	Any minor	S.D. Codified Laws § 34-23-16
	Alcohol or drug abuse treatment	Any minor	S.D. Codified Laws § 34-20A-50
	Mental health treatment	18+, married or emancipated	S.D. Codified Laws § 27A-15-1
Tennessee	STD testing/treatment	Any minor	Tenn. Code Ann. § 68-10-104(c)
	HIV testing/treatment	Any minor	Tenn. Code Ann. § 49-6-1008(a)
	Family planning	Any minor	Tenn. Code Ann. § 68-4-107
	Alcohol or drug abuse treatment	Any minor	Tenn. Code Ann. § 63-6-220
Texas	STD testing/treatment	Any minor	Tex. Fam. Code Ann. § 32.003
	Alcohol or drug abuse treatment	Any minor	Tex. Fam. Code Ann. § 32.003
Utah	STD testing/treatment	Any minor	Utah Code Ann. § 26-6-18(1)
	Blood donation	18+	Utah Code Ann. § 15-2-5
Vermont	STD testing/treatment	12+	18 Vt. Stat. Ann. § 4226
	Alcohol or drug abuse treatment	12+	18 Vt. Stat. Ann. § 4226
Virginia	STD testing/treatment	Any minor	Va. Code Ann. § 54.1-2969(D)(1)
	HIV testing/treatment	Any minor	Va. Code Ann. § 32.1-36(C)
	Family planning (not sterilization)	Any minor	Va. Code Ann. § 54.1-2969(D)(2)
	Alcohol or drug abuse	Any minor	Va. Code Ann. § 54.1-2969(D)(3)
	Blood donation	17+	Va. Code Ann. § 54.1-2969(F)
	Mental illness	Any minor	Va. Code Ann. § 54.1-2969

Continued

TABLE B.5 Continued

State	Condition or Disorder	Age	Statute
Washington	STD testing/treatment	14+	Rev. Code Wash. § 70.24.110
	HIV testing/treatment	14+	Rev. Code Wash. § 70.24.017
	Family planning	Any minor	Rev. Code Wash. § 9.02.100(1)
	Alcohol or drug abuse treatment	13+	Rev. Code Wash. § 70.96A.095(1)
	Mental health treatment	13+ if inpatient or outpatient, or 12+ if treatment by Department of Social Services	Rev. Code Wash. §§ 71.34.030, 71.34.042
West Virginia	STD testing/treatment	Any minor	W.V. Code § 16-29-1(b)
	HIV testing/treatment	Any minor	W.V. Code § 16-3C-2(a)(3)
	Family planning	Any minor	W.V. Code § 16-29-1(b)
	Alcohol or drug abuse treatment	Any minor	W.V. Code § 60A-5-504
Wisconsin	STD testing/treatment	Any minor	Wis. Stat. §§ 252.11, 48.023
	Alcohol or drug abuse treatment	12+	Wis. Stat. § 252.10
	Mental health care	14+	Wis. Stat. § 51.14
Wyoming	STD testing/treatment	Any minor	Wyo. Stat. § 35-4-131
	HIV testing/treatment	Any minor	Wyo. Stat. § 35-4-130
	Family planning	Any minor	Wyo. Stat. § 42-5-101
	Blood donation	18+	Wyo. Stat. § 12-1-101(e)

TABLE B.6 FOLLOWS

TABLE B.6 Regulation of Research with Children and Adolescents in State Custody: Responses from Child Welfare or Social Services Personnel

State	Contact
Alabama	Dr. Page Walley, Commissioner, Department of Children's Affairs
Delaware	Peter S. Feliceangeli, Deputy Attorney General
	Patricia M. Hearn, Office of the Secretary, Department of Services for Children, Youth and their Families (DSCYF)
Florida	Gladys E. Cherry, Director, Family Safety, Department of Children & Families
	Sue Ross, Chief, Children's Mental Health, Department of Children & Families (DCFS)
Illinois	Mark Testa, Director, Children and Family Resource Center
Louisiana	Eileen Fourroux, Program Specialist, Office of Community Services

Findings

No state regulations; follow federal government.

No statutes or policies relating to health care research involving children in state custody.

DSCYF provides services to children who experience abandonment, abuse, adjudication, mental illness, neglect, or substance abuse; does *not* permit involvement of children in their care in medical research.

Statutes address confidentiality of records and requirements for researcher access for abuse/neglect studies; must sign privacy agreement; requires approval of Department of Health's IRB, the Review Council for Human Subjects (RCHS) (Florida Statutes, Ch. 39.202), which tracks federal regulations.

RCHS's review procedures are available at http://www.doh.state.fl.us/execstaff/rchs/index.html.

Florida's DCFS has its own IRB (with Federalwide Assurance (FWA)) to review applicable protocols; follows *Belmont Report* and federal regulations (according to its FWA application), approved May 2003.

All research involving wards of the state and former or current recipients of services from the Department of Children and Family Services (DCFS) must be approved through the DCFS IRB; additionally, a state-appointed guardian must approve research involving any ward of the state.

Non-personally identifying information may be released to a professional, university professor, or graduate student for "bona fide professional, academic, or scholarly research in the field of child welfare services" (La. R.S. 46:56F(5)(a)); identifying information (except identifying information in abuse & neglect cases) may be released with written approval of the Department, and the child's representative, and if the research has been approved by IRB (46:56F(5)(b)). Contact with client/former client is permissible, if it "will not have a detrimental effect on the client," if the client or his or her legal guardian consents in writing, and if the research is of value to the Department (46:56F(6)).

Office of Community Services (OCS) policy: Except for identifying information, the OCS State Office must preapprove access to foster care records, records of abuse/ neglect investigations, and child welfare services records by external investigators (the latter cannot be undergraduate students) –(Policy 1-550). If investigators desire access to identifying information/clients, they must submit a written request to OCS State Office. Financial incentives cannot be used to recruit participants; written certification from researcher's IRB is needed. The following are also required: the research must have no detrimental effect on client, written consent of client/legal guardian, and the research must be of value to department (Policy 1-550).

The agency's procedure for research proposal requests: Requests are reviewed on the basis of potential benefits to knowledge development in child welfare field, relevance

Continued

TABLE B.6 Continued

State	Contact
Louisiana (continued)	
Maine	Michael Norton, Director, Division of Public Affairs/Quality Assurance, Bureau of Child and Family Services (BCFS), Department of Human Services (DHS)
New Hampshire	Philip F. Nadeau, Department of Health and Human Services (DHHS)
	Bernie Bluhm, DHHS, Division of Children, Youth, and Families (DCYF)
New Jersey	Sudha Tiwari Kantor, Esq., Director, Office of Legal, Policy, and Legislative Affairs, Department of Human Services (DHS)

Findings

to OCS priorities, demands placed on OCS resources, potential for adverse impact on subjects/families, and the soundness of research design and procedures. If the researcher seeks direct contact with clients, full committee (of OCS) review is required.

Identifying data are released only if it is absolutely necessary for advancing knowledge development and OCS programs, the IRB had provided written approval, and the IRB has a written plan for long-term protection of identifying information released in connection with research. Identifying information is given only to the principal investigator (PI) and co-PIs to the extent necessary and not to research assistants or others involved in the research; they must also sign confidential agreement that carries with it criminal penalties if that information is released (agency procedures were provided in an e-mail from Ms. Fourroux).

No policies specifically address medical research, but there are policies on confidentiality and medical treatment orders; allows optional disclosure of nonidentifying information for "bona fide" research and identifying information with commissioner's prior approval; cannot contact subject directly without subject's consent through DHS before such contact (MRSA Title 22, sec. 4008.2.f).

BCFS policy: BCFS given legal mandate to make informed decisions regarding care and treatment for children in DHS custody (Child and Family Services Manual, Policy V.I-5) for treatment for "immediate risk of injury." When a child is in DHS custody, DHS gives consent; if a child is in voluntary care of DHS, consent is given when the child receives "generally accepted treatment" and there is "reasonable cause to believe that parents or custodians would object" and parents/custodians are not available to consent (Child and Family Services Manual, Policy X.A.).

Research requires approval by/must be conducted under auspices of an IRB.

N.H. statute prohibits release of confidential files or other identifying information to researcher, except when DCYF contracts with researcher to evaluate its programs/ impact on families (then it reports only non-identifying outcomes) (see RSA Sec. 170-G:8-a).

No state laws/regulations/general policies. DHS has specific policy for "social welfare research." Child abuse/neglect research must be "bona fide research" by "bona fide researcher" to seek information "absolutely essential to purpose of research," must include individual or parent/legal guardian consent (Policy 604.1), must follow Program Evaluation Unit protocols, and obtain written consent of Division of Youth and Family Services (DYFS) director.

If DYFS believes that the research is useful, the researcher can avoid consent requirements by entering "consultant employee" arrangement (Policy 604.3). The researcher cannot use DYFS to contact former clients or use DYFS as intermediary to get children enrolled in research unrelated to DYFS (state custody) involvement, e.g., for market research (Policy 604.4).

Continued

TABLE B.6 Continued

State	Contact
New Mexico	Linda Carlisle, Juvenile Justice Division (JJD) Data Analysis Unit, Children, Youth & Families Department (CYFD)
North Dakota	Krista Andrews, Esq., Department of Human Services
Oklahoma	Linda Smith, Director, Division of Children and Family Services
Rhode Island	Kevin Aucoin, Administrator, Department of Children, Youth and Families (DCYF)
South Carolina	Mary C. Williams, Director, Division of Human Services, Department of Social Services
South Dakota	Virginia Wieseler, Office of Child Protection, Department of Social Services
Tennessee	Mary Jane Davis, Assistant General Counsel, Department of Children's Services (DCS)

Findings

JJD policy prohibits medical, pharmaceutical, or cosmetic experiments with clients in CYFD custody or under juvenile probation supervision; however, superintendent or chief Juvenile Justice Probation and Parole Officer (JPPO) may apply for access to a "special medical procedure" (including research or experimental procedure) for client on the basis of appropriate medical personnel/supervising physician referral; must meet ethical, legal, and medical treatment standards and submit written consent between client and client's parent/guardian/custodian and treating physician.

Director of JJD, with approval of medical director, Office of General Counsel, and secretary of CYFD may allow data collection from clients and analysis of data as part of research study if benefits CYFD clients, prevents client identification, and a confidentiality agreement restricting use of data by third parties is signed (JJD General Procedures, PR 11 Medical Research on Clients; note that scope is limited to JJD).

No state laws/regulations addressing research with children in state custody. Department policy requires IRBs (in general) to review research and to track federal regulations (policy emphasizes that federal regulatory protections apply to all children, including those in state custody).

Generally, research with children is not done; evaluations are done. However, the University of Oklahoma, which does most of the evaluations, follows the recommendations of its IRB.

No state laws or agency regulations specific to children's consent and research (particularly if a child is in state custody).

DCYF practice is to require written parental or legal guardian consent before dissemination of personally identifiable information; does not require parental consent for non-personally identifying data (e.g., demographics of children in care).

Proposals should be reviewed by staff development and legal counsel, identifying any DCYF resources affected; ultimately up to director or his/her designee to approve request to share information

Person engaged in bona fide research may have access to records on child abuse and neglect, subject to director's permission and with limits as director may impose (S.C. Code of Laws sec. 20-7-690(B)(17)).

Does not allow medical research with children in custody.
Not aware of cases/statutes that address this issue.
In general, both parental and state consent (since child in state custody) required for medical treatment.

Has in place a research review committee (RRC), under DCS's director of policy, planning, and research, to decide on appropriateness of all research requests; applies to research involving use of human subjects or access to confidential records/data. Director of policy, planning, and research appoints RRC if researcher seeks access to

Continued

TABLE B.6 Continued

State	Contact
Tennessee (continued)	

Findings

department records/reports/data, confidential records normally requiring informed consent (e.g., medical records), or human subjects directly.

Director of policy, planning, and research reviews requests for information/data not in public domain but not involving access to departmental records (less stringent review). RRC bases review on factors typical of federal IRB reviews, and IRB review/approval is required when federal law requires such (e.g., greater than minimal risk to children); researcher must agree to give DCS research results for review/comment before publication or dissemination.

Prohibited from approval is research "that uses juveniles for medical, pharmaceutical, or cosmetic experiments, or use of medications such as stimulants, tranquilizers, or psychotropic drugs administered for purposes of . . . experimentation and research" (DCS Policy 6.1, B.8). However, this policy does not apply if the medications prescribed as clinically indicated are used as part of therapy, or if medical procedure is medically necessary even though it is not part of general program of medical experimentation (DCS Policy 6.1, B.8).

Informed-consent policy is being updated. The draft version gives parents the legal right to consent to medical treatment for their child, unless parental rights are terminated; DCS is authorized to consent to ordinary medical treatment by virtue of court order granting it legal custody, but "best practice is to involve the parent(s) in the child's treatment and to facilitate the parental role in giving informed consent" (draft DCS Policy 20.24); presumes that children ages 14+ have the maturity to consent to medical treatment but is determined on a case-by-case basis; youth ages 16+ with serious emotional disturbances have the same legal rights as adults in outpatient and inpatient mental health treatment decisions, i.e., they can consent to treatment mental health conditions (draft DCS Policy 20.24, B.7); parental consent is not required for drug abuse, prenatal care, STD care, or contraceptive use.

Health administrator of youth development center or community residential facility may grant use of health records for research if precautions are taken to disguise identities of subjects and the researcher agrees not to disclose identity of youth subjects or material that might have direct adverse effect on youth (DCS Policy 20.25, C.2.c).

Important distinctions are based on what type of "guardian" is acting on behalf of child: that is, is state officially the legal guardian or guardian just in sense of being "legal custodian" (meaning no termination of parental rights); this would affect who may speak on behalf of the child/consent to research and treatment (see TCA 37-5-103, which defines "legal custodian" as person/agency given legal custody by court order, whose physical custody includes right to make ordinary medical treatment decisions [subject to limits of order granting custody and remaining rights/ duties of parents]). As matter of agency policy, DCS tries to get parental consent when feasible and in child's best interests.

Privacy Memorandum (from M. J. Davis to DCS Health Insurance Portability and Accountability Act of 1996 (HIPAA) Privacy Workgroup, April 16 2003) specifies that the parent is not the minor's personal representative with regard to health

Continued

TABLE B.6 Continued

State	Contact
Tennessee (continued)	
Utah	Navina Forsythe, Supervisor, Data Research Reporting Unit, Division of Child and Family Services (DCFS)

Findings

information when state law does not require consent before minor can obtain health care services and minor consents (e.g., STD care, physician finds minor "sufficiently mature" to make health care decisions and minor consents); furthermore, Tennessee common law (judge-made law) presumes all minors ages 14+ have the capacity to make informed health care decisions ("Rule of Sevens"), referred to as "mature minor exception" (see *Cardwell v. Bechtol*, 724 S.W.2d 739, 1987).

DCFS research representative to Department of Human Services (DHS) IRB and DCFS director must review and approve research; generally, review tracks federal regulations, but also requires research to be in the best interests of DCFS and DCFS clients and the results to be of potential benefit to DCFS and DHS (Procedure on Foster Children in DCFS Custody Involvement in Research, Dec. 2002). DHS IRB reviews are pursuant to federal regulations and state laws on family educational rights and privacy act (UCA sec. 63-2-101-909), reporting abuse/neglect/exploitation (UCA sec. 62A4a-403), and HIPAA.

Informed consent for children in DCFS custody procedures: DCFS caseworker for child consults with foster parents (adoptive parents if the research involves adoptive children) and may contact therapists, school personnel, and others who work with the child to see if the child may participate; if participation is approved, caseworker signs informed consent; if the child is under 18 and the goal is to return the child home or to place the child in the custody of a relative or if parental rights are not terminated, parents/relatives must be consulted and give permission. If they give permission, they sign a consent form; if they object, the child cannot participate. If the child has the "maturity to understand the implications of participating in research," the child is consulted. If the child agrees, the child signs an assent form unless he or she is 18+, in which case he or she signs the consent form; if the child does not agree, the child does not participate and the researcher must contact the Office of Guardian ad litem (if one is appointed) and give the guardian ad litem (GAL) a description of the research project; if GAL expresses concerns, the child cannot participate (Procedure on Foster Children in DCFS Custody Involvement in Research, Dec. 2002).

More thorough procedures contained in DHS's Policy and Resource Manual: Institutional Review Board, Policies and Procedures, Policy 01-10 (effective Feb. 24, 2003), which explains that an appropriate authority within DHS reviews the procedures; depending on the nature and source of proposed research, the authority could be (1) an appropriate division director (e.g., director of DCFS) or (2) an appropriate division director and DHS IRB. If the research involves pharmaceuticals or biomedical devices, another layer of review applies. Any research by an external researcher would require DHS IRB review.

No children under guardianship or custody of DCFS, Division of Substance Abuse and Mental Health, Division of Youth Corrections, or Division of Services for People with Disabilities may participate in study involving use of placebo (DHS Policy and Resource Manual, Policy 01-10).

Continued

TABLE B.6 Continued

State	Contact
Washington	Michael Garrick, Ph.D., Executive Secretary, Washington State IRB
Wisconsin	Kitty Kocol, Administrator, Division of Children and Family Services, Department of Health and Family Services

SOURCES: The information presented in the table is drawn from inquiry (by mail, e-mail, and follow-up calls) of state child welfare and related departments. The initial query letter was sent in June 2003, and the responses are those received as of October 23, 2003.

Findings

No state law or policies pertain directly to research involving children and adolescents.

The IRB follows advice of local assistant attorney general, based on state laws related to consent.

No specific state policies on research other than statutes/regulations related to confidentiality and, if applicable, any federal guidelines/regulations under which it is funded.

Depending on nature of research request and "type" of children involved, will negotiate with researcher on individual basis for each study: might allow direct access to children or data systems or, alternatively, might permit indirect access through Department.

NOTES

1. U.S. Department of Health and Human Services. *Protection of Human Subjects in Research*. Washington, D.C.: U.S. Government Printing Office, 1991 (codified at 45 CFR Part 46). The regulations and a list of all agencies adopting the Subpart A (the Common Rule) may be found at http://ohrp.osophs.dhhs.gov/humansubjects/guidance/45cfr46.htm (accessed May 6, 2004).

2. 45 CFR 46, Subpart D.

3. 34 CFR Part 97 (Protection of Human Subjects) and Part 98 (Student Rights in Research, Experimental Programs, and Testing). The Protection of Pupil Rights Amendment (PPRA), codified at 34 CFR Part 98, requires schools and contractors that receive funding from the U.S. Department of Education to obtain written parental consent before minor students are required to participate in any U.S. Department of Education-funded survey, analysis, or evaluation that reveals certain information, including mental and psychological problems potentially embarrassing to the student and his or her family; sexual behavior and attitudes; and illegal, antisocial, self-incriminating, and demeaning behavior. PPRA also seeks to ensure that parents can review such surveys, analyses, or evaluations before their minor child's participation. Subsequent legislation (No Child Left Behind Act) required that schools must provide directory information to military recruiters upon request and allowed parents to refuse their child's participation in certain additional information collection activities. More information is available on the U.S. Department of Education's website. Available at: http://www.ed.gov/offices/OII/fpco/ppra/index.html (accessed August 28, 2003) and http://www.ed.gov/policy/gen/guid/fpco/ppra/parents.html (accessed May 6, 2004).

4. See, e.g., *Standard Operating Procedures. Guidance on the Inclusion of Children in Research*, Johns Hopkins University Committee on Human Research (which explains four categories of risk under "additional protections" for child subjects with reference to federal regulations). Available at: http://www.jhsph.edu/chr/Childrens_guidelines.pdf (accessed June 24, 2003); *Informed Consent Guide for the Institutional Review Board* of the University of Southern California Health Sciences Campus, November 2, 1999 (which provides informed-consent requirements based on DHHS and FDA regulations, including the consent and assent procedures for research with children). Available at: http://ccnt.hsc.usc.edu/irb/irb.html (accessed June 23, 2003).

5. 45 CFR 46.402(a) (emphasis added).

6. 45 CFR 46.402(e).

7. Taussig HN. 2002. Risk behaviors in maltreated youth placed in foster care: a longitudinal study of protective and vulnerability factors. *Child Abuse & Neglect* 26:1179–1199 (study examining protective and vulnerability factors in foster care youth); Child Welfare League of America. National Fact Sheet 2003: Making Children a National Priority. Available at: http://www.cwla.org/advocacy/nationalfactsheet03.htm (accessed October 23, 2003) (citing evidence that children whose families do not receive appropriate treatment for alcohol and other drug abuse are more likely to end up in foster care, remain in foster care longer, and reenter foster care once they have returned home than are children whose families do receive treatment).

8. English A. 1995. Guidelines for adolescent health research: legal perspectives. *Journal of Adolescent Health* 17:277–286; Santelli J, et al. 2003. Guidelines for adolescent health research. A position paper for the Society of Adolescent Medicine. *Journal of Adolescent Health* 33(5):396–409; Hartman RG. 2002. Coming of age: devising legislation for adolescent medical decision-making. *American Journal of Law and Medicine* 28:409–453; Broome ME, Stieglitz KA. 1992. The consent process and children. *Research in Nursing & Health* 15:147–152.

9. See, e.g., Ariz. Rev. Stat. Ann. 44-132.

10. See, e.g., Ind. Code Ann. 16-36-1-3; Maine Rev. Stat. Ann. Tit. 15, 3506A.

11. See, e.g., Calif. Fam. Code 7002(c), 7120-7122; N.C. Gen. Stat. 7B-3500.

12. See, e.g., *Connecticut Office of Legislative Research (OLR) Research Report 2002-R-0008* (emancipation of minors under common law). Note also that emancipation likely also released parents from debts arising from their children's decisions. See, e.g., Support of Minors and Emancipation, State of Michigan, 37th Circuit Court, Family Division Justice Center, April 2000; Conn. Gen. Stat. Sec. 46b-150(d)(a) (emancipation order allows minor to "consent to mental, dental, or psychiatric care, without parental consent, knowledge, *or liability*" (emphasis added); W.Va. Code 49-7-27 (parents or custodians of emancipated minor not obligated to provide care of financial support); Wy. Stat. 14-1-202(a)(iii) (emancipation terminates parental tort liability for minor).

13. Conn. Gen. Stat. Sec. 46b-150(d)(a).

14. Md. Code Ann., Est. & Tr. Art. 13, sec. 503(c) (a minor 15 or older may contract for annuities or life insurance for self).

15. For explicitly including right to make health care decisions among legal effects of emancipation, see Calif. Family Code sec. 7050(e)(1) (effects of emancipation include minor's capacity to "consent to medical, dental, or psychiatric care, without parental consent, knowledge, or liability"); Conn. Title 46B, Ch. 815t sec. 46b-150d(a) (emancipated minor may "consent to medical, dental, or psychiatric care, without parental consent, knowledge, or liability"). But see, e.g., Md. Code Ann., Est. & Tr. Art. 13 sec. 503(a) (a married minor may buy/sell property if spouse of age); Md. Code Ann., Est. & Tr. Art. 13 sec. 503(c) (at age 15 an individual may contract for insurance); Md. Code Ann., Est. & Tr. Art. 13 sec. 503(b) (a minor in the military can enter real estate transactions); N.C. Gen. Stat. 7B-3507 (final decree of emancipation gives the minor or petitioner the "same right to make contracts and conveyances, to sue and to be sued, and to transact business as if the petitioner were an adult").

16. A. Campbell, personal communication (with Abigail English, JD, Director, Center for Adolescent Health & The Law), August 5, 2003.

17. See, e.g., W.Va. Code 16-30-3(o) (which defines a "mature minor" as "a person less than eighteen years of age who has been determined by a qualified physician, a qualified psychologist or an advanced nurse practitioner to have the capacity to make health care decisions).

18. *Restatement (Second) of Torts*, sec. 892A, cmt.b (1979).

19. But cf. *Novak v. Cobb County-Kennestone Hospital Authority*, 849 F.Supp 1559 (N.D. Ga. 1994), *aff'd* 74 F.3d 1173 (11th Cir. 1996) (which declined to recognize mature minor exception pursuant to O.C.G.A. sec. 31-9-7).

20. See, e.g., Id. Code 39-4302; Ark. Stat. Ann. 20-13-104, 20-9-106, 20-9-60; Miss. Code Ann. 41-41-3.

21. Ala. Code 22-8-4.

22. Calif. Family Code 6922 (applies only to minors age 15 years or older who are living apart from their parents and managing their own affairs); Oregon Rev. Stat. 109.640.

23. S.C.C.A. 20-7-280 (for health services other than operations, unless the operation is deemed essential to the health and the life of child).

24. See, e.g., Colo. Rev. Stat. 13-22-103; Ind. Code Ann. 16-36-1-3; 22 Maine Rev. Stat. 1503.

25. See, e.g., Va. Code Ann. 54-2969.

26. For further discussion of the extent and limits of minor medical decision-making, see Stenger RL. 1999/2000. Exclusive or concurrent competence to make medical decisions for adolescents in the United States and United Kingdom. *Journal of Law and Health* 14(209):208–241.

27. Santelli J, et al. 2003. Guidelines for adolescent health research: a position paper for the Society of Adolescent Medicine. *Journal of Adolescent Health* 33(5):396–409.

28. See, e.g., 25 Tex. Admin. Code 405.409 (which requires minor's assent for research of mental health patients); 25 Tex. Admin. Code 414.758 (special conditions for greater-than-minimal-risk research and research with minors); 25 Tex. Admin. Code 414.754 (which provides special rules for research with persons involuntarily committed to Texas Department of Mental Health and Mental Retardation facilities); Va. Code Ann. 32.1-162.16, 32.1-162.18, 32.1-162.19, 12 Va. Admin. Code 5-20-10, 5-20-100, 35-180-10 (research connected with Department of Health and Department of Mental Health facilities must adhere to special requirements for nontherapeutic, greater-than-minimal-risk research); V.C.A. 32.1-16.16 (in which nontherapeutic research is defined as having no reasonable expectation of direct benefit to the physical or mental condition of the subject); Calif. H&S Code 24178 (A.B. 2328, signed September 11, 2002, as Chap. 477, which allows for surrogate consent to research in certain situations); Calif. H&S Code 111530 (which requires parental/guardian consent and minor assent if the child is age 7 years or older for experimental use of drugs with minors); 15 Calif. Code Regs. 1454 (which provides specific rules for clinical research with juveniles in the state corrections system); Del. HSS Policy Memo No. 55 (July 1992) (clients served by Delaware Health & Social Services may not be research subjects unless the Human Subjects Review Board approves the research and the research is compatible with DHHS [federal] regulations); D.C.C. 21-2047 (the guardian of an incapacitated person may not consent to experimental treatment or research); D.C. Code 6-1969 (a parent or guardian may act as a legally appointed representative (LAR) for experimental research with mentally retarded individuals); Ohio Admin. Code 5122-28-05 (which considers a parent or guardian of a minor to be the LAR for research subject to the authority of the Department of Mental Health); Ohio Admin. Code 5122-28-05(A)(4) (consent age of 18 for research subject to Department of Mental Health regulation); Code of Maine Regs. 14-193-001(XI); 14-142-001(XI) (for children receiving services from Bureau of Children with Special Needs, clinical research laws require full written informed consent, assent by minors over age 12, approval of clinical director for off-label use of FDA-approved drug, Research and Experimental Review Board review, and compliance with federal DHHS regulations; a special review process is required if research with minors presents greater than minimal risk).

29. This link was made in a prominent report issued by the National Commission for the Protection of Human Subjects of Biomedical and Behavioral Research, which recommended allowing minor consent to research when the research is conducted in or relates to the types of care to which minors can consent in the treatment context. National Commission for the Protection of Human Subjects of Biomedical and Behavioral Research. 1977. *Report and Recommendations: Research Involving Children*. DHEW publication (OS) 77-0004. Washington, D.C.: U.S. Government Printing Office.

30. See, e.g., English A. 1995. Guidelines for adolescent health research: legal perspectives. *Journal of Adolescent Health* 17:277–286; Nelson RM. 2001. Nontherapeutic research minimal risk, and the Kennedy Krieger Lead Abatement Study. *IRB: Ethics & Human Research* 23(6):7–11.

31. See, e.g., *Cohen v. Bolduc*, No. SJC-08544 (Mass. 01/11/2002) ("We conclude that, absent an express limitation by the principal in the health care proxy itself, the proxy statute does not prevent an agent from making that treatment decision, provided the principal does not object."). Available at: http://caselaw.lp.findlaw.com/scripts/getcase.pl?court=ma&vol=sjcslip/8554&invol=1.

32. *Cardwell v. Bechtol*, 724 S.W. 2d 739, 743-4 (Tenn. 1987) (citations omitted). The *Cardwell* case is preeminent among recent cases in its clear enunciation of the origins of and reasoning behind the "mature minor" exception, as well as its explanation, cited here, of the flexibility of the law in adapting to changing conditions and the openness to a context-sensitive interpretation of actions in the absence of specific relevant legislative enactments. For a further discussion of *Cardwell*, see text accompanying notes 82–84, infra. Complicating

matters, however, states may choose to remove this flexibility in interpretation in the face of silence by explicitly superseding common law through statutory means. See, e.g., N.C. Gen. Stat. 7B-3509 (which supersedes the common law of emancipation, other than by marriage).

33. 45 CFR 46.402(b).

34, For useful suggestions for developing guidance to clarify "assent" and "consent" in research with children, see Broome ME, Stieglitz KA. 1992. The consent process and children. *Research in Nursing & Health* 15:147–152. See also American Academy of Pediatrics. 1995. Informed consent, parental permission, and assent in pediatric patients. *Pediatrics* 95:314–317; Wendler D, Shah S. 2003. Should children decide whether they are enrolled in non-beneficial research? *American Journal of Bioethics* 3(4):1–7 (which argues that the "assent" threshold should be set at age 14 and that a "dissent" requirement should also be adopted for nonbeneficial research).

35. See, e.g., National Institutes of Health (NIH) Policy and Guidelines on the Inclusion of Children as Participants in Research Involving Human Subjects, released March 6, 1998. Available at: http://grants1.nih.gov/grants/guide/notice-files/not98-024.html (accessed June 23, 2003) (for grant proposals received by NIH after October 1, 1998, the website sets forth policy and guidelines for inclusion of children (defined as youth up to age 21) to encourage NIH-supported research with children); Best Pharmaceuticals for Children Act, January 4, 2002 (P.L. 107-109) (which extends the pediatric exclusivity provision of the Food and Drug Administration Modernization Act of 1997 (P.L. 105-115), which sunset on January 1, 2002, through 2007; note that the exclusivity provision provides marketing incentives to manufacturers that conduct drug studies with children by extending patent protection for 6 months in return for such studies); Regulations Requiring Manufacturers to Assess the Safety and Effectiveness of New Drugs and Biological Products in Pediatric Patients (FDA Pediatric Rule), 21 CFR sec. 201, 312, 314, 601, 63 FR 66632, December 2, 1998 (which requires manufacturers of certain products to provide sufficient data and information to support directions for pediatric use for the claimed indications). Note that the Pediatric Rule was struck down in October 2002 by a federal court as exceeding FDA's statutory authority (*Association of American Physicians and Surgeons, Inc. v. United States Food and Drug Administration*, Civil Action No. 02-02898 (Dist. Ct. D.C., October 17, 2002); however, DHHS worked with Congress to pass similar federal legislation requiring pharmaceutical companies to conduct clinical drug trials with children (see Bush Administration will Seek New Legislation for Mandatory Pediatric Drug Testing, DHHS Press Release, December 16, 2002. Available at: http://www.hhs.gov/news/press/2002pres/20021216c.html (accessed June 23, 2003)). The Pediatric Research Equity Act of 2003 was signed into law on December 5, 2003.

36. See, e.g., Md. Health-General Article Cod. Ann. Sec. 13-2001 et seq. (2002).

37. *Grimes v. Kennedy Krieger Institute, Inc.*, 366 Md. 29, 782 A.2d 807 (2001) (hereinafter *Grimes*); see also Mastroianni A, Kahn JP. 2002. Risk and responsibility: ethics, *Grimes v. Kennedy Krieger*, and public health research involving children. *American Journal of Public Health*.92(7):1073–1076.

38. 45 CFR 46.409.

39. 45 CFR 46.409(a).

40. 45 CFR 46.409(b).

41. A. Campbell, personal communication (with Mary Jane Davis, Asst. General Counsel, Tennessee Department of Children's Services), July 21, 2003. Tennessee's Department of Children's Services is currently revising its informed-consent policy to clarify this presumption of parental consent authority. TN DCS Policy 20.24, eff. 02/01/00, rev'd. 05/09/03 (draft copy on file with author).

42. *Pierce v. Society of Sisters*, 268 U.S. 510 (1925) (which upholds the liberty interest of parents to direct upbringing and education of children); *Parham v. J.R.*, 442 U.S. 584 (1979) (which states that parents' liberty interests in raising children extends to decisions over whether

to institutionalize children with mental illness, although parental discretion is not absolute). It is also worth noting that in the *Parham* decision, the U.S. Supreme Court determined that there did not need to be a separate process for initial admission decisions for inpatient commitment of children for children who were wards of the state (versus children whose natural parents sought admission). In so holding, the Court stated that, "Since the state agency having custody and control of the child in loco parentis has a duty to consider the best interests of the child with respect to a decision on commitment to a mental hospital, the State may constitutionally allow that custodial agency to speak for the child, subject, of course, to the restrictions governing natural parents" (*Parham*, 442 U.S. 584, 619).

43. See, e.g., Utah Department of Human Services IRB. *Procedures & Instructions for Researchers. Department of Human Services Resource Manual*, eff. February 24, 2003 (copy on file with author).

44. A. Campbell, personal communication (with Dr. Page B. Walley, Commissioner, Alabama Department of Children's Affairs), June 16, 2003.

45. See, e.g., Utah Department of Human Services IRB. *Procedures & Instructions for Researchers. Department of Human Services Resource Manual*, eff. February 24, 2003; State of Tennessee Department of Children's Services. *Research Proposals. Administrative Policies & Procedures*: 6.1, eff. February 1, 2000, rev'd. November 1, 2001 (copy on file with author).

46. Maryland Department of the Environment. Lead Poisoning Prevention Program. *Childhood Blood Lead Surveillance in Maryland. 1999 Annual Report.* Released February, 2001. Available at: http://www.mde.state.md.us/assets/document/LeadCoordination/leadreport99.pdf (accessed August 11 2003.

47. Maryland Department of Health and Mental Hygiene. Community and Public Health Administration. Center for Maternal and Child Health. Childhood Lead Screening Program. *Targeting Plan for Areas at Risk for Childhood Lead Poisoning.* May 2000. Available at: http://www.fha.state.md.us/och/html/stp.html (accessed August 11, 2003).

48. Maryland Department of the Environment. *Annual Report 2000*, p. 53. Available at: http://www.mde.state.md.us/assets/document/AboutMDE/annualreport.pdf (accessed August 11, 2003).

49. *Grimes* at 807.

50. *Grimes* at 818, 819, 842.

51. Id. at 819.

52. For interesting discussions of the merits and the ramifications of the decision, see Kopelman LM. 2002. Pediatric research regulations under legal scrutiny: *Grimes* narrows their interpretation. *Journal of Law, Medicine & Ethics*;30:38–49; Glantz LH. 2002. Nontherapeutic research with children: *Grimes v. Kennedy Krieger Institute. American Journal of Public Health* 92(7):1070–1073.

53. *Grimes* at 816–817.

54. Id. at note 6.

55. Id. at 850.

56. Nelson RM. 2001. Nontherapeutic research minimal risk, and the Kennedy Krieger Lead Abatement Study. *IRB: Ethics & Human Research*23(6):7–11, 8–9.

57. *Grimes* at 853 ("not in best interest of any healthy child to be intentionally put in a nontherapeutic situation where his or her health may be impaired, in order to test methods that may ultimately benefit all children").

58. See, e.g. Alliance for Human Protection. **A landmark decision by Maryland's highest court ... Infomail.** August, 20, 2001. Available at: http://www.researchprotection.org/infomail/0801/20.html (accessed June 20, 2003).

59. Kopelman LM. 2002. Pediatric research regulations under legal scrutiny: *Grimes* narrows their interpretation. *Journal of Law, Medicine & Ethics*,30:38–49; Nelson RM. 2001.

Nontherapeutic research minimal risk, and the Kennedy Krieger Lead Abatement Study. *IRB: Ethics & Human Research* 23(6):7–11.

60. See, e.g., University of Maryland Baltimore County IRB. Requirements for Research Involving Children. Updated March 11, 2002. Available at: http://www.umbc.edu/irb/Children.htm (accessed June 21, 2003).

61. Md. Health-General Code Ann. Sec. 13-2001 et seq. (2002).

62. A. Campbell, personal communication (with Jack Schwartz, Assistant Attorney General, State of Maryland), June 20, 2003.

63. *Grimes* at 862.

64. See, e.g., Sharav VH. 2003. Children in clinical research: a conflict of moral values. *The American Journal of Bioethics* 3(1):1–81. Available at: http://www.bioethics.net/journal/infocus/pdf/sharav.pdf (accessed February 25, 2004).

65. For more information on the Willowbrook scandal, see Bonita L. Weddle, *Mental Health in New York State, 1945–1998: An Historical Overview*. New York State Archives: New York. Available at: http://www.archives.nysed.gov/includes/g/researchroom/c_rr_health_mh_hist.html (accessed June 23, 2003).

66. NY Cons. Law Services Pub Health sec. 2442.

67. *T.D. v. N.Y. State Office of Mental Health*, 165 Misc. 2d 62, 626 N.Y.S.2d 1015 (1995).

68. *T.D. v. N.Y. State Office of Mental Health*, 228 A.D.2d 95 (1996) (hereinafter *T.D.*).

69. Id. at 100.

70. Id. at 123.

71. Id. at 124.

72. Id. at 120; see also *Grimes* at 817.

73. *T.D.* at 124-5, citing NYCRR 527.10(e)(3)(iii).

74. See, however, 45 CFR 46.408(c) (which allows the waiver of parental permission if it is not a reasonable requirement for the subjects involved, e.g., abused and neglected children). This federal regulation allows for protection of minors by waiving parental consent, so long as another mechanism is in place for their protection and it is in accord with state and local law. The New York court suggests—at least for studies with abused or neglected children that are not federally funded and that are nontherapeutic and present greater than minimal risk— local commissioners of health are the appropriate, and necessary, consenting authorities; surrogate consent or a waiver of "guardian" consent is not appropriate. *T.D.* at 124–125.

75. The court argues that the OMH regulations' surrogate consent provisions are unacceptable for greater-than-minimal-risk nontherapeutic research in light of earlier treatment-related holdings and the state's interest in child health and welfare as *parens patriae*, suggesting such research may lead to the same result at "denial of necessary medical treatment" (Id. at 124).

76. See, e.g., *Grimes* at 840 and *T.D.* at 127.

77. *Grimes* at 855; see also *T.D.* at 122–123 (need for notice and judicial review).

78. *In re the Matter of Rena*, 705 N.E.2d 1155, 1157 (Mass. App. Ct. 1999). See also *In re E.G.*, 549 N.E.2d 322 (Ill. 1989) (Jehovah's Witness case in which the Illinois Supreme Court applied substituted judgment standard to see whether a minor was sufficiently mature to make informed decision); *In re Swan*, 569 A.2d 1202 (Maine 1990) (the state's highest court holds that evidence of the wishes of a minor with the capacity to weigh risks and benefits in refusing life-sustaining treatment is an important factor). But c.f. *In re Application of Long Island Jewish Medical Ctr.*, 557 N.Y.S.2d 239 (Sup. Ct. 1990) (the court orders a transfusion for a 17-year old over his objection under the *parens patriae* doctrine, without consideration of "mature minor" framework, another example of New York's conservative approach).

79. *In re Rena* at 1156–1157.

80. Id. at 1157.

81. Id. at note 2, citing Mass. G.L. c. 112, sec. 12S.

82. *Cardwell v. Bechtol*, 724 S.W. 2d 739 (Tenn. 1987).

83. Id. at 745.

84. Id. at 749 ("for the jury to determine whether the minor has the capacity to consent to and appreciate the nature, the risks, and the consequences of the medical treatment involved"). In this case, the court ruled that the minor, a female 5 months shy of 18 years of age, had the capacity and maturity to consent to treatment for a herniated disk.

85. See Stenger RL. 1999/2000. Exclusive or concurrent competence to make medical decisions for adolescents in the United States and United Kingdom. *Journal of Law and Health* 14(209):208–241.

86. National Commission for the Protection of Human Subjects of Biomedical Research. 1977. *Research Involving Children: Report and Recommendations*. DHEW publication (OS) 77-0044. Washington, D.C.: U.S. Government Printing Office, (which suggests that adolescents' legal ability under state law to consent to certain medical treatments without need for parental permission, indicative of adolescent capacity, should extend to research context for same conditions). See also, Santelli J, et al. 2003. Guidelines for adolescent health research: a position paper for the Society of Adolescent Medicine. *Journal of Adolescent Health* 33(5): 396–409.

87. Mastroianni A, Kahn JP. 2002. Risk and responsibility: ethics, *Grimes v. Kennedy Krieger*, and public health research involving children. *American Journal of Public Health* 92(7):1073–1076; Rogers AS, D'Angelo L, Futterman D. 1994. Guidelines for adolescent participation in research: current realities and possible resolutions. *IRB: Ethics & Human Research* 16(4):1–6, 3–4; Santelli J, et al. 2003. Guidelines for adolescent health research: a position paper for the Society of Adolescent Medicine. *Journal of Adolescent Health* 33(5): 396–409.

88. See Hartman RG. 2002. Coming of age: devising legislation for adolescent medical decision-making. *American Journal of Law and Medicine* 28:409–453. For examples of studies that might benefit the policy-making community, see Bernhardt BA, et al. 2003. Parents' and children's attitudes toward the enrollment of minors in genetic susceptibility research: implications for informed consent. *American Journal of Medical Genetics* 116A:315–323 (which assesses parents' and children's reactions to disease susceptibility research and perceptions of risks and benefits of participating); Oleschnowicz JQ, et al. 2002. Assent observed: children's involvement in leukemia treatment and research discussions. *Pediatrics* 109:806–814 (which examines the role of older children in discussing recent diagnosis of leukemia and treatment options including enrollment in a randomized, clinical trial); Rogers AS, Schwartz DF, Weissman G, English A. 1999. A case study in adolescent participation in clinical research: eleven clinical sites, one common protocol, and eleven IRBs. *IRB: Ethics & Human Research* 21(1):6–10 (which investigates decision-making by IRBs with respect to one common study protocol recruiting minor adolescents for HIV/STD study).

89. See, e.g., Brown K.2003. The medication merry-go-round. *Science* 299:1646–1649; Meadows M. 2003. Drug research and children. *FDA Consumer Magazine* January–February. Available at: http://www.fda.gov/fdac/features/2003/103_drugs.html (accessed March 24, 2003).

90. See, e.g., The Alliance for Human Research Protection (AHRP). Its listserv and website increasingly draw attention to research with children, especially pharmaceutical research; for example, see the recent alert to recent developments in the United Kingdom where the British government disapproved a license for Seroxat (Paxil) for use by children and adolescents based on adverse events in recent clinical trials. GlascoSmithKline [sic] PAXIL Warning Letter to Health Care Professionals. *AHRP News Alert*, June 19, 2003. Available at: http://www.ahrp.org/infomail/0603/19.html (accessed June 23, 2003).

91. 45 CFR Parts 160 and 164 (Standards for Privacy of Individually Identifiable Health Information, implementing requirements set forth in the Health Insurance Portability and Accountability Act of 1996).

92. For a state example of the latter, see Va. Code Ann. 32.1-162.16 (which defines "nontherapeutic research" as that which holds "no reasonable prospect of direct benefit to the physical or mental condition of the human subject."). A point to illuminate: Does "direct benefit" mean benefit to the subject's well-being generally or only specifically to that condition or disorder under investigation?

ADDENDUM B1

Hypothetical Research Studies with Children in State Custody: How Might States Respond?

The following hypothetical research protocols, followed by hypothetical state responses to the regulation of such (based on inquiries made of researchers and regulators in a number of states), may serve to highlight the myriad of approaches applied to research studies involving youth in state custody. They were developed in consultation with researchers focused on the foster care population and were circulated to researchers whose work touches upon these issues in numerous states, as well as representatives of state child welfare departments (or the relevant agencies who regulate such research) for feedback. The comments below are not those of a single respondent; rather, they illustrate the collective wisdom of the respondents; that is, researchers and regulators.

Scenario 1: Behavioral Study

Faculty at a state university's Center for Research in Child and Adolescent Health (the Center) wish to add to their colleagues' work in documenting risk factors for adolescents in foster care. An earlier study from the Center found that adolescents in foster care often have multiple psychosocial and mental health problems that place them at risk for early sexual experiences and HIV infection. The researchers wish to identify such risk factors at early stages to better prevent such later effects. Thus, they propose to target preteens (children ages 9 to 12) in foster care and collect information about substance abuse, sexual activity, maltreatment, and suicidal intent to identify discernible interrelationships among factors that might contribute to early sexual experiences and other HIV-related behaviors (e.g., use of needles to inject illegal drugs). This prospective study will involve 400 youth ages 9 to 12 in foster care. At the onset of the project, children will be given a battery of psychiatric, social, and adaptive functioning measures to gauge mental health risk and protective factors. They will then be monitored for 5 years to identify patterns of behavior. Children will be drawn from multiple sites in four different states.

Was your (foster care/child welfare) office confronted with this situation, or if a similar proposal was brought before it, did it/might it permit these children to participate in the study? Please explain.

More regulatory or restrictive state Obviously, the most restrictive stance would be to bar such research with children in state custody outright. Beyond that, however, there could likely be "exceptions" to the ban (e.g., for "special cause") or a slightly more permissive stance with tight control via departmental regulation.

For example, State A (say) has its own Research Review Board that reviews all requests for conducting research with its client population (by providing access to confidential records or data or direct access to the clients). Its review criteria track those provided for in federal regulations; however, special attention is paid to the "vulnerability" of its subject population, and more invasive research methods (including surveys with highly sensitive information) are scrutinized closely. Informed consent is required: the presumption is in favor of seeking parental consent for children, unless parental rights have been terminated, even though the Department has legal authority for approving "ordinary medical care" for children in its custody. If parental rights are not terminated and if parents are not causing harm to their children, their objection to research will bar their child's participation. Additional review and reconsent are required if there are any changes in the protocol; similarly, reconsent is required if the custodial status of the child changes (e.g., the child is placed with a new foster parent).

Or consider State B, in which requests for direct access to child clients is subject to court approval. It is further stipulated that the caseworker for each child must consent on the child's behalf, as well as obtain the child's assent.

Less regulatory or restrictive state Falling closer to the less restrictive end of the continuum, State C allows research, including access to confidential data and direct client access, if the research protocol is approved by the researcher's own IRB. The researcher must sign a confidentiality agreement and agree not to include personally identifying information in subsequent research reports. Consent for client participation is generally given by the Department of Children & Families (DCF) acting as the custodian for the children. Although the Department's regulations focus on confidentiality, it is expected that research that targets the needs of children in state custody and the needs of the DCF and also that DCF's resources (e.g., staff) will not be stretched in complying with research.

Scenario 2: Research Tied to Clinical Needs

In the early years of HIV infection, there was no treatment for the disease. Many babies who were born infected were placed in foster care because their mothers were too sick to care for them, and most mothers died before the babies' first birthday. When zidovudine (AZT) began to be tested in studies with adults, many pediatric HIV physicians wanted to do clinical trials with HIV-infected children, including these babies, since nothing else was available to save their lives.

Was your (foster care/child welfare) office confronted with this situation, or if a similar proposal was brought before it, did it/might it permit these children to participate in the study? Please explain.

More regulatory or restrictive state States A and B, which were slightly more permissive of noninvasive research, prohibit medical or pharmaceutical experimentation and thus choose to bar this research. As this is far beyond what they consider "ordinary care and treatment" for pediatric populations, they are that much more cautious about enrolling children under their custody, who face their own host of vulnerabilities.

Less regulatory or restrictive state State C is also highly concerned by this hypothetical research and would require ample showing of cause or medical justification for the treatment methods contained within the protocol; that is, there must be some physician documentation that the testing is being conducted with all pediatric populations, not simply those in foster care, and that it is medically warranted and not purely an experiment without some data backing AZT's use. Furthermore, the children's prognoses must be sufficiently poor as to balance the risks of the research. Close monitoring by the host institution's IRB is also expected. Consent will be required by each caseworker, who will act somewhat like an ombudsperson for his or her clients.

Overall Comments: Conducting Research in a State of Flux

Based on a query of noted researchers in the field, as well as a sampling of the opinions of regulators from select (larger) states, it seems that the more likely approach to the inclusion of wards of the state in research cannot be depicted as either black or white (i.e., as routinely permissive or routinely negative), but rather resembles shades of gray. That is, researchers likely face a continuum of permissibility, based on the county or local atmosphere, the population involved (including age), the risks inherent in the study, whether the study has a medically indicated or therapeutic" connection (e.g., treatment, say, with a new anti-HIV medication for youth is available only within the context of research protocol) or seems more purely research based or experimental, etc. As the research risks increase (e.g., in the AZT study described above), it is more likely that the research will be prohibited or at the very least subjected to much greater regulatory scrutiny and monitoring, whereas survey research and the like might be approached more favorably, with fewer restrictions. Children who are wards of the state (e.g., in juvenile detention facilities or psychiatric institutions) are more likely to be excluded from participation than children in physical custody of the state (e.g., foster care).

The lack of black-and-white approaches is not necessarily a problem; in fact, it likely represents the best course given the need for individualization of studies to match individual or local community needs. Such flexibility is also in keeping with the federal government's emphasis on local review, notably, through the IRB structure. However, this results in a situation of uncertainty for researchers, who are advised to build rapport with local regulators and routinely confer with these regulators—as well as ethics and legal counsel—to ensure that a proper balance is maintained between research needs and the protection of vulnerable children and adolescents.

C

HEALTH CARE PRIVACY AND CONFLICT-OF-INTEREST REGULATIONS RELEVANT TO PROTECTION OF HUMAN PARTICIPANTS IN RESEARCH

In addition to regulations aimed explicitly at the protection of human participants in research, other statutes, regulations, policy statements, and guidelines may also contribute to such protection. Regulations on the privacy and confidentiality of personal health information and the disclosure and management of financial conflicts of interest in research are briefly discussed below.

PRIVACY, RESEARCH PROTECTIONS, AND HIPAA

As one of the criteria for institutional review board (IRB) approval of research, Subpart A requires IRBs to determine "when appropriate, [that] there are adequate provisions to protect the privacy of subjects and to maintain the confidentiality of data" (45 CFR 46.111(a)(7)). For research involving only medical records or stored biological samples, the primary issue in protecting research participants involves threats to privacy.

In April 2003, new regulations on privacy went into effect under the

Health Insurance Portability and Accountability Act of 1996 (P.L. 104-191), commonly referred to as HIPAA. The main target of HIPAA was not researchers but health care providers and health insurance plans. In general, the law requires that covered providers and plans

    1.   notify patients or plan members of their privacy rights and how their protected personal health information can be used without special authorization;
    2.   obtain authorization from individuals, under certain circumstances, before releasing information for other purposes;
    3.   secure patient records so that those who should not have access to them do not; and
    4.   create policies and procedures to implement the law.

Under HIPAA, parents usually act as "personal representatives" of the child for the purposes of receiving the required notice of privacy rights, signing authorization for the release of protection information, and obtaining access to information about the child. HIPAA does not require the provision of any information to children and is generally silent on institutional responsibilities to children.

The law does not require permission from patients for health care providers, health plans, and health care clearinghouses to use information as part of their normal activities of providing health care or administering health benefits. For other purposes, including research, the law requires a specific, written authorization for covered organizations to release personal information that is protected under the law. If information is stripped of elements that would allow an individual to be identified, providers and health plans can provide it without written authorization. Some other exceptions to the authorization requirement are also permitted, for example, for certain activities related to preparations for research (e.g., identifying potential research participants by identifying individuals with relevant diagnoses or other characteristics).

Institutional review boards (IRBs) have been concerned about how the requirements under HIPAA might interact with their responsibilities for considering protections for privacy and confidentiality in research. Some questions involve the relationship between informed consent for research and HIPAA authorization for the release of personal health information. As explained in a National Institutes of Health (NIH) document describing the privacy rule, "an *authorization* focuses on privacy and states how, why, and to whom the [personal health information] will be used and/or disclosed for research. An *informed consent* . . . provides research subjects with a description of the study and of its anticipated risks and/or benefits,

and a description of how the confidentiality of records will be protected"
(NIH, 2003b, p. 11, emphasis added).

For research purposes, HIPAA provides that an IRB (or a specially
created Privacy Board, usually for institutions that do not have IRBs) may
waive the requirement for authorization under certain conditions. Among
other conditions, the research must involve no more than minimal risk,
include a plan for protecting the information, and be impractical to undertake without the protected information and the waiver of the authorization
requirement.

The law requires IRBs to review waiver requests, but it does not require
IRBs to review authorizations required under HIPAA. Because the authorization is often part of the consent form for the research, IRBs do review the
authorizations that are part of these forms.

Among researchers studying adolescents, there is some concern that
parents may have access to information about adolescents that would otherwise be held confidential. The final HIPAA regulations defer to state laws
on parental access to the health records of minors. The regulations do not
themselves protect the privacy of this information (Nicoletti, 2003).

Independent of HIPAA, NIH has created Certificates of Confidentiality
that can be issued to research institutions to cover research projects that
collect sensitive information about research participants that might damage
them if disclosed (NIH, 2003a). The purpose of the certificates is to protect
the privacy of research participants by protecting investigators and institutions from being compelled to release identifying information in any federal, state, or local civil, criminal, administrative, legislative, or other proceeding. (The certificates do allow for the provision of information for
DHHS audits and as required by the Federal Food, Drug, and Cosmetic
Act.) Projects must have IRB approval and meet other requirements.

FINANCIAL CONFLICT OF INTEREST

*The public must trust that investigators make [research] deci-
sions solely on the basis of their professional judgment, without
regard for personal gain. Financial conflicts of interest may undermine that trust.*

Lo et al., 2000, p. 1618

A 2002 IOM report on integrity in scientific research defined a conflict
of interest in research as existing "when [an investigator] has interests in the
outcome of the research that may lead to a personal advantage and that
might therefore, in actuality or appearance, compromise the integrity of the
research" (IOM/NRC, 2002, p. 38; see also IOM, 2003). As the financial
rewards from many kinds of biomedical research have increased and as

investigators and research institutions have increasingly sought to participate in reaping those rewards, policymakers, ethicists, and others have become more concerned that conflicts of interest will compromise science and harm research participants. Although these concerns do not, in general, differ as when they involve adult or pediatric research, they are part of the broad context for considering the strengths and limitations of current regulatory protections for research involving children.

Potential avenues for managing, reducing, or eliminating identified or possible conflicts of interest in research vary depending on the nature and the seriousness of the conflict. Options include public disclosure of significant financial interests, relinquishing by investigators of such interests by investigators, independent monitoring of research, changes in the research plan, or changes in the investigators involved in some or all of the research. Most academic and similar institutions have conflict-of-interest policies that govern a variety of activities, including research. The National Bioethics Advisory Commission has recommended that academic institutions be more actively involved in managing investigators' and IRB members' conflicts of interest (NBAC, 2001).

In 1995, the NIH and the National Science Foundation (NSF) published policies on investigator financial conflicts of interest involving research funded by these agencies (NIH, 2000).[1] A recent review by NIH of institutional conflict-of-interest policies revealed considerable variation and some deficits, particularly in the clarity of policies for reporting conflicting interests (NIH, 2002). The review did not attempt to assess the implementation of the policies and did not single out any deficits related specifically to pediatric research. FDA rules do not require the disclosure of information until after the research has been completed and a sponsor submits a marketing application (GAO, 2001; see also, draft guidance from the FDA on financial relationships and interests in research [FDA, 2003]). Although federal rules do not require IRBs to assess investigator financial conflict of interest and many institutions lodge all responsibility for such assessments elsewhere, some institutions have adopted policies that require disclosure of such conflicts to IRBs and, less commonly, to research subjects (Lo et al., 2000).

In 2001, the General Accounting Office (GAO) reported that about one-quarter of IRBs consider financial arrangements between investigators

---

[1]The NIH and NSF policies require institutions receiving funds to (1) maintain a written, enforced policy on financial conflict of interest; (2) inform research investigators of that policy, the associated reporting responsibilities, and the related federal regulations; and (3) report to awarding offices the existence of any conflicting interests and ensure that the interests have been managed, reduced, or eliminated in accordance with the regulations.

and research sponsors (GAO, 2001). In addition, most major scientific journals require disclosure by authors of financial conflicts of interest as a condition of publication.

An IOM committee recently recommended that reviews of possible conflicts of interest involving investigators, primary research staff, and IRB members should be conducted by a committee specifically created for that purpose. Furthermore, the body should be "shielded from institutional pressures or influence" and should transmit its findings to the IRB. The committee also recommended the establishment of an *external* body to review potential institutional conflicts of interest in research and report the findings to the IRB (IOM, 2003).

The focus of conflict-of-interest discussions is usually on the individual investigator or on the commercial sponsors of research. Academic institutions may also have conflicts of interest relevant to research undertaken by their members. For example, medical centers and other research institutions are increasingly involved in profitable partnerships with industry and may receive substantial income from patents and royalties resulting from the research.

No federal regulations apply directly to *institutional* conflicts of interest. In interim guidance on financial relationships in clinical research, the U.S. Department of Health and Human Services has, however, observed that institutions "should not lose sight of the need to manage their own conflicts of interest as well" and that "[t]he financial interest of the institution in the successful outcome of the trial could directly influence the conduct of the trial, including enrollment of subjects, adverse event reporting or evaluation of efficacy data (OHRP, 2001). In the latter case, the guidance suggests that institutions consider having independent investigators conduct a trial if the institution has a financial stake in the outcome.

REFERENCES

FDA (Food and Drug Administration). 2003. Draft financial relationships and interests in research involving human subjects: Guidance for human subject protection. *Federal Register* 68:15456–15460.

GAO (Government Accounting Office). 2001. Biomedical Research: HHS Direction Needed to Address Financial Conflicts of Interest. *Report to the Ranking Minority Member, Subcommittee on Public Health, Committee on Health, Education, Labor, and Pensions, U.S. Senate.* [Online]. Available: http://www.gao.gov/new.items/d0289.pdf [accessed March 11, 2004].

IOM (Institute of Medicine). 2003. *Responsible Research: A Systems Approach to Protecting Research Participants.* Washington, DC: The National Academies Press.

IOM/NRC (National Research Council). 2002. *Integrity in Scientific Research: Creating an Environment That Promotes Responsible Conduct.* Washington, DC: The National Academies Press.

Lo B, Wolf LE, Berkeley A. 2000. Conflict-of-interest policies for investigators in clinical trials. *New England Journal of Medicine* 343(22):1616–1620.

NBAC (National Bioethics Advisory Committee). 2001. *Ethical and Policy Issues in International Research: Clinical Trials in Developing Countries, Volume I.* Bethesda, MD: NBAC. [Online]. Available: http://www.georgetown.edu/research/nrcbl/nbac/clinical/Vol1.pdf [accessed January 27, 2004].

Nicoletti A. 2003. Teens, confidentiality, and HIPPA. *Journal of Pediatric and Adolescent Gynecology* 16(2):113–114.

NIH (National Institutes of Health). 2000. *Financial Conflicts of Interest and Research Objectivity: Issues for Investigators and Institutional Review Boards.* Bethesda, MD: NIH. [Online]. Available: http://grants.nih.gov/grants/guide/notice-files/NOT-OD-00-040.html [accessed March 11, 2004].

NIH. 2002 (July 18). *Financial Conflict of Interest: Objectivity in Research.* [Online]. Available: http://grants1.nih.gov/grants/policy/coi/nih_review.htm [accessed March 11, 2004].

NIH. 2003a (July 21). *Certificates of Confidentiality: Background Information.* [Online]. Available: http://grants1.nih.gov/grants/policy/coc/background.htm [accessed March 11, 2004].

NIH. 2003b. *Protecting Personal Health Information in Research: Understanding the HIPAA Privacy Rule.* Bethesda, MD: NIH. [Online]. Available: http://privacyruleandresearch.nih.gov/pdf/HIPAA_Privacy_Rule_Booklet.pdf [accessed March 11, 2004].

OHRP (Office for Human Research Protections). 2001. *Draft Interim Guidance: Financial Relationships in Clinical Research: Issues for Institutions, Clinical Investigators, and IRBs to Consider When Dealing With Issues or Financial Interest and Human Subject Protection.* Washington, DC: U.S. Department of Health and Human Services. [Online]. Available: http://ohrp.osophs.dhhs.gov/humansubjects/finreltn/finguid.htm [accessed March 11, 2004].

D

GLOSSARY, ACRONYMS, AND LAWS AND REGULATIONS

GLOSSARY

Accreditation. A voluntary certification that institutions, programs, or facilities have adhered to a set of standards for the protection of human research participants as determined by a nongovernmental organization.

Active treatment. Therapy intended to affect a patient's condition in a clinical trial; not a placebo or monitoring only.

Adverse event. An occurrence that causes harm to a patient or research participant or that has the potential to do so. Regulations related to the protection of human subjects focus on serious and unexpected adverse events.

Age of majority. The age designated by state law at which individuals can enter into contracts, consent to medical care, and make other crucial decisions in their own right.

Assent. A child's affirmative agreement to participate in research.

Assurance of compliance. A formal declaration of an institution's commitment to the protection of human subjects. Pursuant to Section 491 of the Public Health Service Act, 42 U.S.C. 289, and to human subjects protection regulations at 45 CFR 46.103, institutions engaged in human subjects research covered by U.S. Department of Health and Human Services (DHHS) regulations and conducted or supported by DHHS must submit a written assurance of compliance satisfactory to the secretary.

Benefit. A positive or valued outcome of an action or event. Benefits resulting from research participation may be physical, psychological, or social.

Blinded. A design feature of clinical trials in which information about whether research participants are in the experimental or control arm is withheld from participants only (single-blinded trials) or both participants and researchers (double-blinded trials).

Certificate of Confidentiality. Certificates issued by the National Institutes of Health to research institutions to protect the privacy of research participants involved in sensitive research by protecting investigators and institutions from being compelled to release identifying information in any federal, state, or local civil, criminal, administrative, legislative, or other proceeding.

Clinical research. Commonly viewed as research that uses human participants to test the safety or effectiveness of medical interventions, especially drugs, or to study the diagnosis or pathophysiology of diseases, disorders, or injuries. More broadly conceived, it "includes all studies intended to produce knowledge valuable to the prevention, diagnosis, prognosis, treatment, or cure of human disease" which involve direct interactions with child participants in research (IOM, 1994a, p. 35). Disease, in this context, can be interpreted to include disorders and injuries.

Commensurate. Reasonably similar to (procedures that prospective research participants ordinarily experience).

Common Rule. The general term for Subpart A of federal regulations protecting human subjects in research as it applies to the U.S. Department of Health and Human Services (45 CFR 46) and 16 other federal agencies.

Compensation. A payment for the time and inconvenience involved in research participation.

Condition. A specific (or set of specific) physical, psychological, neuro-developmental, or social characteristic(s) that an established body of scientific evidence or clinical knowledge has shown to negatively affect children's health and well-being or their risk of developing a health problem in the future.

Conflict of interest. Any financial or other personal interest in the outcome of a research study that may, in actuality or appearance, compromise the objectivity of a researcher and the integrity of the research being conducted.

Consent. An autonomous decision made by an individual with the legal and cognitive capacity to choose voluntarily participate in research.

Control group. The group in a clinical trial that does not receive the experimental intervention.

Data and safety monitoring board. An independent committee charged with periodically reviewing and comparing safety and outcome data collected during a study to determine whether a trial should continue as originally designed, should be altered, or should be terminated.

Data monitoring committee. The term that the Food and Drug Administration and the International Conference on Harmonisation use instead of *data and safety monitoring board.* See *Data and safety monitoring board.*

Determination letter. Correspondence issued by the Office for Human Research Protection that describes findings of an investigation, which may include findings of noncompliance and listing of corrective steps to be taken.

Direct benefit. A tangible positive outcome of an event or action.

Emancipated minor. A person under the age of majority who is granted adult rights by a court on the basis of the maturity of the minor and the minor's need for adult status, usually determined through certain actions, marriage, military enlistment, or being self-supporting and living independently.

Experimental. Unproven or investigational intervention.

Guardian. An individual who is authorized under applicable state or local law to give permission on behalf of a child to participation in research.

Harm. A hurtful or adverse outcome of an action or event, whether temporary or permanent. Harms resulting from research participation may be physical, psychological, or social.

Human research participant protection program. A program consisting of a set of organizational structures, policies, and procedures that apply to a particular research protocol or group of protocols. Specific components may differ depending on the characteristics of a particular study.

Human subject. "A living individual about whom an investigator (whether professional or student) conducting research obtains (1) data through intervention or interaction with the individual, or (2) identifiable private information. Intervention includes both physical procedures by which data are gathered (for example, venipuncture) and manipulations of the subject or the subject's environment that are performed for research purposes)" (45 CFR 46.102(f)). The preferred term in this report is *human research participant.*

Incentive payment. A payment that is intended to attract research participants, that is not linked to expense reimbursement or compensation for time spent in research, and that exceeds a token amount.

Institutional review board (IRB). A group of qualified individuals charged under federal regulation with protecting the rights and welfare of people involved in research in accord with federal regulations. IRBs review and approve plans for research involving humans.

International Conference on Harmonisation. An organization created to develop universal guidelines and requirements for scientific and technical aspects of product registration. Members include regulatory authorities and experts from the pharmaceutical industries of Europe, Japan, and the United States.

Mature minor. A minor who has not reached the age of majority (as defined by state law), but is—as directed by state law—subjectively assessed as being capable of giving the same degree of informed consent for health care purposes.

Minimal risk. A risk associated with research in which the probability and magnitude of harm or discomfort anticipated are not greater in and of themselves than those ordinarily encountered in daily life or during the performance of routine physical psychological examinations or tests of normal, average, healthy children.

Minor increase over minimal risk. A slight or small increase in the potential for harm or discomfort beyond the minimal risk level that is allowed for healthy, normal average children.

Multicenter trial. A clinical trial that is undertaken at multiple sites using a common protocol.

Off-label use. Use of a drug or medical device for a purpose, dose form, patient group, or other use not approved by the Food and Drug Administration for use as indicated on the product label.

Parent. A child's biological or adoptive parent.

Parental permission. Decision made by a parent(s) or guardian with legal authority to allow a child to participate in research.

Participant. Preferred description of human subjects in research.

Pharmacodynamics. The study of the effects of a drug on the body.

Pharmacokinetics. Study of how medicines are absorbed, distributed in, and eliminated from the body.

Phase 1 clinical trial. Initial test of a drug or other intervention with humans. For drugs, Phase 1 trials typically assess tolerability, bioavailability, and pharmacokinetics with a small group of healthy, adult volunteers.

Phase 2 clinical trial. Clinical testing that usually involves a larger group of participants and an assessment of efficacy as well as further evaluation of safety and adverse effects. These trials typically involve participants with a particular disease or condition.

Phase 3 clinical trial. Rigorous controlled clinical studies that extend efficacy and safety testing to a larger number of research participants who usually are randomly assigned to receive the intervention or a standard treatment or placebo.

Placebo. An inactive substance (e.g., a sugar pill) or a sham action (e.g., an injection of sterile water) used with a control group as part of a Phase 3 clinical trial.

Protocol. A document that describes the purpose, design, methods, organization, and other key features of a research study.

Reimbursement. A payment for out-of-pocket expenses directly related to research participation.

Risk. A potential harm or the potential of an action or event to cause harm.

Serious adverse event. An unwanted outcome, which may or may not be related to an experimental intervention, that involves death, hospitalization (new or extended), disability, birth defect, or another major medical event that may jeopardize a research participant and require intervention to prevent one of the above outcomes.

Standard treatment. A treatment currently in use that is believed to be effective.

Subpart A. Federal regulations providing for general protections of human subjects in research (the basic policy of the U.S. Department of Health and Human Services for the protection of human research subjects). See also *Common Rule*.

Subpart D. Federal regulations providing for special protections of child participants in research. The regulations have been adopted only by the U.S. Department of Health and Human Services, the U.S. Department of Education, the Central Intelligence Agency, and the Social Security Administration.

Therapeutic misconception. The belief that the purpose of research is to treat a disease or condition rather than to generate scientific knowledge.

Ward. A child who is placed in the legal custody of the state or other agency, institution, or entity, consistent with applicable federal, state, or local law (21 CFR 50.3q).

ACRONYMS AND ABBREVIATIONS

AAHRPP	Association for the Accreditation of Human Research Protection Programs
AAP	American Academy of Pediatrics
ACHRE	Advisory Committee on Human Radiation Experiments
AMA	American Medical Association
CDC	Centers for Disease Control and Prevention
CFF	Cystic Fibrosis Foundation
CIOMS	Council for International Organizations of Medical Sciences
COG	Children's Oncology Group
DHEW	U.S. Department of Health Education and Welfare
DHHS	U.S. Department of Health and Human Services (formerly U.S. Department of Health Education and Welfare)
DSMB	data and safety monitoring board
FDA	Food and Drug Administration
GAO	General Accounting Office
HIV	human immunodeficiency virus
ICH	International Conference on Harmonisation
IND	Investigational New Drug
IOM	Institute of Medicine
IRB	institutional review board
NAS	National Academy of Sciences
NBAC	National Bioethics Advisory Committee
NCHS	National Center for Health Statistics
NCI	National Cancer Institute
NHRPAC	National Human Research Protections Advisory Committee
NICHD	National Institute for Child Health and Human Development
NIH	National Institutes of Health
NRC	National Research Council
OHRP	Office for Human Research Protections (formerly Office for Protection from Research Risk)
OIG	Office of Inspector General
OMH	Office of Mental Health
OPRR	Office for Protection from Research Risk
PPRA	Protection of Pupil Rights Amendment
SACHRP	Secretary's Advisory Committee on Human Research Protections
STD	sexually transmitted disease
TDN	Therapeutic Development Network
USDA	U.S. Department of Agriculture
WMA	World Medical Association

LAWS AND REGULATIONS

P.L. 87-781. The Drug Amendments of 1962. This act expanded the scope of the Food and Drug Administration's authority by including provisions that required investigators to obtain a subject's consent to participation in research unless it was not feasible or was not in the subject's best interest.

P.L. 93-348. National Research Act of 1974. This Act explicitly provided for the creation of institutional review boards (IRBs) to review biomedical and behavioral research that involved humans. It established and directed the National Commission for the Protection of Human Subjects of Biomedical and Behavioral Research to identify ethical principles for research involving humans, specifically, to consider research involving vulnerable individuals, including children, prisoners, and those with mental disabilities.

P.L. 105-115. Food and Drug Administration Modernization and Accountability Act of 1997

P.L. 106-310. Children's Health Act of 2000. This legislation requires the Food and Drug Administration to bring its regulations into conformity with Subpart D to provide special protections for children participating in research.

P.L. 107-109. Best Pharmaceuticals for Children Act of 2002. The broad purpose of the legislation was to improve the safety and efficacies of drugs for children. One key provision renewed incentives for pharmaceutical manufacturers to test drugs in studies with children to establish safe doses of medications that had been approved as safe and effective for adults. The legislation also requested a study by the Institute of Medicine of research involving children.

P.L. 108-146. Pediatric Research Equity Act of 2003. This legislation grants authority to the Food and Drug Administration to require pediatric studies of certain drugs to ensure their safety and efficacy for children.

21 CFR 50. The Food and Drug Administration policy on the Protection of Human Subjects.

21 CFR 56. The Food and Drug Administration policy on institutional review boards.

45 CFR 46. The U.S. Department of Health and Human Services policy on Public Welfare, the Protection of Human Subjects.

   Section 404. Research not involving greater than minimal risk.

   Section 405. Research involving greater than minimal risk but presenting the prospect of direct benefit to the individual subjects.

   Section 406. Research involving greater than minimal risk and no prospect of direct benefit to individual subjects, but likely to yield generalizable knowledge about the subject's disorder or condition.

Section 407. Research not otherwise approvable that presents an opportunity to understand, prevent, or alleviate a serious problem affecting the health or welfare of children.

E

COMMITTEE BIOGRAPHICAL STATEMENTS

Richard E. Behrman, J.D., M.D. (*Chair*), is Executive Chair of the Education Steering Committee of the Federation of Pediatric Organizations. He is also Clinical Professor of Pediatrics at the University of California, San Francisco, and the George Washington University, Washington, D.C. He is a member of the Institute of Medicine (IOM) and has chaired several IOM committees, mostly recently, one that developed recommendations to improve palliative and end-of-life care for children with life-threatening diseases. His areas of special interest include perinatal medicine, intensive and emergency care of children, the provision and organization of children's health and social services, and related issues of public policy and ethics. Dr. Behrman is editor-in-chief of the *Nelson Textbook of Pediatrics*. He previously held positions as senior vice president of medical affairs at the Lucile Packard Foundation for Children's Health, chairman of the boards of the Lucile Packard Foundation for Children's Health and the Lucile Packard Children's Hospital and director of the Center for the Future of Children. Prior to holding these positions, he served as vice president of Medical Affairs and dean of the School of Medicine at Case Western Reserve University and earlier served as professor and chairman of the Departments of Pediatrics at Case Western Reserve University and Columbia University.

Arthur L. Beaudet, M.D., is chairman and the Henry & Emma Meyer Professor, Department of Molecular and Human Genetics and professor of pediatrics and molecular and cellular biology, Baylor College of Medicine, Houston. His research interests include the genetic basis underlying cystic fibrosis, metabolic disorders, and several other diseases. Dr. Beaudet was codiscoverer of a gene for Angelman syndrome, a chromosome 15 disorder that causes serious mental retardation and physical disabilities. He is studying the role of genomic imprinting and epigenetics in causing disorders such as autism. He is an editor of *The Metabolic and Molecular Bases of Inherited Disease*. Dr. Beaudet is a member of the IOM and has served on the National Research Council Panel on Scientific and Medical Aspects of Cloning and the IOM Roundtable on Research and Development of Drugs, Biologics, and Medical Devices.

Russell W. Chesney, M.D., is Le Bonheur Professor and chair of the Department of Pediatrics at Le Bonheur Children's Hospital, as well as a codirector of the Center for Pediatric Pharmacokinetics and Therapeutics at the University of Tennessee, Memphis. Dr. Chesney is principal investigator for the Pediatric Pharmacology Research Unit, 1 of 13 units in a network of the National Center for Child Health and Development. He previously was a professor of pediatrics at the University of California, Davis. He is editor of the journal *Pediatric Nephrology* and past president of the American Society of Pediatric Nephrology. Dr. Chesney serves as president of the Association of Medical School Pediatric Department Chairs, president of the American Pediatric Society, and in 2000 was chairman of the board of the American Board of Pediatrics. His ongoing research interests include the regulation of renal amino acid transport; inherited renal tubular disorders; and the physiology, biochemistry, and clinical application of vitamin D metabolites to childhood disorders of bone and mineral metabolism.

Francis Sessions Cole III, M.D., is vice chairman of the Department of Pediatrics, the Park J. White, M.D., Professor of Pediatrics, and professor of cell biology and physiology at the Washington University School of Medicine and director of the Division of Newborn Medicine at St. Louis Children's Hospital. He is a member of the Society of Pediatric Research, the American Society for Clinical Investigation, and the American Pediatric Society. Dr. Cole served on the IOM Committee on Palliative and End-of-Life Care for Children and Their Families. His research interests focus on the molecular basis of the susceptibility of the newborn infant to infection and, more recently, on the contribution of genetic variation in the surfactant protein B gene to the risk of respiratory distress syndrome in newborn infants.

Deborah L. Dokken, M.P.A., is a family health care advocate and consultant in family-centered care. She is a member of the Institutional Ethics Forum at Children's National Medical Center in Washington, D.C. She and her husband are the parents of three children born prematurely, one of whom survives. Her first child, who died at the age of 5 months, was enrolled in a clinical trial. Ms. Dokken is a coinvestigator with a multisite research project led by the Education Development Center, Boston, that seeks to improve inpatient care for children with life-threatening medical conditions. She was the cofounder of a nonprofit, community-based organization, Partners in Intensive Care, and was a founding member of the Parent Partners Group in the neonatal intensive care unit at the George Washington University Hospital in Washington, D.C.

Celia B. Fisher, Ph.D., is the Marie Ward Doty University Chair, director of the Center for Ethics Education, and professor of psychology at Fordham University, New York City. She has served as chair of the American Psychological Association's Ethics Code Revisions Task Force, the New York State Board for Licensure in Psychology, and the Society for Research in Child Development Committee for Ethical Conduct in Child Development Research. Dr. Fisher is a member of the Secretary's Advisory Committee on Human Research Protections (U.S. Department of Health and Human Services) and is also a member of the Data Safety and Monitoring Board at the National Institute of Mental Health (NIMH). Dr. Fisher has written commissioned papers on the ethics of research with mentally impaired and vulnerable populations for the President's National Bioethics Advisory Commission and for NIMH on the ethical conduct of research involving ethnic minority children and adolescents.

Angela R. Holder, J.D., LL.M., is professor of the practice of medical ethics at the Center for the Study of Medical Ethics and Humanities at the Duke University Medical Center. She was formerly clinical professor of pediatrics (law) at the Yale University School of Medicine. At Duke, among other responsibilities, she oversees the development of educational materials on research ethics for clinical investigators. She served on the IOM Committee on Effects of Medical Liability on Delivery of Maternal and Child Health and the Committee on Palliative and End-of-Life Care for Children. Her research interests include legal and ethical issues related to children and adolescents in the health care system, human subjects research, and confidentiality of medical information. She is the author of *Medical Malpractice Law and Legal Issues in Pediatrics and Adolescent Medicine*. She is a past president of the American Society of Law and Medicine.

Loretta M. Kopelman, Ph.D., is chair and professor, Department of Medical Humanities, at Brody Medical School, East Carolina University. She serves on eight editorial boards and was president of the Society of Health and Human Values and founding president of the American Society for Bioethics and the Humanities. She edits the research ethics section of the

Encyclopedia of Bioethics. She has edited or coedited six books, including *The Rights of Children and Retarded Persons, Ethics and Mental Retardation*, and *Children and Health Care: Moral and Social Issues*. Her research interests include the ethics of research design and the rights and welfare of children, mentally retarded individuals, and research subjects.

Susan Z. Kornetsky, M.P.H., C.I.P., is director of Clinical Research Compliance in the Department of Clinical Investigation at Children's Hospital Boston. Her responsibilities include directing an institutional review board (IRB) administrative office, assisting investigators in protocol development, and ensuring compliance with all federal and state regulations pertaining to human research. She is a member of the Secretary's Advisory Committee on Human Research Protections and earlier served on the National Human Protection Advisory Committee and is past president of the Applied Research Ethics National Association. Ms. Kornetsky is a member of the Board of Public Responsibility in Research and Medicine and the Association for the Accreditation of Human Research Programs. She serves as faculty for IRB 101, an educational effort to bring IRB training to individual institutions.

Robert M. Nelson, M.D., Ph.D., is associate professor of anesthesia and pediatrics at the University of Pennsylvania School of Medicine and the Children's Hospital of Philadelphia. He is also the senior fellow at the Center for Bioethics, University of Pennsylvania. He serves as chair of the Committees for the Protection of Human Research Subjects at the Children's Hospital of Philadelphia. He is former chair of the Committee on Bioethics of the American Academy of Pediatrics. Dr. Nelson is a member of the Food and Drug Administration Pediatric Advisory Subcommittee, serves as a consultant to the Office of Human Research Protections, and was a member of the Pediatric and Informed Consent Working Groups of the National Human Research Protections Advisory Committee at the U.S. Department of Health and Human Services. His research involves the use of focus groups and individual interviews to explore the views of parents and children about research participation.

David G. Poplack, M.D., is the Elise C. Young Professor of Pediatric Oncology; head, Hematology/Oncology Section, Department of Pediatrics, Baylor College of Medicine; and director, Texas Children's Cancer Center, Houston. He is principal investigator for the College's Pediatric Pharmacology Research Unit, 1 of 13 units in a network of the National Center for Child Health and Development. Dr. Poplack is coeditor of the book *Principles and Practice of Pediatric Oncology*, now in its fourth edition. Before going to Baylor, he was deputy branch chief of the Pediatric Branch of the

National Cancer Institute and head of the Clinical Pharmacology and Experimental Therapeutics Section. His research has focused on the development of innovative therapies for childhood leukemia and other pediatric cancers.

Bonnie W. Ramsey, M.D., is director of the Cystic Fibrosis Therapeutics Development Network Coordinating Center with the Children's Hospital Regional Medical Center, which was created to coordinate a network of cystic fibrosis care centers, resource laboratories, and interpretive centers involved in clinical trials. She is also professor of pediatrics at the University of Washington School of Medicine, vice chair for Research, and associate director of the Core Center for Gene Therapy in Cystic Fibrosis and other genetic disorders at the University of Washington School of Medicine. She was a member of the IOM Committee on Assessing the System for Protecting Human Research Participants.

Diane Scott-Jones, Ph.D., is professor of psychology at Boston College, where she serves on the Institutional Review Board and on the Responsible Conduct of Research Committee. Her research interests include family processes, child and adolescent development, and developmental processes in African-Americans and other ethnic groups. She previously was professor of psychology at Temple University and spent 2 years at the National Science Foundation, where she started a grants program in child learning and development. She is a fellow of the American Psychological Association and the American Psychological Society. She is a member of the MacArthur Foundation Research Network on Successful Pathways through Middle Childhood. She is past editor of the *Journal of Research on Adolescence* and is currently associate editor of the journal *Urban Education* and editorial board member of the *Journal of Social Issues*. She served on the American Psychology Association's Task Force to revise its Ethical Principles for Research with Human Participants and on former President Clinton's National Bioethics Advisory Commission, which produced six reports on research ethics and bioethics. She is currently chair of the Research Ethics Committee of the Society for Research in Child Development; Advisory Board member of Harvard University's Murray Research Center, which archives longitudinal data sets; and participant in a new National Institutes of Health-funded project to develop the course Ethical Issues in Behavioral Health Research.

Stephen P. Spielberg, M.D., Ph.D., is vice president of health affairs and professor of pediatrics and of pharmacology and toxicology at Dartmouth College. He also is the dean of Dartmouth Medical School. He is adjunct professor of pediatrics, medicine, and pharmacology at Thomas Jefferson

University and adjunct professor of pediatrics at the Robert Wood Johnson Medical School. Previously, he served as vice president of pediatric drug development at Johnson and Johnson Pharmaceutical Research and Development, was professor of pediatrics and pharmacology at the University of Toronto and at Johns Hopkins University, and was at Merck Research. He represents the pharmaceutical industry on the Food and Drug Administration Pediatric Advisory Subcommittee and was the rapporteur for the Pediatric International Conference on Harmonisation Initiative to harmonize pediatric drug development regulations among Europe, Japan, and the United States. Dr. Spielberg served on the National Research Council Subcommittee on Reproductive and Developmental Toxicology. His research interests include mechanisms of idiosyncratic adverse drug reactions, human pharmacogenetics, and pediatric clinical pharmacology.

INDEX

A

Accreditation, 198-199, 243-245, 394
Acetaminophen, 67
Acne research, 80, 185
Adolescent Medicine HIV/AIDS Research
    Network, 262, 264
Adolescents. *See also* Assent; Emancipated
    minors; Mature minors; Wards of the
    state
    comprehension of research participation,
      183-185
    consent process for, 8, 9, 154, 156, 171-
      172, 192-194, 200-201, 204, 206,
      207, 322
    decisional maturity, 186, 325
    defined, 62, 64-66
    developmental physiology, 62, 65-66
    enrolled in clinical trials, 87
    medical examination components, 124
    payment for participation, 10, 213, 218-
      219, 227
    pharmacokinetics in, 70
    privacy issues, 158, 187, 205, 323, 327
    runaways and throw-aways, 200
    waiver of parental permissions, 354-362
Adverse events. *See also* Harm
    defined, 106, 394
    in ethical principles, 46
    examples of, 28-29, 82, 234
    monitoring, 37, 105, 106-107
    in placebo-controlled trials, 142
    reporting requirements, 105, 106-107,
      231
    serious, 398
Advisory Committee on Human Radiation
    Experiments, 48, 164, 165
Advocates and advocacy for participants,
    154-155, 159, 208, 328-329, 339
Age of consent
    for medical care, 4, 94, 156, 325-326,
      354-362
    for research participation, 94, 326-328
Age of majority
    defined, 394
    state laws, 94, 104, 322-323, 342-343
Agency for Health Research and Quality, 90
AIDS, 78
Alabama, 104, 325, 340, 342, 344, 347,
    354, 364-365
Alaska, 340, 342, 344, 347, 354
Albert Einstein College of Medicine, 271
Alexander, Leo, 46 n.9, 47 n.10
Allergy and Asthma Network, 194, 221
Allergy research, 80
Altruism, 164, 165, 167, 168, 170, 191
American Academy of Pediatrics, 60, 65-66,
    120, 140, 161, 221, 251

American Cancer Society, 80
American Law Institute, 325 n.8
American Medical Association (AMA), 45
    n.7, 46 n.9, 223
American Pediatric Society, 254
Anesthesia research, 168, 183
Antibiotics, 50, 76
Anticancer agents, 66, 71-72, 73, 80, 106
Anticonvulsants, 69
Antidepressants, 27, 60
Antihistamines, 71
Arizona, 340, 342, 344, 347, 354
Arkansas, 340, 342, 344, 347, 354
Arthritis, 77
Assent. *See also* Consent process; Informed
    consent; Parental permission
    age appropriateness of process, 7, 8,
        156, 171-172, 173, 179-180, 183-
        185, 192-193, 205-207
    cognitive development and, 179-180,
        205-206
    comprehension of research participation
        and, 7, 28, 42, 131-132, 181-193,
        205-206
    defined, 51 n.13, 101, 146-147, 156,
        327, 394
    discretion in documenting, 207
    ethical principles, 40-41, 50, 84, 148, 192
    experience of illness and, 131-132, 189-
        190
    forms, 193, 206, 207
    historical evolution of policies, 50, 51
        n.13
    information to be provided, 206
    legal requirements for, 3, 104, 151-153,
        156-157, 182, 191, 204
    motivations for, 164, 165, 167, 168,
        170, 191
    "mutual pretense" process and, 191
    parental influence, 187, 190-191, 204-
        205
    payment for participation and, 189, 211
    for placebo-controlled trials, 140
    procedures for seeking, 148, 149-151,
        156, 172-173, 205-207
    purpose of research and, 171
    recommended improvements in, 20, 203-
        205
    waiver of, 156
    withdrawal from trials, 183, 187-188,
        190, 197

Association for the Accreditation of Human
    Research Protection Programs, 244
Association of American Medical Colleges,
    244 n.2
Association of American Universities, 244
    n.2
Association of Medical School Pediatric
    Department Chairs, 221
Assurance of compliance, 95, 110, 235,
    242, 394
Asthma research, 77, 80, 167, 168-169, 191
Astrocytoma, 80
Atopic dermatitis, 77
Australian studies, 170, 172, 174, 186
AZT, 108

B

Bartholome, William, 43
Bayley Scales of Infant Development, 125
Beaumont, William, 45 n.7
Beecher, Henry, 35, 39, 50, 248
Behavioral studies, 384-385
Belmont Report, 40-41, 43, 52-53, 93, 110,
    255
Benefits of research, 1, 25-26, 58. *See also*
    Risk-benefit assessment
    collateral or indirect, 132
    defined, 115-116, 395, 396
    direct, 42, 132-133, 136, 154, 158, 204,
        218, 396
    ethical principles relating to, 40-44, 45
        n.7, 47
    expectations of, 150, 151, 164, 165,
        167, 169, 170, 398
    to other children, 115-116, 126-127,
        149 n.2
    peripheral, 149 n.2
    potential, 115, 116, 133-134
    prospective long-term studies, 39
Benzyl alcohol, 67
Bernard, Claude, 45 n.7
Best Pharmaceuticals for Children Act of
    2002, 2, 30, 68, 89, 106 n.3, 233,
    400
Bilirubin, 69
Boston University, 48
Brazelton Neonatal Behavioral Assessment
    Scale, 125
Breast cancer, 171
Brokowski, Carolyn, 182

C

Caffeine, 70

California, 325, 340, 342, 344, 347, 354

Canada, 168, 173

Cancer research, 66, 71-72, 73, 77, 80, 81, 87, 88, 162, 170, 174, 175, 182, 189-190, 218

Cardiac disease, 67, 77, 87-88, 89

Center for Drug Evaluation Research, 55

Centers for Disease Control and Prevention, 161

Centers for Education and Research on Therapeutics, 90

Central Intelligence Agency, 95, 100, 321

Cerebral palsy, 77

Cherokee Nation, 116

Children. *See also* Assent

    cognitive development, 179-180

    comprehension of research participation, 7, 183-185

    defined, 63-64, 101, 154, 321

    enrolled in clinical trials, 87

    in foster care, 321, 322 n.2, 328

    as interpreters for parents, 199

    mortality rates, 80

    neglected or abused, 154, 200, 328, 329, 335

    outcome measures in, 76

    pharmacokinetics in, 69, 70

Children's Health Act of 2000, 53, 54, 96, 100, 233, 400

Children's Hospital Boston, 220-221

Children's Hospital of Pittsburgh, 271

Children's Oncology Group (COG), 71-72, 81, 88, 108, 261

Chloramphenicol, 27, 70

Chronic granulomatous disease, 80

Clinical investigation, definition, 33, 165 n.5

Clinical Investigation of Medicinal Products in the Pediatric Population, 111, 217

Clinical practice innovations, 32

    "radically new" procedures, 32

Clinical research. *See also* Clinical trials; Pediatric drug research

    benefits of, 25-26

    challenges, 59, 74-87

    clinical care distinguished from, 34, 150

    as complex, high-stakes enterprise, 35-36

    context for, 59-62

    definitions, 33-34, 395

    experimental, 33, 396

    importance of, 29

    infrastructure, 83, 86-87, 92, 238

    multidisciplinary, 86

    organization and administration, 36

    policies and procedures, 36

    resources, 36

    on stored biological specimens, 83

    structures, 36

    therapeutic vs. nontherapeutic, 33-34, 50, 331-337

    unethical practices, 28, 331-332

Clinical trials. *See also* Multicenter trials; Pediatric drug research

    active treatment, 394

    administering interventions and measurements, 78-79

    behavioral considerations, 79

    blinded, 151, 170, 395

    children's rules for, 188

    control groups, 81, 108, 117, 139-142, 151, 396, 397

    cooperative research groups, 71-72, 81, 87, 88, 91, 108

    costs, 35, 83, 275

    crossover studies, 81, 142

    data on children's participation, 87-88

    designing and conducting, 2-3, 74-87, 91-92, 142-143

    developmental considerations, 67, 71-72, 82

    direct-benefit characterization, 34

    disease-specific, 81

    effect of participation on outcomes, 150

    of emergency care, 87, 92, 155, 203

    enrollment and retention of participants, 80, 87-88, 217-218, 220, 223-224

    expertise of investigators in pediatrics, 3, 63, 78-79, 91-92, 93-94, 99, 136, 142-144, 244, 250

    facility appropriateness, 78, 92, 136, 143

    family-centered care, 84-85

    with healthy children, 27, 50, 117

    with ill children, 27, 160, 170, 197-198

    long-term monitoring and evaluation, 82-83, 92, 275

    minority participants, 87-88

    outcome measures, 75-78

perceptions and expectations of
  participants, 150, 151, 164, 165 n.5,
  168, 170, 398
Phase 1, 72, 73, 133, 170, 397
Phase 2, 73, 397
Phase 3, 73, 397
placebo-controlled, 81, 108, 139-142,
  155, 159, 164-165, 329-330, 398
progress reports, 99
prospective studies, 27
protocols, 398
quality-of-life interventions, 172
randomized controlled, 81, 159, 164-165,
  168
recruitment practices, 217-218, 220,
  223-224
registry, 88, 242
small study populations, 80-82, 91, 142
standard treatment, 398
suspension or termination, 194, 229,
  234, 236
with wards of the state, 385-386
withdrawal from, 174, 183, 187-188,
  190, 197, 215
Collins, Frances, 193
Colorado, 325, 340, 342, 344, 347, 354
Common Rule (45 C.F.R. Part 46, Subpart
  A), 320-321
  agencies adopting, 54, 95
  criteria for research approval, 3, 97, 99
  defined, 395
  exempted research, 53, 97, 99-100
  expedited review, 53, 100, 117
  historical evolution of, 52-53
  informed consent, 53, 97
  institutional assurances and
    responsibilities, 95, 96-97
  institutional review boards, 97-99
  minimal risk standard, 117, 121
  vulnerable populations, 52
Compliance oversight
  accreditation perspective, 11, 21-22,
    243-245
  adverse event reporting, 105, 106-107, 231
  assurance of compliance, 95, 110, 235,
    242, 394
  of child participants in research, 29, 55,
    234-239
  citations of noncompliance, 236
  concerns about, 230-234
  of conflicts of interest, 232

critical reports on, 231-234
data limitations and needs, 10-11, 230,
  233, 234, 238-239, 240, 242, 243
determination letters, 29, 235-236, 396
by FDA, 56-57, 60 n.1, 105 n.3, 234,
  236-238, 239
"for-cause" investigations, 232, 235
of foreign research, 56-57, 232-233
of human research, 230-234
monitoring, 37, 105, 106-107
"not-for-cause" evaluations, 232, 235
by OHRP, 232, 234, 235-236, 239, 241-
  242, 396
progress in, 29, 55
quality improvement perspective, 11,
  235, 241-243
recommendations, 21-22, 238-239, 247-
  248
reporting requirements, 105, 106-107,
  231
suspension or termination of research,
  194, 229, 234, 236
voluntary actions by institutions and
  sponsors, 11, 238, 240-245
Comprehension of research participation.
  See also Assent; Consent process;
  Informed consent; Parental
  permission
adolescents, 183-186
and assent, 7, 28, 42, 131-132, 181-193,
  205-206
children, 7, 183-185
cognitive development and, 179-180,
  205-206
competency standards, 185
in crisis situations, 7, 169-170
and decision making by parents, 166-178
experience with illness and, 131-132,
  171, 189-190
format of presentation and, 181, 184
harms and benefits, 42, 163-164, 183-186
interpretation of terms, 165 n.5
parents, 159-178
purpose of research, 150, 164-165, 183-
  186, 398
readability of forms, 160-163, 195, 206
research needs, 208
rights of participants, 174, 183, 184,
  187-189, 197
therapeutic misconception, 7, 150, 151,
  164, 398

Condition, defined, 128-129, 130
Conference on Social Responsibility in Pediatric Research, 48
Confidentiality
  assurances in consent process, 193
  Certificate of, 395
  ethical principles, 40
  genetic studies and, 28
  harm from violation of, 115, 116
  for minors, 158, 187, 323, 327
  regulations, 53, 388-390
  translators and interpreters and, 199
Conflict of interest
  compliance oversight, 238
  defined, 395
  financial, 35
  finders' fees as, 223
  nonfinancial, 35
  physician recruitment of own patients as, 35-36, 223
  regulations, 390-392
Connecticut, 340, 342, 344, 347, 355
Consent process. *See also* Assent; Informed consent; Parental permission
  accreditation standards, 244
  for adolescents, 8, 9, 154, 156, 171-172, 192-194, 200-201, 204, 206, 207, 322
  adverse events and, 107
  advocates and independent research monitors, 154-155, 159, 202-203, 328-329
  age appropriateness of, 7, 8, 156, 171-172, 173, 179-180, 183-185, 192-193, 205-207
  assessment of participant's understanding, 166
  benefit and risk descriptions, 150-151, 154, 160, 163-164, 166, 184, 199-200
  collaborative model of decision making, 173, 174-175, 209
  community consultation and public disclosure, 155
  continuous model, 171, 175, 177, 188-189, 192, 197-198
  in crisis (acute-care) situations, 7, 169-170, 171, 175, 186, 192, 196, 197-198, 218
  for emancipated and mature minors, 9, 157-158
  for emergency care trials, 87, 155, 175, 203
  family physician's influence, 7, 152, 168, 173-175, 177, 213
  family systems perspective, 172-173, 196, 203-205, 209
  form design and content, 149-150, 153-154, 156, 160-163, 166, 181, 182, 184, 191, 193, 194, 198, 206, 207, 217, 222
  for future use of stored tissue samples, 83
  historical evolution of, 45-47, 48, 49-50
  interpreters and translators, 177, 180, 198-199
  investigator training for, 208
  involvement of children in, 7-8, 40-41, 148, 149-151, 156-157, 171-173, 192, 205-207
  IRB policies and practices, 7, 8, 140-141, 149-151, 156, 157, 158-159, 162-163, 193-195, 196, 201-203, 207
  language and cultural considerations, 8, 175-176, 177, 180, 198-199, 206-207
  litigation concerns and, 150, 152, 331-334
  for multisite studies, 162-163, 194-195
  outcome information presented in, 163-164
  payment discussed in, 9, 215, 217, 222, 224-225
  purpose of research presented in, 50, 84, 150-151, 159, 164-165, 182-186
  quantitative information about outcomes, 163-164, 173
  questions for parents to ask, 12, 177-178
  recommended improvements in, 8, 18-21, 151, 166, 191, 195-209
  regulatory requirements, 3, 4, 9, 48, 153-154, 400
  research directions, 208-209
  rights of participants explained, 174, 183, 184, 187-189, 197, 199
  state laws and litigation, 201, 330-339
  structure of, 8, 172-173, 196, 203-205, 209
  treatment vs. research participation, 161, 164-165, 174

type and amount of information, 157, 172-173, 174

undue influences on, 9, 173, 174, 213-214, 215, 216, 221

verbal presentation of information, 7-8, 156, 161, 166, 175, 181, 188-189, 194-195, 196, 207

views and results of, 168, 174, 175-176

waiver of parental permission, 9, 19-20, 154-155, 200-203

for wards of the state, 158-159, 200-201, 209

Consortium of Social Science Associations, 244 n.2

Control groups, 81, 108, 117, 139-142, 151, 396, 397

Cooperative research groups, 71-72, 81, 87, 88, 91, 108

Corticosteroids, 69, 71

Cosmetic surgery, 185

Council for International Organizations of Medical Sciences, 56-57, 127, 139, 217, 222, 256

Crossover studies, 81, 142

Cyclosporine, 27

Cystic Fibrosis Foundation, 88, 178, 218, 221, 262

Cystic fibrosis research, 75, 76, 77, 87, 108-109, 193, 271

Cytochrome P-450 1A2, 70

D

Data and safety monitoring boards
composition of, 109
defined, 396
expertise in pediatrics, 37, 108, 252-253
federal regulations, 97, 107-110
independence of, 109, 110
responsibilities of, 108-109, 140

Data monitoring committees. See Data and safety monitoring boards

Declaration of Helsinki, 33 n.4, 49-50, 57, 110, 111, 139

Delaware, 340, 342, 344, 347, 355, 364-365

Denver Developmental Screening Test II, 125

Developing countries, 57, 67

Diabetes research, 55, 65, 77, 87, 169, 184, 189, 190, 218, 271

Didanosine, 110

Diethylene glycol, 67

Disease, defined, 33

Disorder, defined, 128

District of Columbia, 340, 342, 344, 347

Dornase alpha (Pulmozyme), 76

Drug Amendments of 1962, 400

Drug research. See also Pediatric drug research
costs, 35

Drugs. See also specific drugs and classifications of drugs
developmental issues, 60, 61, 65-72, 81
dosing schedules and errors, 68, 69-70
excipient safety, 67-68
extrapolation from adult studies, 2, 26-27, 43, 58, 60, 68-69, 71, 91
half-life, 69-70
labeling information for pediatric use, 60, 90-91
misbranding, 67 n.6
off-label use, 60-61, 67, 74, 397
Phase 1 trials, 397

E

Economically disadvantaged persons, 10, 42-43, 46, 122, 213, 214, 224, 331-332, 333

Emancipated minors
conditions for establishing, 323, 344-346
consent, 104, 157-158, 324
defined, 157, 323, 324, 325 n.10, 396
mature minors distinguished from, 325, 327-328
state laws, 323-324, 344-346

Engelhardt, Tristram, 43

Ethical principles
adverse events, 46
AMA code, 45 n.7
Belmont Report, 40-41, 43, 52-53, 93, 110, 213
beneficence and nonmaleficence, 40-44, 45 n.7, 47
Declaration of Helsinki, 33 n.4, 49-50, 57, 139
education and training in, 268-270
foreseeable benefit of research and, 44
for future use of stored tissue samples, 83
historical evolution of, 44-53

implementation, 85
informed consent and assent, 2, 40-41,
    45-47, 48-49, 50, 84, 147-149, 192
justice, 41, 42-43, 57, 122, 129-130
nonbeneficial research and, 42, 43
Nuremberg Code, 46-47, 49
payment for participation, 41, 213-215
physician-patient relationship and, 44
placebo-controlled trials, 139-142
for research involving children, 7, 43,
    51, 52-53, 93, 101, 183-185, 188
respect for persons (autonomy), 40-42
in review of protocols, 48-49
and trust, 25
UNESCO guidelines, 56 n.17
European Agency for the Evaluation of
    Medicinal Products, 111
European research, 175
Exempt research, 53, 99-100
Expedited review, 53, 99-100

                        F

Federal agencies. *See also individual*
    agencies
    education and guidance for IRBs and
        investigators, 268-270
    policy development, guidance, data
        collection, and research, 273-274
    roles and responsibilities, 15-16, 18, 23,
        267-274
    under Common Rule, 54 n.1
Federal Food, Drug, and Cosmetic Act, 48,
    67, 152, 230
Federal rules and regulations. *See also*
    Common Rule; Compliance
    oversight; Food and Drug
    Administration rules and policies;
    National Institutes of Health policies;
    Subpart D
    adverse event reporting, 105, 106-107
    ambiguity in, 4, 94, 102-103, 106, 114,
        230, 231, 232
    applicable research, 230, 247
    for assent, 3, 104, 151-153, 156-157,
        182, 191, 204
    assurance of compliance declaration, 97,
        110, 394
    for continuing review, 99
    data and safety monitoring boards, 107-
        110

data monitoring committees, 105, 107-
    110
foreign research, 56-57, 110
historical evolution of, 52-57
minimal risk defined in, 115
for parental permission, 3, 152-155,
    193
payment for participation, 215-217
Federation of American Societies of
    Experimental Biology, 244 n.2
Federation of Pediatric Organizations, 86
Fetal research, 52
Florida, 340, 342, 344, 348, 355, 364-365
Fluoxetine (Prozac), 60
Food and Drug Administration
    Modernization and Accountability
    Act of 1997, 89, 400
Food and Drug Administration rules and
    policies
    adverse event reporting requirements,
        106, 107
    age categories, 63, 64, 65
    compliance oversight, 60 n.1, 67 n.6, 88,
        91, 105 n.3, 106-107, 108, 233, 234-
        235, 236-238
    conformity with Subpart D, 5, 53, 95,
        100, 400
    data monitoring committees, 108
    on foreign research, 110, 111, 233
    Good Clinical Practices Program, 55, 68,
        234-235
    guidance on research involving children,
        255
    incentives for pediatric drug research, 2,
        27, 90-91
    for informed consent, 48, 94, 154, 400
    on institutional review boards, 400
    Investigational New Drug Application,
        56, 111, 152
    Office of Pediatric Therapeutics, 238
    Office of Science and Health
        Coordination, 234-235
    for parental permission, 9, 154, 155,
        201-202, 203
    payment guidelines for participants, 216,
        217, 227
    on pediatric drug trials, 2, 71, 73, 75-
        76, 90-91
    on placebo-controlled trials, 139 n.8
    protocols referred to Commissioner,
        102, 116, 134

recommended roles and responsibilities, 18, 23, 269

regulations, 3, 4, 9, 53, 54, 95-96, 100, 193, 230, 321, 400

review and monitoring program, 105, 106-107, 236-237

Forced expiratory volume at 1 sec (FEV₁), 76

G

"Gasping syndrome," 67

Gelsinger, Jesse, 55, 234

General Clinical Research Centers, 261

Genetic Alliance, 221

Genetic research, 75, 80, 116, 171, 182, 186, 193, 253

gene therapy trials, 28, 39, 55, 105, 109, 150, 234, 271

Georgia, 340, 342, 344, 348, 355

Germany, 46

Glantz, Leonard, 44

Glucuronyl transferase, 70

Gonorrhea, 45

Good Clinical Practices Program, 55, 68, 234-235

Good manufacturing practices, 68

Gorman, Richard, 90

"Gray baby syndrome," 70

Guardians, 101, 154, 217, 321, 396

Guideline for Good Clinical Practice, 110-111

H

Harbor-UCLA Medical Center, 271

Harm. *See also* Adverse events; risk

defined, 114-115, 396

discomfort as, 115, 140

duration and magnitude considerations, 123, 126, 128, 134

identification of, 26

instances of, 67

prospective long-term studies, 39

unanticipated problems, 107

Hauerwas, Stanley, 43

Hawaii, 340, 342, 344, 348, 355

Health Insurance Portability and Accountability Act of 1996, 94, 388-390

Hemophilia, 123

Hepatitis, 50

Hess, Alfred F., 46

Hexachlorophene, 69

Hippocrates, 40

HIV research and testing, 88, 108, 171-172, 194, 262, 264, 271

Hohmann, Elizabeth, 239

Human Genome Project, 28, 39

Human research participants protection program

components or modules, 37

core functions, 37

defined, 396

ethical principles, 39-44

historical evolution of policies, 52

implementation challenges, 28, 29-30, 37-38

for multicenter trials, 37, 39

systems perspective, 36-39

Human subjects

defined, 34, 396

Hyaline membrane disease, 27

I

Ibuprofen, 167

Idaho, 340, 342, 344, 348, 356

Illinois, 340, 342, 344, 348, 356, 364-365

Immunosuppressive agents, 27

In vitro fertilization, 52

Indian Health Service, 116

Indiana, 325, 340, 342, 344, 348, 356

Infants

defined, 63

experiments on orphans, 46

functioning and behavior, 125

instances of harm to, 67, 70

low-birth-weight, 82, 88

outcome measures in, 76

pharmacokinetics of drugs, 69-70

premature, 1, 26, 27, 58, 63, 67, 69, 75, 78, 80, 82, 87, 88

well-child examination components, 124

Informed consent. *See also* Assent; Comprehension of research participation; Consent process; Parental permission

age of majority, 4, 94, 104, 154, 156, 325-326, 354-362

defined, 146, 395

by emancipated and mature minors,
157-158
ethical principles, 2, 40, 45-47, 48-49,
147-149
exempted research, 53, 97, 99-100
federal regulations, 53, 97, 151-153,
231
general conditions for, 51, 116, 148-
149, 190
informational requirements for, 159
for long-term studies, 83
parental permission distinguished from,
148-149, 159, 198-200
for placebo-controlled trials, 139, 140-
141
reading levels and readability of forms,
160-163
Institute of Medicine, 30, 233, 234, 243,
246, 251
Institutional review boards
central review model, 265-266
community and family input to, 14-15,
254
composition, 35, 96, 97, 253-254
consent policies and practices, 7, 8, 143-
144, 156, 157, 158, 193-195, 321,
327
continuing review by, 99, 107
database and information system, 266,
267
defined, 396-397
documentation of decisions and
checklists, 55, 105, 134, 267, 242,
257-259, 260-261
expedited review, 53, 100, 117
foreign, 56
guidance on research with children, 15,
255-258, 268-270, 273
historical evolution of, 48-49, 51, 52
inspections of, 108
minimal risk interpretation, 118-121
monitoring adverse events, 107-108
multicenter protocol review, 255, 261-
266
Native American, 116
payment policies, 216, 217-218, 219,
220-221, 224-225, 261
pediatric expertise on, 251-261
qualifications of members, 14, 22-23,
37, 76-77, 86, 97-99, 158, 244, 248,
251-255, 321

recommendations, 14, 15, 18, 22-23,
138, 253, 258, 266
referral of protocols to the DHHS
Secretary or FDA Commissioner,
102, 103, 116, 134, 137 n.6, 270-
273
regulatory framework, 96-97, 97-99,
101, 321, 400
roles and responsibilities, 13-15, 28, 49,
51, 53, 96-97, 105 n.3, 106, 108-
109, 138, 232, 247, 251-267
sharing information about decisions, 55,
105, 134, 267, 274-275
supplemental policies and guidance, 258,
261
variability in decisions, 262-265
waiver of parental permission, 19, 84
written basis for judgments, 6, 134
Intelligence tests, 125
International Conference on Harmonisation,
33 n.4, 56, 63, 71, 111, 139, 156-
157, 217, 396, 397
International Covenant on Civil and
Political Rights, 49 n.12
*International Ethical Guidelines for
Biomedical Research Involving
Human Subjects*, 111
International research, regulation of, 56-57,
110, 232-233
Interventions, defined, 34
Intraocular lens replacement, 61
Investigators and research teams
child life specialists and child
psychologists, 79
consent policies and practices, 20, 84,
193-195
cultural sensitivity, 84
expertise in pediatrics, 3, 20, 63, 78-79,
91-92, 93-94, 99, 136, 142-144,
244, 250
inspections of, 108
minimal risk interpretations by, 118-121
payments to, 222-223, 227-228
progress reports, 99
recommendations, 19, 250
roles and responsibilities, 12-13, 35, 84,
99, 142-143, 248-251
training and retention of, 86-87, 250
Iowa, 340, 342, 344, 348, 356
Ivy, Andrew, 46, 47 n.10

J

Jenner, Edward, 45
Jewish Chronic Disease Hospital Study, 331-332
Johns Hopkins University, 332
Joint Commission on the Accreditation of Healthcare Organizations, 244
Jonsen, Albert, 53 n.14

K

Kansas, 340, 342, 344, 348, 356
Kennedy Krieger Institute, 331-332
Kentucky, 340, 342, 344, 349, 356-357
Kernicterus, 69
Kidney disease, 92
Koski, Greg, 229

L

Lamivudine, 110
Lasagna, Louis, 47
Lead abatement studies, 330-331
Legally authorized representative, defined, 101
Legislation. *See also* Regulatory framework for protection; *specific statutes*
    incentives for pediatric research, 89-90
Leukemia, 26, 66, 75, 80, 82, 87, 88, 106, 169, 184
Lilly, Joseph, 169
Lilly, Maureen, 58
Lippincott, Sarah, 191-192
Long-term studies
    implementation, 83
    importance, 82
Louisiana, 340, 342, 344, 349, 357, 364-367

M

Maine, 325, 340, 342, 344, 349, 357, 366-367
Maryland, 328, 331-334, 339, 340, 342, 345, 349, 357
Massachusetts, 336, 340, 342, 345, 349, 357
Maternal and Child Health Bureau, 89

Mature minors
    abortion law, 336
    consent to research, 104, 158, 203, 204, 206, 323
    consent to treatment, 336-337, 347-352
    defined, 325, 397
    emancipated minors distinguished from, 325, 327-328
    state laws, 324-325, 336-337, 347-352
    status events for consenting to health care, 347-352
McCormick, Richard, 43
Measles, 1, 26, 45
Medical Device User Fee and Modernization Act of 2002, 60 n.1
Medical experiment, 165 n.5
Medical research, 165 n.5
Medical study, 165 n.5
Mentally ill, institutionalized persons, 42-43, 50, 51 n.13, 334-336
Methylphenidate (Ritalin), 60
Michigan, 340, 342, 345, 349, 357
Midazolam hydrochloride (Versed), 89
Minimal risk
    "daily life" reference, 5, 118, 121, 126
    defining, 5, 115, 117-126, 397
    developmental status or age considerations, 122, 124, 126
    discomfort as, 115
    ethical principles, 47
    exemption or expedited review, 53
    for healthy children, 5, 117, 120, 121-125, 126
    for ill children, 120, 122-123
    investigator and IRM interpretation, 118, 120-121
    moral and social implications, 5, 120-121
    and no benefit to participant, 84, 103, 127
    procedures categorized as, 123, 134-136
    psychological tests, 125
    recommended interpretation, 5-6, 126
    relativistic interpretation, 5, 121-122, 126, 127
    routine examination standard, 4, 124-125
    socially allowable risks, 123
Minnesota, 340, 342, 345, 350, 357
Minor increase over minimal risk standard
    benefit standard, 6, 115-116, 130, 328-329
    commensurate procedure criterion, 128, 131-132, 395

defining, 118, 120, 126-128, 397
disorder or condition criterion, 6, 128-
    131, 395
recommendations, 130-131
research-only procedures, 137
Minorities, 175
Mississippi, 104, 340, 342, 345, 350, 358
Missouri, 340, 342, 345, 350, 358
Montana, 340, 342, 345, 350, 358
Mothers of Asthmatics, 221
Multicenter trials
    consent process, 162-163, 194-195
    defined, 397
    enrollment and retention of participants,
        84
    in foreign countries, 110
    implementation of protective policies,
        28, 37, 39
    need for, 92
    protocol review, 261-266
    reporting adverse events, 107
    risk categorization in, 120
    size of study populations, 81
    state regulation of, 4-5
    variable review of, 261-266
Mumps, 1

N

National Academy of Sciences, 25
National Association of State Universities
    and Land Grant Colleges, 244 n.2
National Bioethics Advisory Commission
    (NBAC), 32-33, 34, 35, 56, 83 n.8,
    113, 117, 136-137, 223, 232-233,
    248
National Cancer Institute, 87, 108, 162, 265
National Center for Health Statistics
    (NCHS), 63, 64
National Commission for Quality
    Assurance, 244
National Commission for the Protection of
    Human Subjects of Biomedical and
    Behavioral Research, 6, 33 n.4, 40,
    43, 51 n.13, 52, 53, 93, 101, 125,
    126, 127, 129, 131-132, 134, 136,
    138, 139, 154, 156, 200, 201, 268-
    269, 400
    Belmont Report, 40-41, 43, 52-53, 93,
        110, 255
    Research Involving Children, 52-53, 255

National Conference of State Legislators,
    338
National Governors Association, 338
National Health Council, 244 n.2
National Human Research Protections
    Advisory Committee (NHRPAC),
    122, 123, 127, 129, 131, 135, 269
National Institute of Allergy and Infectious
    Diseases, 88
National Institute of Child Health and
    Human Development (NICHD), 88,
    89
National Institutes of Health policies, 178,
    234
    age categories, 64
    Certificate of Confidentiality, 395
    Clinical Center, 47-48, 52, 222
    clinical research curriculum grants, 86
    historical evolution of, 47-48, 52
    incentives for research, 2, 27, 52, 91-92
    IRB database and information system,
        266, 267, 275
    for monitoring data and safety, 105, 108
    notification of institution's
        noncompliance, 236
    parental permission, 155
    on payment for participation, 219-220,
        222, 227
    prospective studies of
        immunosuppressive agents, 27
    recommended roles and responsibilities,
        23, 269
    regulations applicable to, 95, 97
National Research Act of 1974, 52, 400
National Research Council, 30
Native Americans, IRBs, 116
Navaho Nation, 116
Nebraska, 104, 340, 342, 345, 350, 358
Nebulized albuterol, 60
Nelson, Robert M., 211
Nelson Textbook of Pediatrics, 63, 64, 65
Neonatal Research Network, 88
Neonates, 63, 69, 70, 124, 168, 175. *See
    also* Infants
Netherlands, 167
Nevada, 340, 342, 345, 350, 358
New England Medical Center Hospital, 271
New Hampshire, 341, 342, 345, 350, 358,
    366-367
New Jersey, 341, 342, 345, 350, 358-359,
    366-367

New Mexico, 341, 342, 345, 351, 359, 368-369
New York, 334-336, 339, 341, 342, 345, 351, 359
New Zealand studies, 167-168
North Carolina, 341, 342, 345, 351, 359
North Dakota, 341, 342, 345, 351, 359, 368-369
Nuremberg Code, 46-47, 49, 152
Nutrition research, 184

O

Obesity, 77, 80
Office for Human Research Protections, 53 n.15, 136
    central IRB review model, 265-266
    compliance oversight by, 55, 99, 216, 229, 232, 233, 234, 235-236, 239, 396
    determination letter, 216, 396
    guidance on research involving children, 255
    payment guidelines, 215-216
    quality improvement initiative, 235, 241-242
    recommended roles and responsibilities, 6, 18, 23, 136, 155, 202, 203, 239, 269, 270, 272
Office for Protection from Research Risks, 55
Office of Management and Budget, 239, 241
Office of Public Health and Transfer, 55
Ohio, 341, 342, 345, 351, 360
Oklahoma, 341, 342, 345, 351, 360, 368-369
Oregon, 325, 341, 342, 346, 351, 360
Organ transplants, 27
Otitis media, 80
Outcome measures
    age-appropriate, 75-77
    consent and quantitative information about, 163-164
    death, 75
    defining, 75-78
    developmental appropriateness, 76-77
    normative data, 78
    pain scales, 77
    physical or cognitive functioning, 76-77

quality-of-life, 77
surrogate measures, 75-76
survival after diagnosis and disease-free survival, 75
Oversight of regulations. *See* Compliance oversight

P

Pain assessment and management, 77, 79
Parental permission. *See also* Assent; Consent process; Informed consent
    compensation and, 331
    comprehension level and, 7, 42, 131-132, 159-178, 198-200
    conditions/disorders not requiring permission for treatment, 354-362
    crisis-driven decision making, 169-170, 171
    decision-making process, 166-178
    defined, 101, 146, 397
    ethical principles, 148
    exceptions to requirements for, 324
    expectations of benefit and, 151, 164-165, 167, 169-171, 199-200
    experience of illness and, 171
    family physician's influence, 7, 168
    federal regulations, 103-104, 152-155
    forms, 193
    by guardians, 49-50, 146, 154, 396
    informational requirements for, 159-160
    informed, 198-200
    informed consent distinguished from, 148-149, 159
    investigator's undue influence on, 173, 174
    legal requirements for, 3, 151-155, 331-337
    limits of authority, 335
    motivation for decisions, 167-169
    process, 149-151, 175-176
    reading levels and readability of forms, 160-163
    research on decision making, 166-178
    risk-benefit standards, 331-337
    views and results of consent process, 168, 174, 175-176
    waiver of, 4, 9, 19-20, 51, 84, 94, 97, 104, 154-155, 193, 194, 200-203, 321, 335

Parents
  compensation for time and
    inconvenience, 10, 212, 214, 217,
    219, 220, 221, 227, 228, 395
  defined, 101, 154, 397
  incompetent, 154
  influence of children, 187, 190-191,
    204-205
  participation in clinical studies, 34
  questions to ask during consent process,
    12, 177-178
  reimbursement for expenses, 10, 212,
    213, 214, 217, 218, 219, 220, 225-
    226, 398
  responsibilities of, 160
  termination of rights, 329
Participants, defined, 397
Partnership for Human Research Protection,
  Inc., 244
Pattee, Suzanne, 178
Payment for participation
  acceptable types of, 10, 225-227
  to adolescents, 10, 213, 218-219, 227
  amounts paid, 217, 218, 219
  bonuses for completion of study, 217,
    224
  and child's assent, 189, 211
  compensation for time and
    inconvenience, 10, 212, 214, 217,
    219, 220, 221, 227, 228, 395
  ethical concerns, 9, 41, 211, 213-215, 220
  federal regulations and policies, 215-
    217, 220, 227
  to guardians, 217
  incentive payments, 189, 212, 213, 214-
    215, 216, 221, 227-228, 396
  for injuries related to research, 221-222,
    227
  IRB policies and practices, 9, 216, 217-
    218, 219, 220-221, 223, 224-225
  nonfinancial alternatives, 10, 214, 228
  OHRP guidelines, 215-216
  and parental permission, 331
  to physicians' for finders' fees, 222-223,
    227-228
  professional organizations' positions on,
    221
  recommendations for improving, 9-10,
    21, 223-228
  recruitment advertising, 217-218, 220,
    223-224
  reimbursement for expenses, 10, 212,
    213, 214, 217, 218, 219, 220, 225-
    226, 398
  research on use of, 217-220, 227
  and risk-benefit assessment, 132, 216,
    331
  risk-related, 10, 216, 218, 219-220, 221,
    226-227
  token payments or gifts, 212-213, 215
  types of, 212-213, 221
  undue influence of, 9, 213, 214, 221
  waiver of treatment costs as, 221
  written policies on, 9, 222, 224-225
Pediatric AIDS Clinical Trials Group, 88
Pediatric drug research. *See also* Clinical
    research; Clinical trials
  with adolescents, 7, 64-66
  adverse effects by developmental stage,
    67, 71-72, 82
  age-appropriate formulations, 26-27, 61,
    66, 67-68, 73
  with children, 63-64, 69, 76, 78, 79
  commercial value of, 61-62, 89
  costs of, 61
  data monitoring committees, 108
  direct benefits of, 133
  disclosure of findings, 27 n.1, 106, 250
  efficacy trials, 73, 133
  ethical and regulatory standards, 60 n.1,
    62, 63, 85
  incentives for, 30, 59, 89-92
  with infants, 63, 67, 69, 70, 76, 78, 79
  information gaps, 26-27
  labeling for pediatric doses, 89
  long-term follow-up and surveillance,
    71-72, 75, 76, 82-83, 106, 275
  normative data, 75, 76, 78
  patent protection, 89
  payment for participation, 217
  rationale for, 66-72
  reporting adverse events, 106-107
  pharmacodynamics, 66, 71, 72-73
  pharmacokinetic studies, 26-27, 63, 66,
    68-70, 72, 73, 133
  process for, 72-74
  for unique diseases, 67, 72, 73, 78
  waiver of labeling requirements, 90
Pediatric Emergency Care Applied Research
    Network, 155
Pediatric Pharmacology Research Network,
    88

Pediatric Research Equity Act of 2003, 90, 400

PedsQL 4.0 instrument, 77

Pellegrino, Henry, 248

Pennsylvania, 341, 342, 346, 351, 360

Percival, Thomas, 45 n.7

Pertussis, 45, 168

Pharmacodynamics, 71, 397

Pharmacokinetics, 68-70, 397

Phenolbarbitol, 71

Phenylketonuria, 58

Phenytoin, 69

Placebo-controlled trials, 81, 108, 139-142, 155, 159, 164-165, 329-330, 398

Polio, 1, 26

Polycystic ovary syndrome, 65

Pregnant women, 52

President's Commission for the Study of Ethical Problems in Medicine and Biomedical and Behavioral Research, 53-54

Prisoners, 42-43, 52, 159, 231, 321, 328

Privacy issues, 115, 158, 187, 205, 323, 327, 339

Professional societies. *See also individual organizations*
  recommended role of, 250-251

Protection of Pupil Rights Amendment, 321

Prussia, 45

Pseudomonas aeruginosa infection, 109

Psoriasis research, 217

Public Citizen, Health Research Group, 221

Public Responsibility in Medicine and Research, 244 n.2

Public review and comment process, 55

Pulmonary hypertension, 89

Q

Quality improvement
  government initiative, 39, 55, 241-243
  projects as research, 32

R

Radiation experiments, 48, 50

Radiation therapy, 26, 59, 82

Ramsey, Paul, 43

REACH (Reaching for Excellence in Adolescent Care and Health), 262

Recombinant DNA Advisory Committee, 269

Recommendations
  assent and permission process, 8, 18-21, 151, 166, 191, 195-209
  compliance oversight, 10-11, 21-22, 238-239, 247-248
  data collection, 10-11, 23, 238-239, 247-248, 273-274
  federal agency responsibilities, 23, 273-274
  institutional review boards, 14, 15, 18, 22-23, 138, 253, 258, 266
  payment policies, 9-10, 21, 223-228
  risk-benefit assessments, 5-6, 17-18, 126, 127-129, 130-131, 134-136, 138

Recruitment of participants, 217-218, 220, 223-224

Regulatory framework for protection. *See also* Compliance oversight; Federal rules and regulations; State regulatory framework; *specific statutes*
  conflict of interest, 390-392
  historical evolution of policies, 45-54, 151-153, 231
  importance of, 3, 29
  international efforts to harmonise, 56-57
  privacy of subjects, 388-390

Research. *See also* Clinical research; Pediatric drug research
  definitions, 31-33, 114
  quality improvement projects distinguished, 32

Research Involving Children, 52-53, 255

Retinoblastoma, 80

Retinopathy of prematurity, 1, 26

Rhode Island, 341, 342, 346, 351, 360-361, 368-369

Rhode Island Hospital, 271

Risk. *See also* Minimal risk
  defined, 114, 398
  to others, 116
  procedures categorized by, 5-6, 123, 134-136
  reasonableness of, 138-142

Risk-benefit assessment
  algorithm, 117, 119
  basic concepts, 114-116
  clinical equipoise criterion, 138-142

commensurate procedure criterion, 6-7, 128, 130, 131-132, 395
by components vs. whole protocol, 136-138
and consent issues, 131, 140-141, 154, 163-164, 331-337
correlates of health and disease and, 129-130
developmental status or age considerations, 6, 122, 124, 126, 128
direct benefit standard, 42, 132-133, 138
disorder or condition criterion, 6, 126, 128-131, 133, 136, 395
environmental considerations, 133
ethnic, cultural, and religious considerations, 116
foreseeable benefit to others, 126-127
government guidance, 134-136
justice considerations, 122, 129-130, 131
minimal risk standard, 5, 6, 102-103, 117-126, 136
minimization of risk from procedures, 134-136, 142-144
minor increase over minimal risk standard, 102-103, 126-128, 136, 137, 138, 140
no benefit to participant, 84, 103, 127, 130-131, 132-134, 137, 138, 331-337
payment for participation and, 132, 216, 331
placebo-control trials, 139-142
presentation of information in consent forms, 163-164
privacy considerations, 28
prospective long-term studies, 39
recommendations, 5-6, 17-18, 126, 127-129, 130-131, 134-136, 138
regulatory framework, 5, 101-103
required determinations, 117, 118
subjectivity of, 118, 120, 265
vital importance standard, 6, 130, 133-134
Roche, Ellen, 234

S

Sagan, Leonard, 44
Schizophrenia, 27

Secretary's Advisory Committee on Human Research Protections (SACHRP), 6, 18, 122 n.1, 134, 135, 136, 272, 273
Shirkey, Harry, 59
Simone, Joseph V., 66
Sleep research, 55, 271
Smallpox research, 45, 46, 55, 116, 133, 271
Social Security Administration, 95, 100, 321
Society for Adolescent Medicine, 201, 202, 203, 251
Society for Pediatric Research, 221, 251, 254, 270
South Carolina, 325, 341, 342, 346, 352, 361, 368-369
South Dakota, 341, 342, 346, 352, 361, 368-369
Sponsors of research
financial rewards, 35
roles and responsibilities, 274-275
Stanford-Binet Intelligence Scale, 125
State regulatory framework
age of consent for medical care, 4, 94, 104, 156, 201, 322-323, 325-326, 354-362
age of majority, 4, 94, 322-323, 342-343
case law examples, 328, 330-337
education-related research in school settings, 340-341, 344-346
emancipated minors, 323-324
illustrations of state laws, 331-337
mature minor provisions, 324-325, 347-352
recommendations, 4-5
research-specific legislation, 326-328
research-specific regulations, 328-330
uniform guidelines and national discussion, 337-339
wards of the state, 328-330, 364-375, 384-387
Subpart A. *See* Common Rule
Subpart D
age of majority, 322
agencies adopting, 95, 96, 100, 232, 321
ambiguities in, 232
categories of approvable research, 3, 4, 102-103, 117
consent to participate in research, 3, 103-104, 322
defined, 398

definitions, 101
historical evolution of, 53
minimal risk standard, 117, 121
risk-benefit assessment, 101-103, 133-134
Sudden infant death syndrome, 75, 167-168
Sulfanilamide, 67
Sulfonamides, 67, 69
Surfactant therapy, 26, 27
Syphilis, 45

T

Tennessee, 336-337, 341, 342, 346, 352, 361, 368-373
Tetracyclines, 71
Texas, 341, 342, 346, 352, 361
Theophylline, 70
Therapeutics Development Network (TDN), 88, 218, 262
Therapeutic misconception, 7, 150
Tobramycin solution for inhalation (TOBI), 76, 108-109
Toulmin, Stephen, 43
Tuberculosis studies, 46, 195
Tuskegee Syphilis Study, 52, 331
Typanocentesis, 120

U

United Nations, 49 n.12
Education, Social and Cultural Organization, 56 n.17
University of California at Los Angeles, 220, 271
University of Maryland, 332
University of North Carolina, 271
University of Pennsylvania, 28, 55
University of Rochester Medical Center, 321 n.1
University of Washington, 222, 271
U.S. Department of Education, 54, 95, 100, 321
U.S. Department of Health and Human Services policies. See also Food and Drug Administration
adverse event reporting requirements, 106, 107
age categories, 64
compliance oversight, 231-232, 233
criticisms of, 55, 94

on foreign research, 110-111
funding allocations, 90
historical evolution of, 51, 52-53, 54
on investigator qualifications, 99
on payment of participants, 214, 220, 223, 227
protocols referred to the Secretary, 103, 116, 134, 137, 270-273
public review and comment process, 55
regulations on protection of human subjects, 2, 3, 4, 9, 52-53, 94, 95, 96, 100, 102-103, 106, 153, 155, 193, 200, 230, 321, 400-401
U.S. Department of Health, Education and Welfare, 51, 52, 54
U.S. General Accounting Office, 88, 231-232
U.S. Public Health Service grants, 49, 153
U.S. Surgeon General, policy statements, 48-49, 51, 152-153
Utah, 341, 343, 346, 352, 361, 372-373

V

Vaccine research, 26, 27, 45, 50, 55, 116, 133, 161, 168, 183, 271
Vaughn, Andrell, 146
Vermont, 341, 343, 346, 352, 361
Veterans Administration, 222
Virginia, 341, 343, 346, 352, 361
Vulnerable groups
consent laws, 51 n.13, 320, 322, 329-330, 331-337
economically disadvantaged persons, 42-43, 46, 122, 331-332, 333, 337
mentally ill, institutionalized persons, 42-43, 50, 51 n.13, 334-336, 337
prisoners, 42-43, 52, 159, 231, 321, 328
underuse and overuse of, 42-43

W

Wards of the state
consent laws, 104, 158-159, 200, 321, 328-330, 338, 364-375
defined, 101, 398
experimental research on, 50, 338
protocol scenario, 384-387
Washington State, 167, 341, 343, 346, 352, 362, 374-375

Wechsler Intelligence Scale for Children, 125
Wechsler Preschool and Primary Scale of Intelligence, 125
West Virginia, 341, 343, 346, 352, 362
Willowbrook State School, 50, 332 n.15
Wisconsin, 341, 343, 346, 352, 362, 374-375
Women's Health Initiative, 43

World Health Organization, 56 n.17
World Medical Association, 49, 110, 139
Worsfold, Victor, 43
Wyoming, 341, 343, 346, 352, 362

Y

Yasui, Lise, 196